The Challenge of Ageing

A Multidisciplinary Approach to
Extended Care

The Challenge of Ageing
A Multidisciplinary Approach to Extended Care

Edited by

Marion W. Shaw HVC, DipNEd, FRCNA
At one time Principal Adviser, Extended Care Services,
Health Commission of Victoria
Honorary Secretary, Australian Association of Gerontology

Foreword by
R. B. Lefroy AM, MA(Oxon), MB, BS, FRACP, FACRM
Honorary Fellow,
Department of Medicine, University of Western Australia

SECOND EDITION

CHURCHILL LIVINGSTONE
MELBOURNE EDINBURGH LONDON NEW YORK AND TOKYO 1991

CHURCHILL LIVINGSTONE
Medical Division of Longman Group UK Limited

Distributed in Australia by Longman Cheshire Pty Limited,
Longman House, Kings Gardens, 95 Coventry Street,
South Melbourne 3205, and by associated companies,
branches and representatives throughout the world.

© Longman Group UK Limited 1984, 1991

First edition 1984
Second edition 1991
    Reprinted 1993

ISBN 0-443-04357-4

**National Library of Australia Cataloguing in
Publication Data**

The Challenge of ageing: a multidisciplinary approach to
    extended care.

    2nd ed.
    Bibliography.
    Includes index.
    ISBN 0 443 04357 4.

    1. Aged — Care. 2. Geriatrics. I. Shaw, Marion W.
362.6

Produced by Longman Singapore Publishers (Pte) Ltd
Printed in Singapore

Foreword

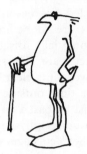

Demographers predict that by the end of the century there will be a considerable increase in the proportion of old people, more particularly those in their 80s, with consequences for the whole of society. Nor can we escape the conclusion that we are witnessing a new biological phenomenon — the survival of the unfittest (Isaacs et al 1972). In the light of these reports it is not surprising to read of 'The Impending Crisis of Old Age: a challenge to ingenuity' (Shegog 1981). The facts which have been illuminated by this spotlight on old age are disturbing; they call for action. But action should be according to carefully considered precepts if crisis is to yield to a reasonable solution. In Australia we need look no further than legislation responsible for the Aged or Disabled Persons Homes Act, or the growth of the nursing home industry — our two major essays in the care of old people — to find examples of inappropriate planning and inadequate results.

There is also a dilemma more fundamental than the problem of appropriate planning. By giving special consideration to old people is there not a danger of isolating them from the rest of society? May we not distort the changes in physical, mental and social function brought about by ageing and damage the opportunity for integration by high-lighting them as separate problems? Should we, in fact, be writing books on the health

care of the elderly with the risk of giving the impression that old people exist in isolation? The tendency towards segregation has already seriously affected old people's lives. In a society which measures success in terms of work achievement and economic gain, compulsory retirement creates a division into those who are useful and those who are not. Rehousing schemes and encouragement to rely on institutional care, which seem to have become part of our culture, are both measures which have tended to divide old people from other age groups. Any response to the crisis which is forecast, any attempt to lay special emphasis on the needs of elderly people, should take into account the dangers of separating them from the rest of society.

In spite of these misgivings, there is undoubtedly a need for planned support of a growing number of people, not because they are old but because they are either disabled or potentially disabled. Providing we recognise this distinction, making disability, not age, the criterion for care, we are less likely to damage the important links which elderly people need with the rest of society; and we are more likely to use our resources to the best advantage.

This book is directed towards the care of an important minority. They are people whose disabilities arise from the territories of mind, body

v

or their social environment. Those concerned are physicians, social workers, nurses, special therapists and others.

They each describe special features of concern; but just as important as their individual contribution is the organisation providing the link which is essential to their efforts. The chapters on Assessment, Restorative Care and the Care Delivery Team underline the special aspects of this branch of medical practice.

But do we really need this group of people setting up as yet another specialty? With the advent of more disabled people will it not be sufficient merely to add to the status quo — the general practitioner, the acute hospital and the nursing home?

It is now over 40 years since the foundation in Britain of the Medical Society for the Care of the Elderly (it later became the British Geriatrics Society which is now searching for another name!). These people came together in the belief that something had to be added to existing medical practice if adequate care was to be provided for disabled elderly people. Every district health administration in that country now has a department of geriatric medicine; there is abundant proof that the old order was insufficient. Whatever the differences between the British and Australian systems of medical practice, there is a good reason to believe that we should attempt to emulate their success in this regard.

The advantages of specialisation in medicine over the last few decades are unquestionable; and yet the spawning of specialties is not always to the advantage of the disabled person. He is, at times, in danger of disintegration when he displays his multiple impairments and disabilities before the various departments of a modern hospital. This is one of the reasons why a particular organisation — a specialty with a difference, one which has breadth rather than depth — is a necessity. In its absence, the person who has a combination of physical, mental or social disabilities, particularly when those changes have been tempered by the process of ageing, is unlikely to receive adequate attention.

Where should this organisation — the geriatric service, the extended care service or whatever it is to be called — be based? This is an important issue from the point of view of its survival as well as its efficiency. Continuing disability has not been a major concern of the acute hospital; ever since the beginning of the voluntary hospital it has been policy to avoid this responsibility and to relegate chronic disease to another place. But this can no longer be regarded as reasonable practice if adequate resources are to be made available to disabled and potentially disabled people. Among those resources are the staff. From the description of their work it is clear that they will spend much of their time outside the hospital; nevertheless, they must be based on the hospital. If we wish to encourage physicians, social workers, nurses and their colleagues to accept the challenge of caring for elderly disabled people, an occupation which has not had the ready appeal or the rewards which belong to other forms of medicine and nursing, we should not continue to deny them a place in the acute hospital. This new membership works both ways: it is also to the advantage of the hospital whose staff often need assistance with the care of the growing number of elderly people in their wards. All general hospitals should have a department which has special expertise concerning people with continuing disabilities.

There are a number of phases in the care of this group of people. Reference is made in this book to some of the more acute episodes, e.g. those concerned with changes in blood pressure, falls, incontinence, etc. Changes in behaviour form an intriguing and important section of the medicine of late life and present a particular challenge to the combined skills of physician and psychiatrist. The phase of rehabilitation or restorative care, depending for its success on the intricacies of a multidisciplinary approach, is given prominence. Care at home is another important facet of the total programme, demanding the integrated attention of a number of carers. This diverse group of activities, preceded always by the important process of assessment, stands — or should stand — in sharp contrast to nursing home care, which in Australia has represented our major activity concerning disabled elderly people. This isolated concentration on the end stage of disease, necessary though it is for some people, has in many ways been a disaster. The care of established disability has too often taken precedence over efforts to prevent it and resources have been improperly used in the absence of a concerted plan of assessment, restorative and home care. A hospital-based team, working in the manner outlined in these pages, will provide the only real opportunity in redressing the balance.

Nursing homes must exist — at least the permanent care phase of nursing must continue. But where and by whom? Should we continue to condone the unfortunate schism that exists between acute and chronic disease? Separate development of acute hospital and nursing home is presently part of our national policy. This apartheid situation has evolved as a legacy of the old voluntary hospital system, in which responsibility for chronic disability was discarded in favour of acute episodic disease. It is likely to continue, to the detriment of disabled elderly people, unless what we now call acute hospitals agree to take on the role of extending their philosophy and their skills in the manner described in this book; and thereby adding the responsibility of continuing care.

This new emphasis on medical practice will not by itself ensure a better deal for the increasing proportion of elderly people predicted by demographers. The opening section of this book reminds us of the numerous facets concerned with a person's well-being; and that the care of elderly people — those, that is, who need care — is more social than medical. Successful ageing is to a large extent a social skill involving a number of adaptations and developments both by the individual and by society. Family relationships, community awareness, a just system of welfare and adequate support for losses sustained by the ageing person are all part of the development. Nevertheless, there remains that important minority of disabled or potentially disabled people who are at present missing out. They will continue to do so unless we develop the kind of practice described in the foregoing pages.

Perth 1991   R. B. Lefroy

REFERENCES

Isaacs B, Livingstone M, Nevelle Y 1972 Survival of the unfittest: a study of geriatric patients in Glasgow. Routledge and Kegan Paul, London

Shegog R F A (ed) 1981 The impending crisis of old age — a challenge to ingenuity. Oxford University Press, Oxford

Preface to the Second Edition

The demand for a second edition of this book is most gratifying as it confirms that the first edition, released in 1984, has been well received and found valuable by a wide readership who, it is hoped, will find further value herein.

It is pleasing also that the contributors to the original version gave their full support to the unenviable task of revision when they met together in April 1989. At that meeting, consideration was given to the many reviews that had been received from within Australia, and from a number of other countries, and the comments, both critical and constructive, were analysed with care.

In this edition greater stress has been laid on the maintenance of health, on the prevention of illness and on other issues such as disease presentation, the management of chronic pain, dual sensory loss — vision and hearing — and, in greater detail, drugs and elderly people.

The main purpose of this book remains the enhancement of a broad understanding of ageing and its implications by health professionals and those concerned with planning, and the provision of support, treatment and care.

No attempt has been made to describe disorders and disease processes in detail, nor the techniques and practice of medical, nursing, social work or other allied health professions as separate disciplines. Textbooks are readily available, of course, for specific disciplines and for specialised areas of knowledge.

An attempt has been made to describe the multiple nature of impairment suffered by a proportion of those who are aged, and to highlight the important underlying principles, which should enable an informed and united approach to be made to medical and psychosocial assessment, and thereby the planning of appropriate action.

The needs of the individual are paramount, and it is important that all health professionals share a common philosophy aimed at the maintenance of health, well-being and optimal independence, together with a clear appreciation of the roles played by others, so as to enable a consistent and coordinated approach in meeting the needs defined.

Readers will find that points of importance are reiterated by various contributors within the context of chapters such as those concerned with assessment and the delivery of services and care. Such repetition should serve to reinforce the vital nature of the approach which is advocated.

In this edition the name of the author or the principal contributor to each chapter is acknowledged at the chapter heading, but as with the first edition, there has been a truly multidisciplinary approach to the text, with the exchange of manuscripts and acceptance of constructive comment. This has helped to maintain consistency in approach, and to enhance understanding among the contributors themselves.

References cited in the text are listed at the end of each chapter together with related reading. A general bibliography is appended at the book's end.

Melbourne 1991   Marion W. Shaw

Preface to the First Edition

Following a College of Nursing Australia Conference in Tasmania in 1979 I met two editors from Churchill Livingstone, Mary Emmerson (now Mary Law) from Edinburgh, and Judy Waters based in Melbourne, and expressed to them the need as I saw it for the production of a book aimed at widening understanding amongst health professionals with regard to disabling and degenerative conditions and their management, and the need to encourage a more positive approach to the maintenance of health and independence particularly in ageing people. I also felt that it was important to demonstrate the purpose and interrelationship of the roles of doctors, nurses, social workers, therapists, the individual client or patient, the family, and the many other people in the community involved in the provision of a system of extended care.

These thoughts were reinforced following the annual Victorian Geriatrics Conference in October of that year, when the speakers met to review and to consider the value of the conference programme. They felt that it was important to build on the papers that had been given by contributing to a book that would enable their ideas to be disseminated more widely.

This book, therefore, is intended as an information source for health discipline students or health professionals, as well as others concerned with the provision of services for elderly people, and through them to widen understanding within the community at large.

I would like to acknowledge the willing cooperation of the many people involved in the preparation, all of whom lead very busy lives. This has been the reason for the long gestation period.

Michael Lindell's contribution is greatly appreciated. He has set the scene by covering environment, and his delightful illustrations add immeasurably to the content of the book. The social environment or the social context of ageing written by Cliff Picton provides the background for the developing theme.

Doreen Bauer helped with structure and editing, as well as by contributing the sections on restorative care, team concepts, domiciliary and residential continuing care; also jointly with John Hurley, the section on stroke. John Hurley and Bernard Worsam dealt with the physiological and medical aspects as well as with the important chapters on drugs and the assessment of need. The chapter covering an area of increasing importance and concern, behavioural disorders in elderly people, was written by Cees Van Tiggelen. Penny Murray-Phillips wrote as an advocate of the value of reality orientation and restorative care for confused elderly people; and Sister Margaret Ryan (Sister of Mercy and a Community Health Nurse) who is currently promoting a community hospice care programme for terminally ill people wrote about the care of those who are dying.

I have had the task of setting the theme, linking the segments, writing on components of care, and the concluding chapter.

It seems appropriate that the friendship and guidance of two people who influenced my own perception of the vulnerability of old people and the special approach required to problem solving and care, should be acknowledged here. One is Dr Lionel Cosin of Oxford with whom I worked for a number of years and whose comments on the early outline of this book were most helpful.

ix

The other, the late Miss Kathleen Sinclair Wilson, pioneered post-basic nursing education to ensure that the needs of elderly people in public hospitals and the community in Victoria were understood.

She also pressed for the inclusion of gerontology and geriatric nursing in the basic nursing programme for student nurses and trainee enrolled nurses. A tardiness in recognising the need for such inclusion still exists.

I trust that this book will help those working in hospitals, in health facilities, in the community and extended care services in general, to work together within a flexible system to enable people to live out their lives in a manner of their own choosing.

Melbourne 1984   Marion W. Shaw

Contributors

Doreen Bauer DipPT GradDipEdAdmin AIMM MAPA
Director of Paramedical Services,
The Queen Elizabeth Geriatric Centre, Ballarat

Edmond Chiu AM MB BS DPM FRANZCP
Associate Professor, Academic Unit for Psychiatry of Old Age, The University of Melbourne

Jennifer Gibbons OAM DipWelfareStud
Special Projects Consultant,
National Centre for Ageing and Sensory Loss, Melbourne

John Hurley MB BS MRCP(UK) FACRM
Director of Medical Services,
The Queen Elizabeth Geriatric Centre, Ballarat

Michael Lindell BArch ARAIA
Architect

Penny Phillips BA BSW(Hons)
Social Worker, Royal District Nursing Service, Melbourne

Cliff Picton BA MSW
Senior Lecturer in Social Work,
LaTrobe University, Melbourne

Sister Margaret Ryan RSM AO RN DipCHN FRCNA

Marion Shaw HVC DipNEd FRCNA

Cynthea Wellings RN BA(Hons) GradDipGeron
Nurse Consultant — Continence, Royal District Nursing Service, Melbourne

Bernard Worsam MB BS FRACP FACRM
Director of Medical Services,
Eastern Suburbs Geriatric Centre, Melbourne

Contents

1. The living environment

Michael Lindell

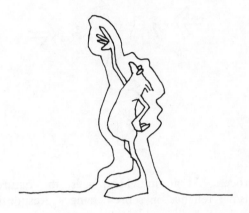

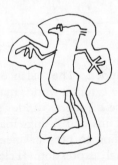

From the instant of conception to the instant of death we each participate in a dynamic interaction with our 'environment'. This word is derived from the French word *'environ'*, to encircle. Our environment does not just encircle us, it envelops us for every second of every minute of our lives. We are, in fact, part of our own environment.

Many elements, some animate, some inanimate, some touchable, some imagined, come together to create this environment. Our senses respond to a multitude of stimuli and from this perceived data a total picture or image is built up of the 'world'. This latter cognitive process differs from individual to individual and changes as we grow older, as our bodies change, as our worlds change, and as our experience develops.

If we are to develop a better understanding of the elusive relationship between humans and their environment we must develop a thorough understanding of the nature of environmental stimuli, the way our senses respond and the way cognitive processes give order to this sensory input.

There are great dangers in generalising or attempting to establish hard and fast rules about human–environment interaction. We each assemble our own ever-changing worlds and there is no 'absolute reality'.

Humans are not just passive observers of their environment; they are participants, modifiers and negotiators. Our senses constantly provide critical information that allows us to react to, and thus interact with our world. We may choose to move, to communicate, or to interfere. In a broad sense this is our 'coping' with our world.

We must know what is happening within ourselves, and around ourselves. The challenge of ageing can be better accepted when an individual and his/her environment is understood as an interactive 'whole' rather than individuals being considered as physiological lumps cast adrift in an environmental sea.

Senses give us information. While sight is obviously of critical importance, other senses are often neglected in the development of built and natural settings. Hearing, taste, touch and smell can all be considered in a truly responsive design

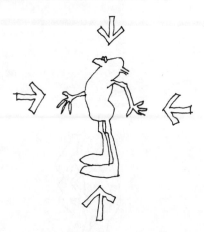

process. As an individual ages, the nature of his/her reliance on senses changes. Responsibly, we must develop places that are laden with stimuli for all senses.

We have available to us many elements which allow us the opportunity to 'tune' or modify our interaction with our environment. Our clothing may be worn for a variety of reasons. It may be for warmth, for protection, for identification or for support. Even the manner in which we wear it communicates information about ourselves to those around us. Our vision may be modified by either dark or corrective glasses, contact lenses or even a monocle.

Each is an option that can be taken up to achieve an end. Jewellery, false teeth, crutches, toupees, hearing aids and other personal effects further mark the individual and possibly enhance his/her capacity to cope with his/her world. Tobacco, alcohol and other drugs are also available to influence our interaction with our world. The social and physical nature of an environment is a major influence on our sense of identity. The

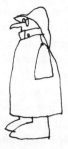

form of a building, its spaces, finishes, textures and relationships can reinforce or erode an individual's identity. In experiencing a building, we do not clearly differentiate between the built and the administrative fabric, we perceive it as a whole. If the goal in a project is to develop his sense of identity, this must be reflected in the design of the building, the administrative systems, the landscaping and the image of the building within the community. The created environment should respect rather than compromise the individual.

Our houses, however formed, are shelters from rain, wind and sun. They may be warmed, they may be cooled. Sound and light may be intro-

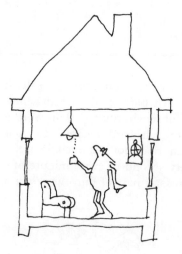

duced or excluded. The balance between the internal and the external worlds may be regulated through the use of doors, windows and louvres. Furniture, curtains and fittings may be included to suit the setting to personal need and further allow individual expression. Telephones, television and radio are options of special significance to the less mobile members of a community.

Humans are gregarious animals and seek to identify with others. The way we cut our hair, shave, dress, drive, eat, talk, walk and sport all reflect on our own image and how we relate to others.

Our responsibility as a community is to create settings that may be changed, that may be used in different ways and are, thus, responsive to varying individual needs. Environmental expression is greatly enhanced by the capacity to move. An individual can clearly express a choice by 'voting with his/her feet'. If we cycle the choice is broadened; if we drive it is further broadened and yet further if we fly. The extent to which we can move is our *range*.

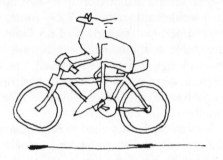

With ageing there is often a shrinkage in range which can lead to isolation. Factors that bear on range include physical and mental capacities, availability of transport and the nature of the physical environment. Barriers can be effective be they touchable or imagined. If an individual is no longer able to wander afar to experience the world, the world and the spectrum of choices associated with it must be brought to the individual. If life in the latter years is to be a challenge, there must be variation, vitality and familiarity within our range.

There is a tendency to be preoccupied with mainly physical elements when considering the

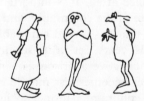

environment. However, the most important part of our world is other people, and with them come social, cultural, territorial and myriad psychological pressures which bear on our intricate interactions.

Understanding the nature of this interaction is the key to developing a 'living environment'. People are the most significant elements in the

worlds of other people. Interaction can take many forms. Contact between people may be by sight, by hearing, by touch or by smell. It may be direct or it may be via another, by electronic means or by a letter. All are valid linkages which give us our community context. The information conveyed in these messages helps us to establish our identity, our worth and our value.

This feedback from the community can be devastating, particularly to older people. Too often they are considered a group of little value, a group who should be retired, a group who the 'non-olds' should care for. The community, despite often being well meaning, is ruthless in its type casting. This attitudinal pressure creates an image or expectation of 'being old' which many people adopt as an appropriate model or role. People who often have little in common apart from longevity are seen as a problem rather than a resource.

Considerable work is now being done on cluster developments that are threaded throughout the community. These offer opportunities for older people, whose blood family has left, to be part of a new family. Such a group need not be just older people. Ideally it is a symbiotic association of individuals. In such settings, all are able to maintain community context and independence, and are challenged to contribute rather than coddled. The term 'disabled' is often used within the community to describe a group of people who move, think or behave differently. The tyranny of designing for the majority of so-called normal people is responsible for disqualifying many from any opportunity to cope, to move and thus to express themselves. What so often happens then, is that the disqualified have no choice but to rely, very obviously, on the qualified. Sadly this

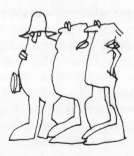

reliance often involves compromise of identity. We all have potentials that may or may not be achieved. It is the responsibility of designers of environments to create settings which offer *all* the opportunity to realise their differing potentials. Thus, the form of the environment can determine the extent to which a disability can create a handicap.

Objective and sympathetic understanding of an individual in his/her total context is the basis of assessment. Such assessment is the foundation upon which treatment or support programmes can be developed.

When humans suffer disabling or degenerative illnesses the opportunity exists to develop the physical, psychological and social environment in such a way as to assist in the restoration of independence and well-being. Individuals must be given the chance to regain as much control over their own destiny as possible.

Privacy is a concept often misunderstood. It is equated with being apart or being alone. However, privacy is not a static state but is ever-changing. At every instant of life, we seek a level of interaction with other people. When we achieve that level an acceptable state of privacy exists. A balance of desired level and achieved level may thus be created in what appears to be an extremely crowded situation. Also, an imbal-

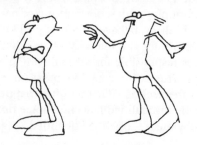

ance may exist where an individual is quite removed from any contact with others. Thus, 'private' is not an appropriate adjective to describe a single bed ward. The room at times may be private but at other times, as is often the case, it is an isolation room.

If an environment is to be developed that is responsive to man's fluctuating interaction needs, it is necessary to create an accessible spectrum of spatial opportunities where a variety of interactions may be experienced. Simply, a choice must be available. So often choice is the first casualty in institutional development.

Too often wards are designed as either single bed or multiple bed. Perhaps there is an option where several beds make up a ward but each has its own defined territory. A day room, no matter how superbly designed, is of no value if it is inaccessible or thought to be inaccessible. A door, even though it may be unlocked, can effectively frighten away a new resident or patient. The 'not knowing' of the space beyond often leads to timidity.

Spaces can be designed to be welcoming; doors are not always essential and initiates may be personally introduced into so-called communal spaces. Rarely do people gather together in large numbers. Usually twos, threes and fours are the most common. Thus, rather than a single day

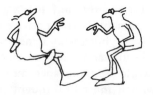

room being the answer, a good case exists for creating smaller spaces throughout a hospital, nursing home or residential complex.

The spectrum of choice must be accessible or it is no choice at all. It is important to consider the structure of the community and its buildings. A building that has served admirably as a family home for 30 years, set in its suburban lot, may become as effective a prison as a moated castle as the owner becomes less mobile and more isolated. The community form and its fabric must

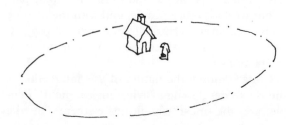

be changed to minimise such problems. A retirement village can become a ghetto in which residents lose community context, unless great care is taken in its structuring and siting.

Our ability to cope with our world is dependent upon our being orientated or knowing where we are and how we relate to others, so that decisions we make in our negotiations of the world are reasonable. Many of the cities, buildings, settings and systems that have been created, make orientation virtually impossible for anyone other than the initiated.

Environments must offer cues that enable us to know our reference points, our landmarks and routes. Differences need to be established to minimise confusion. The reliance on corridors in large buildings contributes greatly to the disorientation so often experienced within. Windows, while important in offering views, are even more important in providing orientation and context. Changes in colours, textures, planes and sounds all can be constructively used to allow people to find their way around. Created environments can support self-expression or they can suppress it. Perhaps the hallmark of an 'institution' is that the individual is made to conform rather than the setting made responsive to his/her needs. An institution is neither a building nor an administrative structure, it is a total setting which reflects

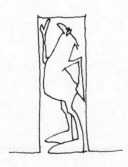

a basic attitude. While generalisations are often made about 'man made' and 'natural' environments, most behavioural settings are a combination of both. Humans developed an understanding of their natural environment and have chosen to modify this world for a variety

of reasons. In our creation of shelters, be they clothing or structures, we have sought to modify the climate and thus create an environment better related to our needs. The structures we have built have also served as 'containers' of activities. As such they have been furnished, decorated and marked in such a way as to enhance the functions to be performed within. Some spaces have been tailored to but one purpose, others to a variety. The trappings used to mark such spaces may be fixed or movable. Buildings, being an integral part of the community fabric, have a symbolic value within a community.

Design is a problem-solving process and thus not only associated with architects, engineers and interior designers. We all have the opportunity to influence part of the environment. The tragedy to date is that not enough has been done to unify the actions of many groups who so often have common goals.

Either deliberately, or by accident, we create *places*. Such places are not just a gathering together of physical elements (Canter 1977). They involve the activities of people and the character of a place is, to a considerable extent, determined by the conceptions held by those using the place. Thus, to achieve a design goal, a process must be developed which is sympathetic to physical form, activity planning and conception development. This can only be undertaken by a team, it is not just an architect's job.

The dynamic nature of communities ensures that rarely, if ever, will a design solution be absolutely appropriate. The challenge is to do better and to be responsive. Data concerning our interaction with our environment are desperately needed, be we young or not young. These data must be in a comprehensible form, so they may

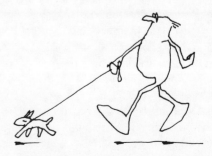

then become a reasonable basis on which to develop future design approaches.

The world is our laboratory and we must heighten our observation and develop approaches to understand better the ways we interact. Rather than looking for rules of similarity let us clarify the ways in which we differ and then develop environments that are based on the premise that we are different rather than identical. We must be extremely careful in designing for the so-called elderly. They are not a race apart.

REFERENCE

Canter D 1977 The psychology of place. The Architectural Press, London

2. The social context of ageing

Cliff Picton

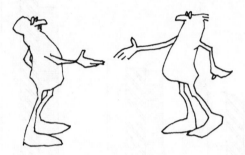

The social context of ageing in Australia is essentially related to the characteristics of the present population variously defined as aged, and the best projections of future trends. In 1987, 10.7% of Australians (1.7 million) were aged 65 years and over. This represents a higher proportion of older people in the population than has ever occurred before. It results from a significant decline in fertility resulting in reductions in numbers in younger age groups and notable increases in life expectancy. Over the last 50 years the expectation of life of both male and female (white) Australians over the age of 60 has increased markedly. Based on 1982 figures, life expectancy at birth stands at 72 years for males and 78 years for females; this compares with 64 years for males and 69 years for females in 1935. Estimates of life expectancy for Aborigines is significantly worse, the best being 61 years for males and 65 years for females, and the worst in country New South Wales at 51 for males and 59 for females (Thomson 1989).

Australia's older population is unevenly distributed across the country with South Australia having the oldest population and Western Australia the lowest proportion of older people.

In line with other developed countries Australia can look forward to a continuing increase in numbers of older people, with those aged 65 years and over reaching 13.4% by the year 2011 and 20% by the year 2031. The fastest rate of increase will occur in the group described as the 'old old', i.e. those 75 years and over. This group is projected to grow from 4.1% of the population in 1987 to 9.2% in 2031; and for the group aged 85 years and over from 0.8% in 1987 to 2.3% in 2031.

Women predominate in these older age groups, representing 58% of the population aged 65 years and over and 73% of those aged 85 years and over (1986 Census). This is in line with a worldwide trend, giving rise to the term 'the feminisation of old age'. As their age increases, so too does the proportion who are widowed.

Figure 2.1 illustrates the percentages of Australia's projected population aged 65 and over, and 80 and over, from 1991 to 2031. In itself, this is not a particularly remarkable projection and the increase will be smaller than in many other industrialised countries and very small compared with some Asian countries, e.g. Indonesia's older population will increase by 134% and Thailand's by 107% by the year 2000. Nevertheless, because Australia has been, hitherto, a predominantly young country in terms of the age structure of the total population, the current highlighting of the ageing phenomenon presents an opportunity and a challenge to social

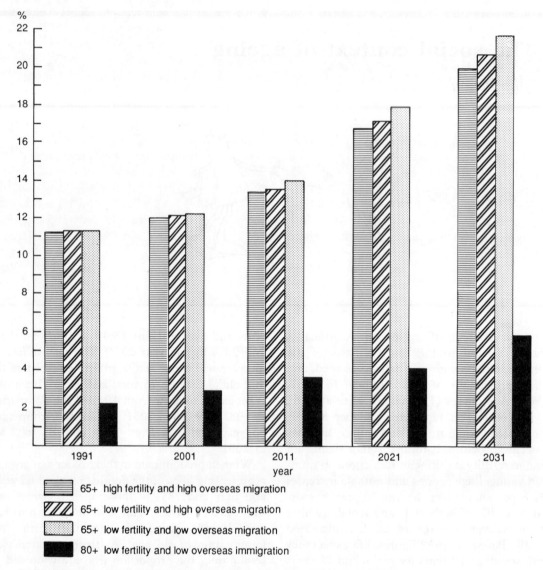

Source: Australian Bureau of Statistics, 1990 Projections of the Populations of Australia,
States and Territories 1989 to 2031. ABS, Canberra

Fig. 2.1 The percentages of Australia's projected population aged 65 and over, and 80 and over, from 1991 to 2031. The demographic assumptions used in making these projections are noted in the key.

policy makers and service providers. The opportunity is to develop policies sufficiently imaginative and flexible to help meet the consequences of a significant shift in the population structure; the challenge is to review existing programmes of health care, social security and welfare to cater more adequately to the needs of a culturally diverse aged population. A population, moreover, likely to contain a greatly increased proportion of physically and mentally frail people who will need better and more varied services than those presently available.

At the outset it is necessary to address the difficult question of what we understand by the concepts of health and welfare for older people. In most countries there are divisions of opinion as to what constitutes an acceptable level of welfare in its broadest sense. The debate is often conducted along ideological lines; on the one hand we have the rugged individualists with their 'stand on your own two feet' philosophy; on the other the advocates of a significant level of state involvement to cushion the weak from the play of forces beyond their control.

Ultimately, of course, decisions about how much or how little to provide will be based on political judgements and economic pressures. Arguments based on notions of altruism and social justice are given little credence especially in times of high inflation and large-scale unemployment. Policy makers will need to be presented more and more with arguments related to the cost-effectiveness of services as well as to the general well-being of older people if an appropriate share of national resources is to be attracted. In this regard, there could be a fortunate coincidence in that many existing resources (in health and welfare) are concentrated in expensive institutional programmes while the growing demands for change point in the direction of community care which is, theoretically, cheaper. That it is also likely to be a more effective way of meeting the needs of those for whom institutional care is neither appropriate nor necessary may be incidental to the framers of national budgets. It is not without significance, however, that in spite of improved assessment techniques, a proportion of placements of older people in nursing homes are thought to be inappropriate.

Another important issue is that of priorities in resource allocations. There are signs in some countries, notably the USA, that taxpayers are in revolt against the seemingly endless upward trend in income taxes. Some politicians see the 'burden' of public health and welfare programmes as an area ripe for cost cutting. Early casualties in this kind of exercise will be those groups traditionally regarded as powerless and stigmatised, including, the old.

Should more emphasis be paid on personal responsibility, or is the state committed to provide health and welfare services to compensate for the 'diswelfares' of industrialisation? Graycar & Kinnear in a recent analysis (1981) argue that: 'This debate is intimately connected with debates about whether allocations should be aimed at adequacy, equity or equality; whether benefits should come as an entitlement or be part of a struggle; whether allocations should focus on self-reliance or dependency'. These issues are at least as much to do with systems of values as with economics.

Viewed against this background and the changes in the characteristics of the aged population there seems to be an urgent need to bring together the economic and the health and welfare perspectives. A willingness to provide care, treatment and support for those older people in need is not only a significant indicator of collective social responsibility; it also recognises certain imperatives within the population of older people. For example, among the consequences of more people surviving beyond the age of 80 are increasing frailty and senile dementia. By planning and rationalising policies and services the effects of these and other conditions may be contained instead of threatening to overwhelm a system insufficiently diverse in range and coverage, and lacking in adequate assessment procedures. In other words, a more efficient use of resources should also mean a more effective meeting of need.

Finding a way of resolving the fundamental dilemma between meeting human need and the allocation of resources in a complex economy is a central problem for policy makers and analysts. Martin Rein (1977) set the dilemma in a social policy context when he wrote:

Conventionally (social policy) is thought to be concerned with redistribution and increasing equality, or at least relieving distress and poverty; economic policy is conventionally thought to be concerned with distribution and increasing output. These distinctions are no longer satisfactory. The scope of social policy is now raising questions about the capacity of the economic system to meet the legitimate demands placed upon it while the political system is not capable of redefining these claims.

In seeking answers to the question, 'How much should the state do for the old?', we have to recognise the constant clashing of values and ideologies. Rein's concept of 'legitimate demands' is in line with the notion of a welfare society — itself a refinement of welfare state, and the old German concept of *Wohlfahrtstaat*. Such concepts have always been attacked by advocates of 'small government' and individualism. Their view of welfare is best summed up by Peter Goldman's description of the British welfare state as 'a mechanism for distributing golden eggs'. The most optimistic scenario given present population trends would be a recognition by governments that a residual approach is austere and stigmatising and that some form of positive discrimination which encourages and supports independence is the best road to integration of the aged. Such a recognition could also pave the way for a more effective use of knowledge, skills and experience of those old people who do not wish to be categorised as retired.

AGEING AND ATTITUDES

Apart from general policy considerations any discussion of ageing and the provision of services must have regard to attitudes. Attitudes and values provide foundations for the beliefs that shape and guide our perceptions of, and responses to, social groups like the aged, the disabled and delinquents. If our responses are based on negative, stereotyped attitudes, the result is likely to be rejection and stigmatisation.

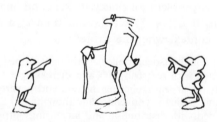

Australian population projections suggest that 16% of our total population will be 60 and over by the year 2001 with a disproportionately high rate among the overseas born. For all countries the social, economic and political implications of these changes are enormous, yet there is widespread confusion, complacency and failure to own up to how little we understand old age. The situation is at once compounded and exacerbated by deeply entrenched ageism which acts as a barrier to action and the development of appropriate policies and programmes. This barrier is frequently experienced by older people and their advocates as a discriminatory practice that tends to exclude or prevent access to a range of services and activities enjoyed without restriction by other age groups.

Ageism

In 1973, Robert Butler and Myrna Lewis used the term ageism to describe 'a process of systematic stereotyping or discrimination against people because they are old, just as racism and sexism accomplish this with skin colour and gender. Old people are categorised as senile, rigid in thought and manner, old fashioned in morality and skills'.

Ageism allows the younger generation to view old people as different from themselves.

Radford (1987), describing the visual, physical and mental derivations of the stereotypes, states 'Ageism is practised by the community, the professions, often most sadly by the elderly themselves if they too come to believe the myths about themselves on which it is built'.

Age discrimination

Age discrimination is a denial, based on chronological age, of equal opportunities on the basis of assumptions that cannot be validated on other grounds. As Equal Opportunity Commissioner Williams notes in her recent report (1989) in Western Australia: 'Discrimination arises because of incorrect assumptions about people's needs and abilities based on their chronological age'.

Since we discovered, albeit belatedly, that older people have opinions they are willing to voice if given the opportunity, the extent of discriminatory attitudes and practices has assumed epidemic proportions. The continuum is long — from employment and insurance to the patronising 'does she have sugar in her coffee' syndrome. Sue Jones (1987), policy officer of the NSW Council on the Ageing, in a position paper on age discrimination provides a wide range of examples to show how discriminatory practices and attitudes permeate almost every aspect of the lives of older people.

Notwithstanding then the likely need for legislation to identify, define and enshrine rights, it seems clear that a more difficult but necessary accompaniment will be the changing of attitudes. In this, the cause will be immeasurably aided by the relatively recent upsurge of confidence in older people in speaking out about their needs and aspirations. The emergence of self-help groups, specific political platforms on ageing, and the rapid spread of self-managed education movements like the University of the Third Age, all present to the general public and government an articulate, educated and astute group of people who are less and less inclined to be ignored, patronised or marginalised.

The empowerment of older people is taking place rapidly. It is being achieved as a result of an alliance between energetic and highly motivated older people and a number of skilled advocates who are not part of their peer group. We are likely to see and hear more and more of them as their confidence grows to match their achievements.

Stereotypes often arise out of fear based on an unwillingness to accept some quality or characteristic in others that we reject in ourselves. When we confront old age we do, in a special sense, confront our future selves. It is understandable that in a society still dominated by images of youth and vitality (even though these images are themselves stereotypes!), some people should develop a negative view of the aged. This is compounded by internal migration patterns that lead to the splitting up of families; and by social services that have tended to segregate and incarcerate the old in institutions.

Of course, stereotypes are grounded in reality. No one can deny that some old people are sick, dependent, poor and lonely. Careful study of the facts, however, puts these people into a total context. But too often we tend to ignore the facts in favour of a distorted view presented by media, advertisers, governments, or even our own prejudices. Attacking a stereotyped view entails presenting a positive image of its opposite. The more older people and their advocates are able to present some of the positives and potential in

ageing the sooner the negative stereotype will diminish.

How do stereotypes affect those they purport to portray? In many ways our systems of social organisation create an environment in which the stereotype becomes the self-fulfilling prophecy. If we force older people to relinquish certain socially significant roles and give them no help or encouragement to seek alternatives, if we ensure that for some the transition from provider and contributor to receiver and observer is abrupt and irreversible, we should not be surprised that some people experience trauma. Some of the most important consequences for these people defined as old have little to do with the processes of ageing per se. They are defined by society often according to a formula no longer relevant. Men commonly retire at age 65. This age was fixed for German male workers by Chancellor Otto von Bismarck in 1889 when the life expectancy was under 50.

Table 2.1 shows how a selection of countries interpret retirement differently.

Although many people look forward to retirement, it is equally true that many wish to continue working beyond the customary retirement age. Participation by men and women aged 60+ in the labour force has been declining since 1966. In 1966, 79.4% of men aged 60–64 were in the labour force; by 1980 this had dropped to 50.1%, a drop of 39.9%. A drop of 52.4% occurred for those aged 65+. Among women aged 60–64, the drop was 12.3% from 15.4% to 13.5%. For those aged 65 and over the drop was 34.1% (**Australian Bureau of Statistics 1980**). Participation in the labour force is a complex matter, as much dependent on government policies, the state of the economy, the number of younger workers seeking employment, as on the older person's wish or capacity. Opportunities are greater for some occupational groups than others, e.g. skilled or professionally qualified workers.

In making provision of services for the aged, whose welfare are we concerned about, theirs or ours? It is reasonable to argue that in seeking to make provision for their health and welfare we are also laying the foundations for our own care in the future. In this sense all welfare activities could be seen as exercises in a paradoxical kind

Table 2.1 Normal pensionable ages in selected countries by sex, 1979

Country and year system enacted	Men	Women
Argentina (1944)	60*	55*
Australia (1908)	65	60
Austria (1906)	65	60
Belgium (1924)	65	60
Canada (1927)	65	65
Czechoslovakia (1906)	60	57
Denmark (1891)	67	67
Finland (1937)	65	65
France (1910)	65	65
Germany, Democratic Republic (1889)	65	60
Germany, Federal Republic (1889)	65	65
Greece (1934)	62	57
Hungary (1929)	60	55
Iceland (1936)	67	67
Ireland (1908)	65	65
Italy (1919)	60†	55†
Japan (1941)	60	55
Luxembourg (1911)	65	60
The Netherlands (1913)	65	65
New Zealand (1898)	65	65
Norway (1936)	67	67
Poland (1927)	65	60
Spain (1919)	65	65
Sweden (1913)	65	65
Switzerland (1946)	65	62
Union of Soviet Socialist Republics (1922)	60	55
United Kingdom (1909)	65	60
United States (1935)	65	65

* Aged 65 for self-employed men and 60 for self-employed women.
† Pension payable at any age after 35 years of contribution.
Source — Adapted from Staples T G 1977 The pensionable age in selected industrialised countries. HEW SSA Research and Statistics Note No. 15, August 26.

of altruism, tinged with self-interest. When we examine the functions of welfare in society we seldom look beyond other people as the intended beneficiaries. Many people, however, do not share the basic premise that some provision should be made. In Australia, as in other countries, concern is expressed from time to time at the extension (or intrusion) of organised welfare, in the broadest sense, into our lives. Fears have been expressed that a widening of the scope of welfare provisions is matched by a corresponding lessening of individual and family responsibility. Someone has even spoken of the old as being 'preyed upon' by welfare. In practice, both views are highly suspect and difficult to sustain.

This brings us back to the ideological debate. Should we see older people as 'deserving' or 'entitled to' a range of services? Many of these people in the 'old old' group have developed a marked capacity for coping after the experiences of economic depressions and two world wars when the range and coverage of social services was less extensive and eligibility criteria more stringent. Those who will be defined as old by the year 2000 will have developed different coping behaviours and expectations. There is every likelihood that they will feel entitled to more than is presently provided. They will also be better educated, more aware of their rights and more confident about making demands on the state for satisfaction. There is another consideration. Australia is moving into an entirely new era so far as the old are concerned. There have never been so many people surviving to a great age. This is a unique phenomenon and it requires new responses and initiatives from governments and service providers. Future generations will judge how well we respond to this challenge.

Perceptions and stereotypes

Ageing is not a homogeneous process, neither is it carried forward by a simple step by step progression. Our perceptions of ageing are amalgams of how we view ourselves on the ageing continuum and how we view those we know or love as they negotiate their own paths. Perceptions are also powerfully influenced by models and images selectively placed before us by the mass media, advertising, or the accident of physical proximity. A vigorous septuagenarian politician directing a nation's affairs is hard to reconcile with patients suffering from senile dementia in a secured geriatric ward. Each, however, is a faithful representation of part of the complex processes we call ageing; each can contribute positively or negatively to our perception of the old, and, perhaps more importantly, to how the old perceive themselves. A recent attempt to integrate people suffering from dementia with other residents in an old people's home led to many asking tearfully 'Will I be like that?'. The subsequent lowering of morale led to the abandonment of the experiment. Service provisions therefore should seek to reflect the long and diverse continuum represented by the aged rather than the narrow, hostile negative stereotype of 'sans everything'.

The cultural diversity of Australia could play an increasingly important part in this more accurate presentation of needs. Next to the State of Israel, Australia has the most culturally diverse population in terms of country of birth. This diversity has already enriched our society in so many ways. Yet it would be easy to forget that the older immigrant often has special needs that must be the target of positive discrimination by governments and service providers. Even though they may have settled well in Australia, it is not uncommon for some people born overseas to revert to their native language and live, as it were, in the past when they become very old. Unless we can help to provide an accepting context for this behaviour to occur within, we will simply add further dimensions to the stereotype. A recognition of their rights and needs, however, could help to break down some of the barriers against those who were born here.

Cultural diversity also serves to present us with other models of how the aged may be more valued and respected than they appear to be in white Australian society.

In 1981 there were 480 000 overseas-born people aged 60 years and over — this represents an increase of 28.5% since 1971. The total number of migrant aged will increase significantly in the future and it is widely projected that 1 in every 4 Australian migrants will be aged 60 years or older in the year 2001. While the Australian population overall is ageing, the ageing of the overseas-born population will continue to be disproportionate, resulting as it does from the patterns of Australian immigration and characteristics of new settlers. Migrant aged persons will increasingly include a wider variety of cultural backgrounds than has hitherto been the case, and future policies and programme developments must be able to cater for increasingly varied needs and expectations.

The most recent data to have specifically sought to understand the particular circumstances of older migrants have been provided by the Australian Council on the Ageing (ACOTA) survey on Older People At Home, conducted in 1981 and published in 1985, and those contained in the Australian Institute of Multicultural Affairs (AIMA) survey data collected in 1984 and published in 1985. The data are limited, in that both the ACOTA and AIMA samples were limited to two major metropolitan areas, with the ACOTA data showing an over-representation of Italian-born migrants and the AIMA data drawn from a sampling of six major migrant communities; nevertheless, the information now available provides a clear picture of significant differences that must be addressed.

In the ACOTA survey, two-thirds of respondents were Australian born. Of the one-third who were immigrant aged, almost half were born in English-speaking countries and half in non-English-speaking countries.

Both surveys found that the majority of older immigrants had spent their productive years in Australia. The AIMA data additionally show that more than 90% of respondents were committed to spending the rest of their lives in Australia.

To summarise the data, we can say that compared with the Australian born and the aged and older people from English-speaking countries, older immigrants from non-English-speaking backgrounds:

- Report high levels of unmet needs
- Indicate lower health status
- Are less aware of existing programmes and services
- Are under-represented in long-term residential care facilities
- Have more difficulties in adjusting to retirement, a less than adequate income and fewer sources of income
- Are more dependent on the support of family

- Have fewer people in their primary network, in their age, linguistic and cultural groups
- Have lower involvement with friends, neighbours and community generally
- Experience social desolation, especially within the institutionalised system, because of communication barriers
- Overall, have an increased need for external support.

Both surveys show the extent to which the needs of older migrants remain unmet. Information about available services is not distributed equally to all Australians — indeed, information distribution within the general community is very poor, thereby doubling the disadvantage to non-English speaking members of the community as what does exist is seldom translated into community languages. The range and quality of services is insufficiently discriminating with regard to the differential needs of migrant communities. These include culture-specific issues such as the sensitivity necessary in regard to care about religious precepts, meal preparation, and most importantly, staff sensitivity to migrant values, expectations and needs.

IMPLICATIONS FOR FUTURE POLICIES

As mentioned, recent government initiatives for older people make little reference to older migrants. Future policies cannot ignore their particular needs. The major issues and concerns have already been identified by researchers, in government reports and by ethnic communities themselves. They include:

- Equity — a fair share of resources regardless of ethnic background.
- Access — equality of access to all services provided for older people.
- Cultural relevance — service delivery should take account of differing cultural values and expectations, with language services that facilitate access and participation.
- Locality — proximity of services to the potential users should be a high priority. However, it should be recognised that ethnic communities are scattered across local government and regional boundaries.

- Community integration — where possible services should be community based rather than institutional.
- Participation — aged members of ethnic communities have the right to participate in the planning and delivery of services designed to meet their needs.

On the service side, it is imperative that our understanding of cultural diversity and differential needs should be reflected in appropriately differentiated responses from the caring professions. The opening chapter of this book includes a special plea for the creation of living environments better related to the needs of older people and to those who support them. This must include a recognition of different needs in such areas as diet, language, religion and the culturally determined hierarchy of relationships based on age and sex. The training and education programmes for doctors, nurses, social workers and others should contain a substantial multicultural element as well as seeking to recruit a culturally diverse group of aspiring professionals. An ability to speak the language of one's patient has been shown to be a powerful reinforcer to professional relationships.

To fully comprehend the needs of old people, governments and the helping professions must acquire an historical–cultural perspective. Attitudes that may appear to clash dramatically will have been formed 70–80 years ago when the social order and the prevailing norms were very different. Yet as research indicates, this does not mean that old people have been left stranded by the outgoing tide. Very old people do represent, in fact, living history, and provide us with important indicators of the rapidity of social and economic change. The process of understanding them simultaneously helps younger people to gain a perspective on contemporary life and offers a way of integrating the old by valuing their knowledge and experience.

This is of course taking an optimistic view. A belief in the capacity of older people in general to respond to their changing developmental and social situations should be a powerful determinant in the debate on resource allocations. The hallmark of successful ageing might be said to represent a degree of acceptance of diminishing functions balanced by an involvement in activities designed to stimulate mentally and physically. All of this needs to be contained in an environment in which old people feel valued, respected for their knowledge and experience and are given opportunities to make choices. Equally, it is the responsibility of governments and service providers to help meet the needs of those who by virtue of age and physical or mental frailty are unable to maintain an independent self-determining existence.

RETIREMENT AND WORK OPPORTUNITIES

Today it is true to state that in most countries in the world (and in all that lay claim to be 'developed') the ordinary person may look forward with reasonable assurance to the achievement of old age. Alongside this phenomenon we must set the revolution that has occurred in the workplace, with mechanisation, automation and rapidly advancing technology affecting the size and composition of the workforce. Compulsory retirement has become a reality for many older workers whether or not they are physically or psychologically prepared for it. Many people fear retirement as a time of enforced leisure, financial hardship and boredom, rather than an opportunity to realise ambitions set aside during their working life.

Worship of work is deeply entrenched in this society. Leisure is often undervalued despite its attractiveness and the possibilities it provides for continuing development and personal enrichment.

Although financial and economic considerations are extremely important to retired persons, perhaps the main challenge is how to achieve and maintain a sense of dignity and purpose after what is commonly thought of as the productive part of life is over. As people differ in temperament, values, skills, education, etc., there will be a wide variety of means of achieving this goal. There is strong evidence that planning for retirement programmes is reaching more people approaching their last years in the workforce. Bodies like the Early Planning For Retirement Association and Colleges of Advanced Education are providing a wide range of short courses on key issues such as finance, health, leisure and nutrition. More and more of the larger employers are bringing such programmes into the workplace and are providing workers with opportunities to attend. Significantly, however, it seems that pre-retirement education is still directed at the professional managerial occupational groups. There is much scope for enlisting the support of the trade union movement to enable the so called blue collar workers to benefit. One organisation, the Australian Council on the Ageing, has begun talks on this matter with the Australian Council for Trade Unions (ACTU).

The question of how the retired will spend their retirement cannot be dissociated from the larger question of a move towards a society in which leisure will play an increasingly important part. The large body of physically active retirees may help to spearhead the transition from a work-orientated to a leisure-orientated society. Planners must consider the fact that the next generation of retired people will be better educated, have more sophisticated skills and wider expectations than those presently retired.

The abruptness with which many people retire, often with little preparation, may have repercussions on their physical and mental health. It is not difficult to imagine what it must mean to a person when the long-established patterns of daily life are disrupted and the whole future plunged into uncertainty. Retirement as viewed by society forces many to acknowledge that the most important part of life is over. Negative effects can be diminished by early planning for retirement especially where it is accompanied by a progressive reduction of working hours.

At a time of rising concern about high levels of unemployment among the young it is not fashionable to argue for the retention of older people in the workforce. Yet, worldwide, this argument is being advanced in the context of older people constituting a significant proportion of the world's economically active population. In developing countries, the average labour force participation rate in 1975 for males aged 65 and over was 53%; for females, it was 17%.

Although many developed nations have shown substantial reductions in older worker participation in the last 30 years, approximately 23% of elderly males in the developed nations, and 8% of elderly females were in the workforce in 1975. These figures together with the economic activities not included in official statistics are only one measure of the current contributions of older people to national economic development. Another factor needing to be taken into account is the wish of many older people to remain economically productive, a factor largely ignored by official economic policies.

Rising dependency rates, a phenomenon affecting countries at many different stages of development, also represent an argument for increasing the rate of participation in the workforce by older people. While some countries have encouraged early retirement by offering attractive retirement options, the economic burden this is placing on their social security systems is increasingly recognised.

The creation of more job opportunities for older people is inextricably a matter of social policy and economic management. Flexible reduction in working hours represents an acceptance that many older people wish to work on a part-time basis. In order to extend this practice new employment options would need to be developed including the provision of low interest loans to encourage self-employment, wage subsidies and other incentives to firms hiring unemployed older workers, and the creation of special workshops. Older people are also a largely untapped resource for providing neighbourhood-based social services needed by their peers and by persons in other age groups. Two such examples already in operation in Victoria are the SPAN Project and the Foster Grandparents Programme. Proponents of the retention of older people in the workforce argue that it is usually easier to persuade existing workers to remain in than to entice the retired to return to employment. Incentives that may be effective in maintaining older worker participation include job redesign (e.g. restructuring a job or work environment in order to maximise the capabilities of the older worker), increased opportunities for part-time work, job sharing, flexible working hours, job training and retraining.

These proposals can only be implemented on a large scale if there are accompanying changes in social and political attitudes to older workers. Trade unions, employers and governments would have to provide safeguards to protect older workers against age discrimination in pay and conditions of employment, as well as the abolition of mandatory retirement practices.

Although the adoption of these and other changes to employment opportunities seems unlikely in Australia in the near future, they must at least be considered as options given an eventual improvement in the economy as a whole. There is considerable evidence that older people are efficient, productive and reliable workers. National educational campaigns would be a *sine qua non* to help overcome inaccurate stereotypes about the capabilities and work performance records of older workers, which in most occupations compare favourably with those of younger workers.

In the short term we are more likely to see an increasing recognition of the potential contribution of older people through the education system and voluntary service. The use of older people as educational aids, while anathema to some teachers, could help to stem the rising tide of illiteracy, encourage the continued practice of arts and crafts now falling into disuse, foster a sense of history in a time of rapid social and economic change, as well as promote intergenerational contacts. The inculcation of an understanding of ageing in the young will have important long-term repercussions for the present cohort of middle-aged people who will be the next generation of the old. A Japanese sociological study (Maeda 1978) indicates that the sense of responsibility towards aged parents and knowledge about ageing are considerably higher among the age group 20–29 years than among the age group 30–39 years. Preparation of the taxpayers of the year 2000 for their prospective responsibilities towards an increased aged population would seem to constitute wise forward planning.

A key factor in the pre- and post-retirement policies for older people should be a recognition of the need for access to continuing or lifelong education. Australia, as a signatory to the recommendations of the United Nations World Assembly on Ageing (The Vienna Plan 1982) endorses this concept: 'Education should form the basis for an ageing policy for, by, with and concerning the ageing. Lifelong education is not merely a means of acquiring knowledge, skills, cultural and spiritual enrichment and personal advancement, but also of acquiring the ability to cope with and participate in the events of daily life'. The Assembly considered educational development as an economic necessity and a right for all human beings 'ranging from literacy to preparation for specific stages of life such as retirement and ageing'.

There is a special need for educational access as a matter of priority for groups such as the following:

• Lone older women such as those recently widowed or deserted and who require retraining and readjustment to their new circumstances in life.
• Blue collar workers aged 55+, recently retrenched and considered too old to rejoin the workforce.
• Older persons of non-English speaking background who need to retain their often deteriorating English.

There is also the need to promote lifelong education as an essential element in the creative use of the increased leisure that retirement offers. One highly successful promotion has been the development in Australia of Universities of the Third Age (Picton 1984).

Universal access to education for children has become an accepted part of life in the developed countries of the world. Increasingly, education beyond the high school or secondary phase has been pursued by a relatively small number of students. Emphasis on the vocational aspects of education has further down-graded the pursuit of knowledge as an end in itself for all but a handful of exceptional scholars. Overall, older, and especially retired, people are numerically under-represented at all levels of the educational system. There are a number of reasons for this under-representation. Many of those who are currently retired would have left school at a very early age, perhaps due to socioeconomic imperatives or the lack of opportunity to pursue education beyond the basic levels. Their experience of the educational system, therefore, was probably unlikely to engender a burning desire to pursue further studies later in life. Not surprisingly, older people in search of educational opportunities in retirement have been found to be predominantly drawn from the professional and managerial classes. Other discouraging factors would include the high cost of further education, difficulty some older people might experience in travelling to and from an academic centre, and the tendency for adult education programmes to run in the evening when some older people may be reluctant to leave home. More pertinent to this discussion, however, is the general absence of the concept of lifelong education and the way in which education has become inextricably linked with the pursuit of academic success in the form of a qualification. The pursuit of knowledge as an end in itself seems to have been an early casualty in the onslaught of intellectual vandalism of recent years. The University of the Third Age concept offers a way out of these difficulties and barriers.

The first University of the Third Age was founded in Toulouse, France, in 1973. There are now close on 200 in Europe, Britain, Latin America and Japan. Their concept is based on three premises: the need for educational institutions, outside those already provided in the mainstream, to meet the previously underestimated requirements of large numbers of older people; the importance of providing mental stimulus and activity for older people as a way of delaying or avoiding the undesirable dependencies of old age (it can even be argued that maintenance of mental activity is cost beneficial to the community by reducing use of health services in later life); and the notion of older people as untapped repositories of knowledge and experience (education is essentially a sharing of knowledge and experience).

In just 5 years this movement has spread throughout Australia and currently (1990) has more than 10 000 older people teaching and learning about 100 different courses.

The creation of more opportunities for volunteer service by older people has many attractions. For the volunteer participants it offers an involvement in activities seen to have value to the community, thus enhancing the self-image of older people as contributors rather than receivers; for governments and service providers it offers a low cost extension of community-based services at a point where need is often most pressing, thus potentially reducing demand for more expensive institutional services.

Volunteer roles for older people are as diverse as the background, work experiences and personal skills of older people themselves. They range from work as friendly visitors and companions to the ill or disabled in their neighbourhood, to work in health care institutions and social welfare agencies such as child care facilities, to providing advisory services to various levels of government.

Governments and voluntary organisations need to develop a policy for linking older people wanting volunteer opportunities with individuals and groups needing their services. It is often said that the potential roles of the ageing in community service are bounded only by the degree of creativity exercised in identifying social needs and matching these with older volunteers' skills and preferences. It is argued that no country can afford to waste such a pool of talents. Volunteer activities can be initiated at the work place through programmes for retired workers, by religious and voluntary organisations and by statutory bodies. The cost of administering such programmes is relatively small compared with professional staff costs, and may require only a part-time coordinator. Depending on the nature of the activity it may be necessary to provide training, out of pocket expenses and transportation.

The system of health care available is a matter of great importance to the old. The frequent changes in the structure of the health care system in Australia in the last 10 years have left many old people confused about their entitlement. How people should contribute to the cost of their health care is a constant bone of political contention. Payment of fees for health care, even though there may be reimbursement later on, probably reduces access to health services for low income old people. A recent report by the International Federation on Ageing (Nusberg 1981) indicated that several countries including France are beginning to raise the proportion of the fee paid by the patient as a cost-saving measure, despite research evidence suggesting that a substantial increase in cost-sharing serves to reduce demand for health care disproportionately among the economically disadvantaged, including the old. In the long run such policies lead to increased use of hospital to treat diseases that might better have been treated at an earlier stage.

This type of policy, and the attitudes underlying it, runs counter to the principle of providing services to meet needs. It is well known that a common failure among older people is the non-reporting of disabling conditions (Williamson et al 1964). This would seem to argue for a sophisticated system of early detection or case finding, a dynamic rather than a reactive system. This view underpins the geriatric service centred on the City Hospital in Edinburgh, Scotland. The philosophy is simple and clear-cut. 'There is no such thing as a non-urgent problem in old age since if an old person is a little unwell today they may be worse tomorrow and by the day after may have developed organ failure with the distinct danger of secondary and multiple system disturbance or collapse' (Williamson 1981).

Here again is a dilemma for politicians and policy makers: what should be the basis for meeting need?

CARING SYSTEMS — PRESENT AND FUTURE

A study of the evolution of caring systems for the aged reveals that organised intervention occurred as social awareness and economic development began to affect families and governments. We should not hark back nostalgically to the good old days when the old enjoyed, as of right, privileges no longer accorded to them in our modern state. They were just as likely then as now to share the poverty, inadequate housing, poor health care and economic insecurity of the families they belonged to. Old age was no guarantee of support as more people became involved in organised labour and the differentiation between work and non-work sharpened.

At the beginning of this chapter we noted the complex interplay of factors entailed in social service provision including altruism and the profit motive. Both have been potent forces in shaping the structure of the aged care systems we have today. The Federal Government (McLeay Committee 1982), as main provider of resources for aged care, has examined the present arrangements for the accommodation of older people who are unable to remain in the community. It is generally recognised that there is an imbalance between residential services and community or domiciliary care. As the numbers of older people grow, it is inconceivable that the economy could support a corresponding increase in the number of institution-based beds. In looking to possible patterns of future services, therefore, it seems likely that there will be a progressive shift in emphasis, as already mentioned, to community-based services.

As in most other areas of health and welfare service provision, programmes for the aged have been developed largely without prior assessment of need other than on a superficial level. Once established, there appear to have been few attempts at systematic monitoring of services to identify levels of effectiveness and efficiency in relation to clearly defined philosophies and goals. This has led to haphazard development that is patchy in coverage and often dictated by needs other than those of the intended beneficiaries. Several official reports in recent years (*Care of the Aged*, Bailey 1978; *Through a Glass Darkly*, Holmes 1977) have pointed to the lack of planning and coordination in the general area of health and welfare. Their recommendations have been largely ignored.

Institutional domination

Institutions have dominated caring systems for a long time. Historically, institutions were established in Britain and Europe, particularly in the 18th and 19th centuries, to house people whose behaviour and/or circumstances were perceived to be problematic. Thus we had the rapid development of houses of correction, bridewells, workhouses, asylums, prisons and hospitals. The often grudging allocation of resources to these facilities reflected the prevailing ethos of laissez faire, as little interference from government as possible. Institutions came to be seen as a way of imposing uniformity, containment and disapproval. Small wonder that they soon became identified in the eyes of the public as places to be feared and avoided. Indeed, in the 19th century, the workhouses, those archetypal institutions, became known as 'the Bastilles of the poor'. Although the English Poor Law System as such did not take root in Australia some of the fear of institutions survives today among the very old who see the larger old institutions as still carrying the stigma attached to them at the beginning of the century.

Traditionally, institutions have failed to differentiate the needs of individuals. The work of Goffman (1961), Jones (1968), Barton (1970) and Miller & Gwynne (1972) has demonstrated the negative effects of prolonged institutional care. Of course there are exceptions — caring communities where the dignity and worth of the individual are respected and independence fostered. Too often, however, the individual has been sacrificed to other imperatives, staff rosters, nursing routines, payment of subsidies for certain categories of care, or outright profit. Ellen Newton's book (1979), *This Bed My Centre*, represents chilling first hand evidence for this.

Another important reason for the continued dominance of institutional care is the system of government subsidies and financial support. Successive Acts of parliament have consolidated the position of institutions by tying subsidies to bed occupancy. Consequently, organisations wishing to attract government funds have, of necessity, put up more buildings.

Although the *Aged or Disabled Persons Homes Act* 1974 has led to the development of many humane and innovative programmes by voluntary organisations, their efforts have to be set alongside the very substantial number of beds provided by the private profit-making sector. Without making any judgement about the control of a significant number of establishments by profit-seeking individuals and companies, it is apparent that the nursing home subsidy system is an encouragement to tie up resources in bricks and mortar. Not only can this practice have deleterious effects on the care of individuals who may not receive appropriate services but there are also serious social policy implications.

Carter (1981) pointed out the domination of the care of the confused aged by the institutional sector and in particular by the private nursing home run for profit. She showed how the system of government funding simultaneously sustained and encouraged private enterprise without giving adequate consideration to the needs of those being accommodated, including alternative forms of care. More recently the Commonwealth Government has introduced Outcome Standards for nursing home care.

Critical to all caring systems is the concept of assessment. This is particularly important at a time of diminishing resources and stringent financial controls. Yet in this area too we find many admissions to institutions being made without appropriate assessment of need or suitability. There is ample evidence that admissions, particularly in the private sector, are often made by friends or relatives or by professionals without prior assessment of the needs and wishes of the older person. In the absence of other alternatives and frequently in the face of the incipient breakdown of the older person's caring family, the availability of a bed can be seized on as the only solution to an urgent and highly stressful situation. The establishment and spread of geriatric assessment teams should result in the solution to this particular problem.

Similarly, inappropriate admissions, resulting from inadequate assessment, can result in unnecessary dependency and a serious waste of scarce resources. It is not enough, however, to criticise the dominance of institutional care merely in terms of its manifest and well documented shortcomings. It can be argued that in the absence of adequate complementary services the institutional sector is doing a reasonable job, and anyway some people will always need that form of care. In the early days of health and welfare provision, the institution often became the repository for social problems because there was

nowhere else; so too, many of our present day institutions for the old have become collection points for people who cannot be contained elsewhere. With the best will in the world an institutional system, unable to differentiate the needs of its patients/residents, unable to function as an open system in exchange with other systems, must take on some of the characteristics of what Miller & Gwynne (1972) have categorised as a warehousing model:

In the warehousing model, the primary task becomes: to prolong physical life . . . The intake into the system is a patient defined in terms of physical malfunctioning. The conversion process entails the provision of medical and nursing care. This provision is facilitated if the inmate, as the object of these ministrations accepts his dependent role in the system . . . To the extent that effective performance of the warehousing task requires the inmate to remain dependent and depersonalised, any attempts by the inmate to assert himself, or to display individual needs other than those arising from his specific disability, are in the warehousing model constraints on task performance. They are therefore to be discouraged

Perhaps the main reason for the continued emphasis on institutional care in Australia is the serious lack of commitment on the part of government and service providers to community care. The present imbalance needs to be transformed progressively into a continuum that includes a sufficient range and variety of forms of care to reflect not only the varied needs of older people, but also the particular skills, treatments and resources offered by different caring systems.

The great majority of older people live in their own homes in the community. When asked where they would like to live, older people almost invariably say 'at home'. Decisions to leave home to enter some form of residential care are often forced on older people because of the absence of adequate, easily accessible community services rather than on some intrinsic benefit offered by admission.

It has been estimated that 1 in 4 admissions to institutional care is inappropriate. The absence of continuing assessment after admission and the frequent lack of rehabilitation programmes mean that admission becomes a one-way ticket. Over time this must mean that some beds are occupied by people who do not need them, effectively blocking the admission of people who do. If it is recognised that admission is the preferred arrangement for some older people, efforts must be directed to achieving a revolving door programme of intermittent care, thereby maximising the use of expensive facilities. At the same time, it should be possible to meet the needs of more older people.

There is now strong evidence from within Australia and overseas that rehabilitation is not only possible but desirable for a number of older people already within the institutional system. One of the most important recommendations of the Jamison Committee (1980) was that States establish suitable rehabilitation centres at each suitable hospital for the rehabilitation of aged patients, and staff were to be adequately trained in geriatric rehabilitation techniques (Rec. 134 p. 22). At one time, disturbing evidence existed that in some private nursing homes older people were kept in bed because they attracted a higher government subsidy. They were also 'easier to look after' which often meant that they were less trouble to the staff who always knew where they were. Not surprisingly many of these people quickly became totally dependent and bedfast. Attempts are now being made by the government department concerned to address such issues, by changing the basis of funding and linking that funding with the assessed care needs of individual patients.

Increasingly, it can be demonstrated that community care works. By community care we mean both caring in the community, domiciliary care where a person is supported in his/her own home by a range of services, and caring by the community through the development of informal networks that support caring by families as well as the individual independence of older people. This approach is geared more purposefully to meeting individual needs in a way that supports the coping capacity of the individual and encourages independence and dignity. Furthermore, it seeks to foster a sense of caring and mutual responsibility in the community. The privatised lifestyle and geographical mobility of some families present problems of loneliness and isolation for people of all ages. The development of a caring community spirit is an important component of social cohesion.

Home and community care programmes

In 1985 the Commonwealth Government inaugurated the Home and Community Care Programme (HACC), a joint Commonwealth–State cost-shared programme. HACC aims to ensure that a range of people, particularly the frail aged, who might otherwise be likely to be admitted prematurely or inappropriately to long-term residential care, are provided with appropriate home and community care services.

Although HACC was a new programme it arose out of four previously provided services — home help, meals on wheels, domiciliary nursing and paramedical services. By bringing these four programmes together, it was hoped to expand existing programmes and encourage innovations.

At the time of introduction there was widespread community support for the HACC philosophy which sought a more appropriate distribution of funds between residential and domiciliary care. In the event there have been structural problems that have yet to be resolved.

REFERENCES

Ageing in a multicultural society — the situation of migrants from non-english speaking countries 1985. Australian Institute of Multicultural Affairs, Melbourne

Australian Bureau of Statistics 1980 The labour force in Australia. Catalogue no. 6204.0, 6203.0

Bailey P 1978 'Care of the aged': consultative arrangements and the co-ordination of social policy development. AGPS, Canberra

Barton R 1970 Institutional neurosis, 2nd edn. Wright, Bristol

Butler R N, Lewis M I 1973 Ageing and mental health. Mosby, St. Louis

Carter J 1981 States of confusion: SWRC reports and proceedings. Social Welfare Research Centre, University of New South Wales, Sydney

Equal Opportunity Commission (Western Australia) 1989 Age discrimination and equal opportunity legislation. Perth

Goffman I 1961 Asylums. Anchor Books, Doubleday, New York

Graycar A, Kinnear D 1981 The aged and the state. SWRC Reports and Proceedings, No. 5. Social Welfare

Research Centre, University of New South Wales, Sydney

Holmes A S 1977 'Through a glass darkly' report of the committee on care of the aged and the infirm. AGPS, Canberra

Jamison Report 1980 Commission of inquiry into the efficiency and administration of hospitals. AGPS, Canberra

Jones M 1968 Social psychiatry in practice: the idea of the therapeutic community. Penguin, Middlesex

Jones S 1987 'Too old' — living with age discrimination. New South Wales Council on the Ageing, Sydney

Maeda D 1978 Ageing in eastern society. In: Hobman D (ed) The social challenge of ageing. Croom Helm, London

McLeay Committee 1982 Sub-committee on accommodation and home care for the aged. House of Representatives, Commonwealth of Australia, AGPS, Canberra

Miller E J, Gwynne G W 1972 A life apart. Tavistock, London.

Newton E 1979 This bed my centre. McPhee Gribble, Melbourne

Nusberg C 1981 Health care for the elderly in other industrialised countries. Background paper prepared by the Institutional Federation on Ageing for the 1981 White House Conference on Ageing, Washington, DC

Older People At Home 1985 Report of a joint survey by the Australian Council on the Ageing and the Commonwealth Department of Social Security, AGPS, Canberra

Picton C 1984 Still learning: Universities of the Third Age and life-long learning. Proceedings of the Menzies Foundation 8: 113–118

Radford A J 1987 Ageism, public prejudice and private preconceptions. Australian Journal on Ageing 6(3): 4–9

Rein M 1977 Equality of social policy. Social Service Review 51: 565–587

Thomson Neil 1989 Aboriginal health: a socio-cultural perspective. In: Lupton G M, Najman J M (eds) Sociology of health and illness: Australian readings. Macmillan, Melbourne

United Nations 1982 Vienna international plan of action on ageing.

Williamson J, Stokoe H, Gray S, Fisher M, Smith A, Stephenson E 1964 Old people at home: their unreported needs. Lancet i: 1117–1120

3. Healthy ageing

Cliff Picton

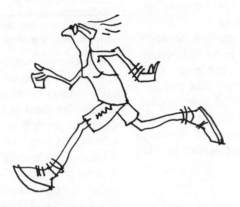

As has been described in Chapter 2, the percentage of the population over the age of 65 years, and in the older age groups beyond 75 years, will continue to increase well into the next century. The percentage of increase will be more dramatic in many other developed and developing countries. It is thus of vital importance to lay stress on the maintenance of health and independence throughout life, and this chapter will address a range of issues with that objective in mind.

NORMAL AGEING

The industrial countries of the world share remarkably similar profiles (Nusberg 1981) with regard to the health and health care needs of their old people. Approximately the same proportion are in some form of institutional care (4–6%). Another 2–4% are bedfast at home. About 12–24% are housebound and walk with difficulty — perhaps 4–8% of this group require a great deal of personal assistance. The remainder, approximately 75% of the older population, are able to get about and need minimal assistance.

In spite of these figures, the popular stereotype of equating older people with physical and mental deterioration persists. Focus on disease and mal-function only serves to foster a blinkered view of the processes of ageing. As Williamson (1981) observes:

Need is not confined to the relatively narrow field of therapeutics but it is expanded to include medical, psychological and social need. Nor is the determination of need confined to the individual old person but it is enlarged to include the needs of the family of which the old person is a member and indeed the needs of their local community insofar as the community is involved in supporting the individual old person.

Thus, we should locate older people in an interacting system consisting of biological, psychological and social elements. Traditionally, policies and programmes have been concerned with the pathological aspects of ageing and this has contributed to our distorted perception. While the part played by disease remains an important one, a pathological model of ageing is an inadequate basis for understanding the complex problems of old people.

Paradoxically, it is much easier to describe pathological conditions than it is to assert what constitutes health and normality. The rate of decline in function from young adulthood varies considerably and the variation continues into old age.

HEALTH MAINTENANCE

Perhaps the most important element in a contented and meaningful old age is the possession of good health. Research and practical experience have shown that health maintenance in the elderly is possible and that disability and disease are not essential components of ageing.

For the elderly, there is a strong link between active life and good health. The more old people participate in a range of activities, the longer they stay healthy. It is generally agreed that policies and programmes for ageing should have regard to the total range of needs of old people — social, psychological, medical and economic. Equally important is the recognition that health in old

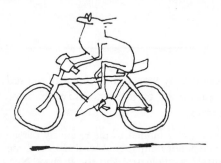

age is largely dependent on conditions of life and the environment, and on the habits of the individual in younger years. Many factors that are important for old age have to be learned during earlier phases of the life cycle.

Recent events, most notably the identification of the health of older people as one of the five initial priorities for the Australian National Better Health Program, indicate a growing recognition of the need to promote health rather than focus on the treatment of illness. The importance of the concept of health promotion was spelled out by the World Health Organization as: 'the process of enabling people, to increase control over, and to improve their health' (Ottawa Charter for Health Promotions, WHO 1988). This represents a significant recognition, inter alia, that older people have an *active* role to play in improving their health status. This concept is an extension of the 'Health for All' Declaration of Alma Ata (1978), which defines primary health care as:

essential health care based on practical, scientifically sound and socially acceptable methods and technology made universally accessible to individuals and families in the community, through their full participation and at a cost that the community and country can afford to maintain at every stage of their development in the spirit of self-reliance and self-determination . . . It is the first level of contact for individuals, the family and community with the national health system (WHO 1978).

A focus on health promotion is designed not only to restore good functioning where problems have already been identified but also highlights the development of behaviours and strategies designed to prevent or delay the onset of conditions inimical to good health. Among the key factors commonly identified in a health promotion approach are nutrition, exercise and relaxation; social interaction and positive self-image; communication and stimulation. These are not listed in order of importance because in general they are interdependent and interactive.

Nutrition

Currently, the Australian community is being bombarded with information (often contradictory) about nutrition. As we learn more about the healthy or deleterious qualities of a range of natural and manufactured food products we are theoretically in a better position than ever before to choose a healthy diet. By contrast, the present generation of older people grew up at a time when there was little information about nutrition and probably little interest. Long held divisions of labour between men and women have produced many older people (particularly men) with few skills in selecting and preparing food and often using inappropriate methods of cooking that are nutritionally unsound.

Lifestyle is an important influence on food intake as well as nutrition. Cooking for one can

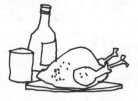

be a lonely chore leading to a lack of interest in food and a decline into poor health. The food packaging and retail industries compound the problem by failing to cater for the reduced need for volume in old age. Smaller packages or individual portions may be hard to find and larger quantities either go to waste or cannot be properly stored.

Simple books on nutrition are readily available, and those published by the National Heart Foundation of Australia are of particular value in this context, as is one prepared by Stewart & Jackson (1988), 'Second Bite of the Cherry', which contains a simple and informative 'healthy diet triangle'.

Social interaction

Social interaction is important at all stages of life but assumes greater significance in old age when failing health, loss of partner and the absence of family and friends may result in social isolation and loneliness. While many older persons find that the retirement years are filled with activities that are extensions or continuations of earlier interests, it is common to find people who do not have ready substitutes for work-related, or family, interactions. Awareness of community facilities

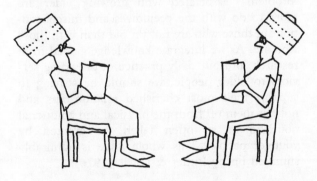

such as libraries, recreation centres and adult education facilities will aid in the selection of something appropriate. Joining a neighbourhood group, a book club or some other social activity not only helps to maintain existing social networks but also provides opportunities to form new friendships. Participation in a lunch club or a day centre may offer the multiple benefits of social contacts, improved nutrition and health

checks with the added bonus of access to a hairdresser and a podiatrist.

Above all it is important to counter the insidious influence of ageist thinking. It is not axiomatic that old age equals declining social interactions and contracting social networks. Those of earlier years may need to be nurtured, augmented or, in some cases, replaced but most older people are perfectly capable of adapting to these changes. Carers, family and friends, as well as professionals, have their roles to play in encouraging the maintenance and development of social contacts to offset losses and changes that may be beyond the individual's control. An awareness of Erikson's (1950) concept of the life tasks of old age as 'ego integrity vs despair' highlights the importance of social interaction for psychological well-being.

The stresses of daily life can often be minimised if mind and body are in a good state of health. Ageing is not without its stresses resulting from both external and internal pressures. Keeping in good shape physically through regular exercise reduces the deterioration of joints and muscles that can accompany lack of use. More and more older people are benefiting from the emphasis on physical fitness so evident in the general community. As well as participating in sporting activities, older people are taking to swimming and walking on a regular basis. Organised walking for pleasure is now well established in most States. Apart from exercising the bodily systems, exercise provides other benefits such as improvements in appetite, reduced susceptibility to minor ailments, and a feeling of well-being and involvement in the wider community. This all helps to promote a positive self-image.

Similar benefits may be derived from relaxation. The world we live in does have many

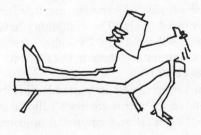

pressures and people of all ages are shown in numerous studies to be exhibiting adverse reactions to stress. It would be a mistake to assume that the mere fact of being retired would make relaxation possible or even easy. Relaxation programmes teaching the techniques that can be

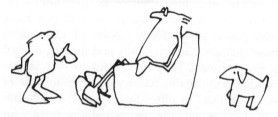

used are becoming increasingly popular alongside yoga and meditation. Greater awareness of the possible benefits from these techniques need to be more widely publicised and specifically aimed at older people.

Communication is the currency of social interaction and the key to forming and maintaining social relationships. Because of the losses associated with ageing some people have reduced opportunities to communicate. Loneliness and social isolation can be precursors to ill-health, both physical and mental. Stimulation for the mind is as important as exercise for the body and older people should be encouraged and helped where appropriate to engage in activities.

SEXUALITY IN LATER LIFE

Until recently it was uncommon to find sexual needs and behaviours in old age discussed in text books on gerontology. The stereotype of old age as a time of decline and decay was extended to exclude any thought of the old having sexual needs let alone enjoying intimacy. Yet as long ago as 1955 Kinsey and his associates showed that relatively healthy older people who enjoyed sex were capable of experiencing it, often until very advanced years. These findings have been confirmed subsequently by other researchers, notably Masters & Johnson (1970) and Butler & Lewis (1976).

Social services, and in particular institutions, have tended to mirror society's callous indifference to the sexual and emotional adjustment of

the aged. Limited awareness, and therefore limited acceptance of older people's sexual needs of expression, has resulted in little support in Western countries for the acknowledgement and enhancement of this part of their lives. On the service side this has frequently placed older people on the same footing as the mentally handicapped and the criminal.

Sexual activity is more prevalent among older people than is popularly assumed. Given reasonable health there is no physiological reason why the pattern of sexual behaviour established earlier in life should not continue in the later years. In fact, the most important factor in the maintenance of sexuality is consistency of active sexual expression. The person who has had an active and satisfactory sex life in earlier years will be most likely to continue in the same vein.

Of course, there are physiological changes and their psychological sequelae which may require modifications to long favoured activities and the learning of new patterns of love making. As Butler & Lewis argue (1976) these need not be barriers to physical and emotional fulfilment in later life.

As we have indicated on a number of occasions elsewhere in this book, some of the alleged 'problems' associated with growing older are more to do with the prejudices and misconceptions of those who are not yet old than with those who are. As we integrate knowledge gained from research into our daily practice of providing services to older people, we should be striving to support their most cherished relationships and not cut them off from the physical and emotional nourishment so often taken for granted by younger people. This whole issue is admirably summed up by Butler & Lewis (1976):

Perhaps only in the later years can life with its various possibilities have the chance to shape itself into something approximating a human work of art. And perhaps only in later life, when personality reaches its final stages of development can love-making and sex achieve the fullest possible growth. Sex does not merely exist after sixty; it holds the possibility of becoming greater than it ever was: It can be joyful and creative, healthy and health-giving. It unites human beings in an affirmation of love and is therefore also morally right and virtuous. Those older persons who have no partners and must experience sex alone need to know that this, too, is their right . . .

DEATH AND LOSS

We have already referred to the stigma that commonly attaches to old age and that is based on misconceptions and sometimes the fear of those not yet old. Death, in spite of the comparatively recent attempts to open up a public debate, is still for many people a taboo subject. Part of the stigma attached to old age may result from the fact that in contemporary industrial societies death is mainly a phenomenon of later life. Kalish (1976) has argued that in other societies where death rates are high, people die at all ages, and death is therefore considered less as an age-specific phenomenon. But in societies with low death rates most people survive into later life. Death, therefore, becomes strongly associated with later life.

Those working with older people often find it hard to cope with the phenomenon of death. How people approach death, their own as well as the deaths of others, depends to some extent on what death means to them. To come to terms with death and learn to accept it emotionally is probably the most difficult task an individual has

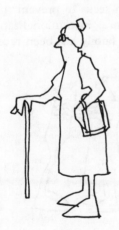

to face. Characteristically, older people fear death much less than the young. Sir William Ferguson Anderson (1971) has noted: 'Seldom does the patient in old age ask if he is going to die, he

may quietly tell his physician this, will prepare himself for and accept death with enviable calmness. It may be that in advanced age this realization is with the elderly and they do not need to put the question in words'.

The two most common reactions to the idea of death are fear and denial. Older people do not appear to be extremely afraid of death, and express fewer death fears than younger people (Kastenbaum 1969, Kalish 1976). Kalish attributes the lower prevalence of death fears in the face of a higher prevalence of actual deaths among the old to three factors:

1. Older people view their lives as having fewer prospects for the future and less value.
2. Older people who live past their own expectations of life have a sense of living on 'borrowed time'.
3. Dealing with the deaths of friends can help socialise older people toward acceptance of their own impending death.

In talking with older people one is often struck by the apparent association between an acceptance of death and the experience of an accumulation of losses — of spouse, friends and contemporaries. Much of the grief work commonly associated with the process of dying is often accomplished, as it were, vicariously with grieving and mourning for significant others. So too there may be less likelihood of the unfinished business associated with death at earlier stages in life. This is not to imply an essentially different grief and mourning process among the old.

Our growing understanding of the effects of loss, the processes of dying and the mechanisms of grief and mourning make it more likely that the older person who is dying will receive a level of supportive care to achieve death with dignity. In particular, the widespread dissemination in books, video tapes and films of the personal experiences of the dying and those who care for them professionally is beginning to demystify death. The spread of the hospice movement is bringing skilled practitioners into close contact with the dying and their families and friends. Ultimately, however, we can best help the dying by coming to terms with our own mortality. In this we have much to learn from the old.

FAMILY AND SOCIAL RELATIONSHIPS

The widely held belief that old people are increasingly neglected and abandoned by their families represents a warning and a challenge to the policy maker and the service provider. Uncritical acceptance of this conventional wisdom could bolster the long established concentration of resources for the provision of institutional care. Service providers, especially those involved in domiciliary care, know that in fact families are the key providers of supportive services. Researchers should be gathering this information to help strengthen the case for more domiciliary and community care programmes.

The stresses and strains felt by the contemporary family are inevitably passed on where there are older relatives. It is generally accepted that the long overdue revolution in the range of educational and employment opportunities for women coupled with the increasing popularity of marriage have virtually dried up the pool of single women who devoted their lives to caring for ageing parents in the earlier part of this century. Family migration and the greater representation of women in the workforce are just two factors diminishing the opportunities for supporting older relatives. The time constraints imposed by having both parents at work may be reflected in the nature and frequency of contacts with the old. Given these constraints, however, it is quite clear that many children and grandchildren perform herculean labours, lovingly and willingly on a regular and sustained basis.

It cannot be denied that some families do not feel duty bound to provide ongoing support for an older relative. This is not a phenomenon of the 1990s nor even an inevitable consequence of the proliferation of government provided services. The nature of the relationship between potential carer and a relative in need of care will be one of the most powerful determinants of whether or not care is provided and for how long. Studies (Isaacs et al 1972, Equal Opportunities Commission Report 1980) have shown how families bear heavy caring responsibilities for frail, ill and dementing relatives because of strong commitment based on a relationship. This caring often carries on for years with little relief from outside agencies either because of inadequate services or because the carer is unaware of the help available, or chooses not to accept it.

In one sense this largely uncharted area of caring is like the submerged part of an iceberg. Our present level of service provision can be hardly described as resting on a firm foundation of knowledge of the extent of need. Too often services for the aged operate on a fire brigade basis arriving on the scene when damage has already been done, often irreparably. If fewer families carried the heavy responsibility of caring they now do, our services would be overwhelmed.

One serious consequence of this situation is the danger that overstressed relatives will break down unless they can be relieved from time to time. Workers in the field of gerontology know that once this type of family support system does break down (MacMillan 1960) it is often impossible to repair it.

There is evidence on a worldwide scale of growing official interest in the role of the family in providing support for its older members. A recent document produced by the International Federation on Ageing (Gibson 1980) as a background paper for the 1981 White House Conference on Ageing stated: 'Partly as a result of humanitarian concerns and partly as a result of escalating long-term care costs, virtually every developed nation seeks to prevent the unnecessary or premature institutionalization of the elderly: And the family has been recognised as a

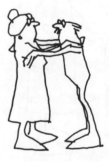

critical factor in helping older persons to remain in the community'.

It is not surprising that this upsurge in interest is linked to economic *and* humanitarian considerations. The increasing numbers and proportions of older people have serious financial implications for all societies. The pressure felt by care-giving relatives is only the epicentre of a shock wave that travels through a nation. Prolonging the capacity of care givers at once addresses the needs and wishes of older people and diminishes the extent of need for more very expensive institutional facilities. A careful analysis of the effects of care giving on the carers, particularly those inducing stress, could provide important policy indicators for community service development. All the present indications are that existing levels of service will need to be extended to complement and support the care giving capacities of families and to discourage the development of unnecessary dependence on family substitute services.

The issue of whether increasing social service provision erodes family caring responsibilities has led to the coining of the term 'the myth of service substitution'. Despite contrary evidence, many policy makers and the general public at large believe that service provision substitutes rather than complements family and community caring. From the family point of view, the issue is important because such an attitude discourages the provision of the very supportive services that could encourage carers, assist them in their efforts, improve the quality of the care they give and extend the length of time they are able to give it.

As yet there has been little systematic research in this area although an Australian study, 'Older People at Home', begun in 1981 by the Australian Council on the Ageing and the Commonwealth Department of Social Security included a major section on carers. Limited evidence from overseas suggests that the availability of public services need not reduce family responsibility. In Denmark, for example, the introduction of a wide range of home help and other community services has not led to decreasing contact with or help to elderly parents by their adult children.

Similarly, if admission rates to institutional care are examined they do not support the family rejection hypothesis. Studies from a number of countries show that the institutionalised elderly are more likely to lack potential family support than the general elderly population because they are childless, unmarried or the sole survivor of a marriage.

Three groups of services are of particular significance — those offering housing assistance, those community/domiciliary services delivered to older people in their own homes and services designed to take some of the pressure off care givers. Australia offers all of these services to a greater or lesser extent but the crucial issue of expansion in one or each of the three areas is closely linked to a general philosophy of caring for the old.

Although multigenerational living is not a common feature of housing occupancy in Australia, many older people enjoy 'intimacy at a distance' with their children. In some countries like Japan and Sweden there are financial inducements to families to house their older members. Social norms and lifestyle seem unlikely to result in similar developments in Australia although the 'granny flat' could become a popular substitute. The development of the concept in Victoria whereby older people can enjoy the security of close physical independence makes the carer's task easier without permanently tying up a valuable resource. When the unit is no longer occupied it can be easily transported to another site.

Community services, such as home help, home nursing, meals on wheels and day care and day hospitals, play an equally important part in keeping older people at home. Although these services do not have the family as their prime focus, their availability can be a major factor in reducing the burden on the family, especially by providing skilled 'back-up' support.

Somewhat paradoxically, the most important services could be said to be those directly ben-

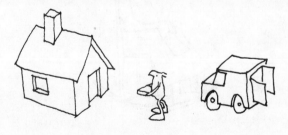

efiting the care givers — usually the family and particularly where the older person is a member of the household. Annis Flew (1980) gives a graphic picture of the nature of the responsibility of caring for an old person suffering from senile dementia. If this is indeed the reality of care in the community, families need all the support they can get. We have some of the necessary services already but they are too few and too thinly spread.

One of the most necessary services for direct care givers is some form of respite care to enable the carer to have a night away from home or a holiday. Although well established in France, Denmark, Germany and Britain this type of care is still not widely available in Australia. Families often find difficulty in locating suitable temporary accommodation.

Night sitting services provide relief for one of the most common problems associated with caring for the frail older person, having to get up frequently to attend to their needs. One of the most remarkable schemes of this type is operated by the City of Stockholm which provides over three hundred thousand hours of night care assistance to older people. A 'go to bed patrol' helps them get ready for bed, and a 'night patrol' returns to give medication and offer other forms of assistance.

The provision of these types of services is a clear indication to care givers of a move beyond the mere rhetoric of family support. As Australian society becomes more aware of the needs of an ageing population, the search for ways to encourage and sustain community care of the elderly will assume greater importance.

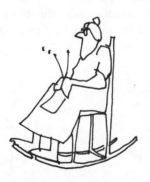

Given that many older people do have families willing and able to give care and support we can examine another issue central to ageing. Part of the stereotype of old age is that it is a time of isolation, withdrawal and loneliness. Policies and programmes have sought to integrate older people in a variety of community settings at the same time endeavouring to foster independence. Dependency of some degree is an almost inescapable concomitant of growing old. Self-reliance is a quality much prized in Australia and this often results in unrealistically high expectations of levels of coping. The provision of a range of facilities and services catering for all points of the continuum from independence to dependence helps break down the stigma of dependency by bringing it within the bounds of normality (and thereby acceptability).

What do older people want, however, and how can their needs and wishes be adequately catered for? The concept of intimacy at a distance has already been mentioned. It reaffirms simultaneously an individual's need for social interaction and the formation of relationships as well as a wish for privacy, self-determination and independence. Much of this will be culturally determined. For example, in 1980 more than 66% of Japan's aged people shared a household with their children while the native-born white Australian will have grown up in a much privatised environment as shown in Table 3.1.

Everyone has some personal view of what constitutes a desirable lifestyle. Social planners and service providers have often imposed on the old, quite arbitrarily, a particular view of what should be appropriate for the later years. To an extent this is inevitable given that it is impossible to introduce sufficient variations in any one service system to match the infinite variety of human nature. Yet more and more researchers are presenting the views of older people showing their dissatisfaction with what they consider to be meagre efforts to meet their individual needs. At the same time pressure groups among older people are forming all over the world. No social system is free from criticism from its intended beneficiaries. One of the strongest criticisms of welfare states, especially as exemplified by Scandinavia, is the rigidity and inflexibility of response

Table 3.1 Non-institutionalised aged population by family status and age, Australia, 1979

Family status	Age group			
	60–64	65–69	70+	Total
Member of a family		Percent		
Couple* with dependent children[†]	4.4	1.6	0.6	2.1
Couple* without dependent children[†]	69.7	63.6	46.0	58.2
Total couples*	74.1	65.2	46.6	60.3
Single aged head with relatives[‡]	4.2	5.3	8.7	6.4
Aged relative of family head	4.0	5.1	9.9	6.8
Total aged persons in families	82.3	75.7	65.2	73.4
Not a member of a family				
Living alone	15.6	21.9	32.3	24.2
Not living alone[§]	2.1	2.4	2.6	2.4
Total aged persons not in family	17.7	24.3	34.8	26.6

Source: Unpublished data provided by Australian Bureau of Statistics from July '79 Survey of Labour Force Status and Characteristics of Families. See bulletin ref. 6224.0 for details of that survey.
* One or both persons being aged (i.e. 60+).
[†] Dependent children and/or other relatives present in family.
[‡] With or without dependent children and/or other relatives present in family.
[§] Living with other (non-related) persons.

to new problems. Calls are increasingly made for greater openness to innovations and encouragement of self-help measures at the individual and neighbourhood levels. A new approach also requires greater real consultations with the consumers of services whose interests and concerns have not always been adequately reflected in policies and programmes.

The same sorts of criticisms are levelled at other systems where the absence of a universal approach to service provision seems to place more older people at risk. Such systems frequently rely heavily on private services provided on a for-profit basis leading to an imbalance in favour of institutional provision.

These sorts of issues have led to consideration of the applicability of notions derived from community development to planning and providing services for old people. Often these seem to have been applied with the same haphazard disregard for the opinions of the old. The spread of housing developments solely for old people, often geographically isolated from health services, shops and public transport, seems largely motivated by considerations of profit. The creation of aged specific communities is a short step from increasing the isolation and stigmatisation of the old.

However, in a democracy, people will seek to exercise choice over their living arrangements. Interestingly, living in this kind of housing development is generally available only to those with considerable financial assets.

We must beware, at the same time, of painting a picture of some idealised, well integrated, multigenerational community. Diversity is not in itself a prescription for harmonious interaction or mutual support. But if the present trend of thought in the direction of community care continues it is surely the diverse community that offers most to the range of older people.

Community constitutes an elusive set of concepts and values. Community of interest is perhaps an essential unifying concept when ageing is the focus of discussion.

Stereotyping and stigmatisation force some old people into a state of isolation that has little to do with geography or physical proximity to other people. It has everything to do with care and concern, relationships and being valued. Living in an environment that has the potential for meeting a range of needs, if required, or wished for, with opportunities for social exchanges would seem to offer reciprocal benefits to older people and others making up any defined community.

The idea of a caring community represents a link between an altruistic wish to care for those in need and the practical management of caring systems. It is interesting that in Europe caring for older people in the community is also known as 'open care' as opposed to institutional or 'closed care'. The increasing support for open care is based not only on a willingness to heed the wishes of older people but also on the desire to promote age-integrated societies.

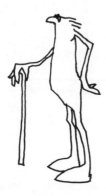

Value judgements about integration take us back to ideological stances on social welfare provision, universal or selective benefits and ultimately to the nature of society itself. Social interaction, potentially at least, raises community awareness about issues and needs. The great policy innovations in the last few decades that have enabled the retarded, the mentally ill and others to gain more acceptance arose out of a growing community tolerance. It became less acceptable to hide them away as their presence in the community gained acceptance. Community awareness is ultimately the key to successful social policy implementation. Heavy reliance on institutional services in Australia has served to bolster the negative stereotype of old age. This is all the more remarkable because of the small size of the institutional population.

Community development means more than just the majority of older people living outside institutions. Those who espouse community development as an instrument of social policy do so in terms of the dynamic potentials for exchanges and transfers between individuals, groups and social institutions. This must include

the potential for cooperation and for conflict because of the key concept of participation and the sharing of power.

Traditionally, the receivers of social services have been seen as beneficiaries, recipients of one-way transfers, often grudgingly made. Over time they have come to accept this status with a passivity bordering on the apathetic. Community development in its many different manifestations has helped to begin to change this situation particularly with the rise of pressure groups.

As pressures build up for community care for older people in Australia, there may well be a parallel pressure for more formalised and meaningful participation by them in decision making. Pressure groups representing the elderly already exert strong political influence in the United States, Sweden, Norway, Germany, France, and The Netherlands.

The International Federation on Ageing (Nusberg 1980) notes:

While there is no conscious adherence to anything like a 'Maslovian' hierarchy of values on the part of Swedish pensioners, the focus of their energies over the past few decades does suggest that once hard-won struggles over increased pensions and improved social services are won, the next order of priorities seems to be in the direction of greater control over or responsibility for policies which have major impact on one's life.

The movement has been slower to gather momentum in Australia although pensioner organisations in particular have been active for many years. To date, most pressure group activity has concentrated on getting pension levels raised. Further politicisation of the old is likely to see a broadening of the range of targets.

Participation can easily become an exercise in rhetoric or window dressing. If older people are encouraged to participate in decisions about services likely to affect their lives, it is essential for policy makers to envisage at what level, with what objectives and with what anticipated outcomes. At its most basic level of definition, participation refers to a process whereby people who do not hold official positions influence decisions about policies and programmes that affect their lives. Arnstein's ladder of citizen participation (Fig. 3.1.) shows clearly how easy it is for the process to be little more than a patronising, placatory exercise.

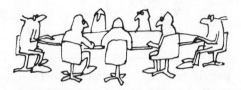

For participation to be meaningful to the old it must be linked to a clear statement of objectives and not merely result in a token aged person on the board of management. Development along the lines of a participation model presents intriguing dilemmas about the reality of exerting influence. As Graycar (1974) has argued about influence in social welfare:

> . . . the service approach is based on concepts which stress the need to provide opportunities for disadvantaged groups to participate in the benefits of society. The *political* orientation on the other hand stresses the need for changing the balance of power so as to empower the disadvantaged to gain a greater measure of the available resources and hence create their own opportunities.

The activities of VOTE (Voice of the Elderly) in New South Wales and South Australia and the promoting of a parliamentary candidate in Victoria on an aged care platform at a recent Federal election suggest the stirring of a political movement. It is no accident that these developments took place in the wake of a well publicised and highly effective visit to Australia by the American 'wrinkled radical' Maggie Kuhn. On the service side, however, there have been few attempts to significantly involve older people in real participation. Passive consumption of services is the norm. The familiar image is one of things being done to, and for, older people; rarely, it seems, are they done with.

Allowing older people to exert influence does not mean asking them what they want and then providing it. There have to be compromises that recognise political and economic realities. However, there is yet to be tacit agreement on the principle of participation. If it is widely accepted it will need to be translated into different levels of involvement that take account of different coping capacities. This would allow for an increasingly flexible range of interactions between service providers and service consumers.

Developments in Europe during recent years could point the way for Australia. An increasingly widespread form of formalised participation is the 'councils of the elderly' at all levels of government. They serve primarily in an advisory capacity examining proposed changes in social security policy, regulations and welfare measures affecting older people. Norway, for example, has established a negotiation and contact committee at the national level on which representatives of relevant government departments and representatives of pensioners serve. All proposed legislation or changes in regulations affecting older people must first be referred to this committee for discussion before they are submitted to parliament.

In Sweden, pensioners' organisations have won the right to have their representatives serving with government officials on 'councils of the elderly' at the municipal, country and national levels. At the municipal level, such councils can influence city planning in its early stages; at the national level, the council has won the right to be consulted on pensions and social policy, as well as other matters concerning older people.

In Germany, some cities have encouraged the formation of 'councils of the elderly' whose rep-

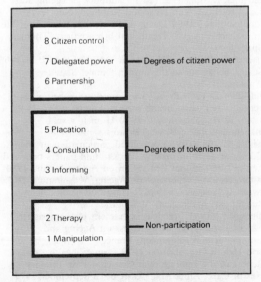

Fig. 3.1 A ladder of citizen participation in the U.S.A. (From Arnstein S R 1971 Journal of the Town Planning Institute 57 (4) April 176–182.)

resentatives are directly elected by older people themselves. In some cases, all persons over 60 are eligible to vote; in others only nursing home residents, and participants in senior and adult day care centres may vote.

If we refer back to Arnstein's ladder of participation (Fig. 3.1.) we can see how most services for older people in Australia are located near the bottom in terms of providing opportunities for voicing opinions or influencing policies. It is often argued that this is inevitable given frailty, dependency, or confusion. How appropriate would it be to involve hospital patients or hostel residents in shaping programmes and regimens? The European models indicate at least a willingness to try. Failure to try can be taken to imply an entirely negative assessment of older people's capacities to make meaningful contributions in areas directly affecting their day to day welfare. A measure of participation encourages people to take responsibility. This leads to a reduction in dependence on others and involvement in shaping the quality of their life.

With advancing age, pathological conditions increase in frequency and require early and accurate diagnosis and appropriate treatment. Moreover, the domestic circumstances of many

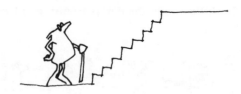

old people render them more vulnerable to risk factors that might have adverse effects on their health, e.g. accidents in the home.

Although some old people suffer from chronic diseases, their overall competence is not necessarily affected. Accordingly, competence and an ability to cope should be the main criteria for assessing an old person's needs. This, of course, demands a corresponding awareness of these factors by health and welfare professionals. The establishment of a geriatric specialty probably leads to better diagnosis, treatment and after care; it promotes research and provides improved opportunities for education and training in long-term care. There is also increasing evidence that the existence of a geriatric unit reduces waiting lists for hospital admissions, lessens the demand for long-term care by preventing reversible deterioration, and prevents the blocking of acute hospital beds.

REFERENCES

Anderson W F 1971 Practical management of the elderly, 2nd edn. Blackwell, Oxford
Butler R N, Lewis M I 1976 The later years: a guide to sexual and emotional adjustment. Sun Books, Melbourne
Equal Opportunities Commission Survey Report 1980 The experience of caring for elderly and handicapped dependents. EOC, Manchester
Erikson E 1950 Childhood and society. Penguin, Middlesex
Flew A 1980 Looking after granny: the reality of community care. New Society 54: 56–58
Gibson M J 1980 Support for families of the elderly: other industrialised notions. Background paper prepared by the International Federation on Ageing for the 1981 White House Conference on Ageing, Washington, DC
Graycar A 1974 Local participation: the Australian Assistance Plan. Australian Social Work 27(3): 5–12
Health for All Committee 1988 Health for all Australians: Report to the Health Targets and Implementation (Health For All) Committee to Australian Health Ministers. AGPS, Canberra
Isaacs B, Livingstone M, Neville Y 1972 Survival of the unfittest: a study of geriatric patients in Glasgow. Routledge and Kegan Paul, London
Kalish R A 1976 Death and dying in a social context. In

Binstock R, Shanas E (eds) Handbook of ageing and social sciences. Van Nostrand Reinhold, New York
Kastenbaum R J 1969 Death and bereavement in later life. In: Kutscher A (ed) Death and bereavement. Thomas, Springfield
Kinsey A C, Pomeroy W, Martin C E, Gebhard P M 1955 Sexual behaviour in the human female. Saunders, Philadelphia
MacMillan D 1960 Preventive geriatrics: opportunities of a community mental health service. Lancet i: 143–1440
Masters W H, Johnson V E 1970 Human sexual inadequacy. Little Brown, Boston
Nusberg C 1980/1981 Formalized participation by the elderly in decision making. Background papers prepared by the International Federation on Ageing for the 1981 White House Conference on Ageing, Washington, DC
Stewart A, Jackson M 1988 Second bite of the cherry. Sun Books, Macmillan, Melbourne
Williamson J 1981 Practical assessment of the geriatric patient Paper given at Congress on Ageing and Communication, Besancon, France
World Health Organization 1978 Primary health care: Report of the International Conference on Primary Health Care, Alma Ata, USSR 6–12 September 1977. WHO, Geneva

4. Physiological ageing

John Hurley

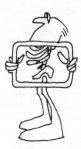

To complement the social context of ageing and healthy ageing, this chapter describes the physiological and accompanying psychological changes that may occur during the normal ageing process. Before thinking about the many ways in which physiological ageing may manifest itself it is important to recall the facts presented in Chapter 3 about healthy ageing. Too often, physiological ageing is viewed negatively, as something to be feared. It needs to be remembered, though, that all individuals do not age at the same rate and neither do the physiological systems. For the majority of people the sum total of the decrements that result from physiological ageing do not add up to major functional losses leading to disabilities. This is the 'good news' of ageing which should be understood by all who work with elderly people and which should be shared with elderly people and their families. The significant physiological ageing changes are summarised in Table 4.1.

SKIN SYSTEM

Environmental influences contribute to the problems of differentiation between physiological and pathological processes in the skin and hair. Exposed skin usually shows the most significant changes, with the epidermis thickening and the dermis shrinking. This is coupled with a progressive decline in the collagen content of the dermis leading to a reduction in skin strength. A loss of subcutaneous fat exaggerates the dermal changes. While the number of blood vessels in the skin decreases, there is usually an increase in vascular hyperplasias such as venous stasis and cherry angiomas. Melanocytes in the basal layers of the epidermis, tend to decrease in number with age but other skin melanocytes tend to increase in size. All of these features of physiological ageing in the skin need to be understood, especially by health care workers involved in the physical handling of frail elderly people. When skin is fragile it has the potential for damage, even with very slight trauma.

The effect of sunlight, especially ultraviolet light, on skin is becoming more understood and appreciated for its potential harm. The degree of pigmentation present in the skin is clearly a significant factor in determining the effect of ultraviolet radiation. It is also thought that skin that tans easily and evenly may have increased, inbuilt protection. Nonetheless, there is clear evidence that ultraviolet exposure and the rate of skin cancer are strongly linked. In countries such as Australia, the skin of elderly people of European extraction may show signs of previous unwise exposure to the sun with hyperkeratotic lesions

Table 4.1 Summary of significant physiological ageing changes

System	Physiological change	Implications	Alleviation
Skin	Decrease in strength and thickness	Possibility of damage, e.g. decubitus ulcer, bruising	Gentle handling
	Decreased skin lipids	Skin dryness	Minimal soap (detergents)
Bone	Progressive bone loss	Potential for fracture increase	Avoid hazards — gentle handling
Muscle	Declining strength	Easily fatigued	Maintain activity
		Tendency to immobility	Progressive strengthening exercise
			Full range mobility exercise
Cardio-vascular	Diminished elasticity of aorta	Pulse and systolic pressure increases	In absence of symptoms and signs of hypertension treatment may be inappropriate for those over 80
Respiratory	Fall in elastic recoil	Decreased vital capacity	Maintain activity
		Increased residual volume	Posture correction
			Breathing exercise
Teeth	Atrophy of gum and bone tissue	Loss of teeth	Dental hygiene
	Reduction of saliva	Nutrition effects	Accurate dental prosthetics
		Cosmetic effects	
Liver	Altered hepatic blood flow and enzyme activity	Affects drug metabolism and clearance	Reduced dosed of certain drugs
			Careful drug monitoring
			Avoidance of long half-life drugs
Kidney	Loss of diurnal excretory pattern	Increasing nocturia	Environmental planning
	Reduced renal blood flow	Reduced excretion of drugs and metabolites	Reduced doses of certain drugs
		Tendency to uraemia	Maintain fluid intake
Bladder	Increased incidence of dysinhibited bladder	Incontinence	Two hourly toileting
			Environmental organisation
Gastro-intestinal	Reduced colonic motility	Constipation	Increase bran in diet
Nervous	Slowed reaction time	Poor performance in functions requiring speed	Allow time for response
			Reduce speed of stimulus
			Reduce number of simultaneous stimuli
			Encourage accuracy
	Diminished reflexes	Especially potential for poor balance	Gait training
			Appropriate walking aids
			Remove household hazards
	Increased threshold for touch awareness	Diminished awareness especially of fleeting touch	Increase strength of stimulus
			Prolong duration of stimulus
	Temperature recognition threshold increased	Potential for injury	Hazard awareness
	Pain threshold increased		Hazard avoidance
	Heat/cold sensation threshold increased	Potential for accidental hypothermia	Hazard awareness
	Decreased sweat glands	Hyperthermia	Careful monitoring in extreme temperatures
			Environmental planning
	Kinaesthesia diminished	Decreased position sense, especially feet	Encourage use of vision
			Organise environment
			Avoid bifocal lenses
	Stereognosis diminished	Difficulty in recognising forms	Encourage visual supplement
	Taste/smell deteriorates	Diminished interest in food	Ensure visual stimulation of appetite
		Decreasing ability to smell smoke	Use of 'smoke detector'

Table 4.1 (cont'd) Summary of significant physiological ageing changes

System	Physiological change	Implications	Alleviation
Nervous cont.	Vision disturbances Increased size of lens Increased density of lens Macular changes	Decreased: accommodation acuity depth perception visual fields adaptation sensitivity glare tolerance colour discrimination	Careful assessment Environmental planning Colour coding Appropriate spectacles Adequate light Reduce glare
		Increased: need of light	
	Hearing disturbances Cochlear degeneration	Progressive loss of hearing Decreased hearing of high pitched sounds initially Speech discrimination difficulties	Hearing aid Face the deaf person Light on face of speaker Speak clearly Do not shout
Central nervous	Reduced brain weight	Impaired memory Dementia	Memory aids
	Altered sleep pattern Reduced REM and phase iv	Difficulty going to sleep More frequent awakenings	Avoid naps near bed time Avoid stimulants: caffeine, alcohol Correct physical discomfort problems Avoid unnecessary sedation

developing. Unfortunately, neoplastic lesions such as basal cell carcinoma, squamous cell carcinoma and malignant melanoma are becoming increasingly common, all related to excessive ultraviolet irradiation. Prevention, through minimising exposure throughout life, must become more fashionable than the previously held notion that a deep tan was a good sign of health.

Another summer hazard for elderly people is the fact that the thermal threshold for skin sweating increases while the sweat output usually decreases. The body has, therefore, less ability to lose heat. This is probably due to a failure of the thermoregulatory component of the autonomic system rather than a change in the sweat glands themselves. Thus, sweating may not be a reliable index of an elderly person's reaction to high temperature. Considerable care should be taken during hot weather to ensure an adequate intake of fluids to assist the body to compensate.

Hair colour usually initially darkens with age and then becomes white or grey. Reduction in the scalp follicle and shaft diameter is common. Loss of hair is usual and is manifested by the progressive thinning of head hair and the absence of body, axillary and pubic hair. In men, though, there may be an increase in the length and coarseness of eyebrow, ear and nasal hair. The

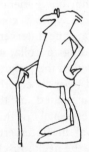

primary significance of these changes lies in the cosmetic effects. Attention ought to be paid to the maintenance of appearance, and thus self-esteem, through the careful management of deteriorating hair.

MUSCULOSKELETAL SYSTEM

Physiologically, there is a progressive loss of calcium from the skeleton but this must be distinguished from pathological osteoporosis which occurs when the reduced bone mineral density is such that bone strength is compromised. Decline in bone mineral density occurs in both sexes at about age 50 with a significant decline at menopause. Progressive loss begins to taper off about 15 years after menopause. The amount of bone loss is dependent, of course, upon the skeleton status at maturity. Because women tend to have less dense bones than men to start with the effect of this decline is seen more commonly in women. It is clear that there is a relationship between oestrogen depletion, occurring at menopause, and loss of bone mineral density but there is no conclusive evidence as yet how this may be used in a preventive way. There is also no conclusive evidence as yet about the role of dietary or supplementary calcium intake in the prevention or treatment of osteoporosis. On the other hand, there is a growing body of evidence that exercise may prevent or delay the onset of osteoporosis through the effects of muscular mechanical stress on bone. There is, further, considerable evidence that bone loss is a complication of immobilisation, bed rest and weightlessness. Exercise must be directed at the bones most likely to fracture — spine, hip and wrist.

Bone loss and osteoporosis may contribute significantly to the phenomenon of vertebral collapse and thoracic kyphosis common in elderly people. In addition, the intervertebral disc becomes fragile, tending to collapse. This is most clearly demonstrated in the progressive decline in height experienced by most elderly people. Problems may be exacerbated in the presence of muscle weakness, especially of the back muscles, and osteoarthritis of the intervertebral joints. In extreme situations, the neck muscles may become too fatigued to support the head erect.

Glycoproteins maintain the fluid content in the tissues but they are progressively reduced in old age causing dehydration of the tissues. Cartilage, which lines the bony surface of the joints, has no direct blood supply, relying for nutrition on these ever-diminishing glycoproteins and the osmosis resulting from alternately applied and released compression. Hyaluronic acid regulates viscosity between tissues. With age, the amount of this acid in the body is reduced resulting in friction between tissues. Hyaline cartilage, which lines the weight-bearing surface of synovial joints, is commonly affected because of depleted hyaluronic acid. These and other biochemical changes may lead to mechanical impairments and, thus, to a growing incidence of degeneration.

Joint structures, especially ligaments and tendons, show a progressive increase in calcification and a concomitant decrease in elasticity. Because overuse and trauma appear to be important contributory elements in joint degeneration it is difficult to distinguish ageing from pathological osteoarthritis. Degeneration may lead to loss of mobility as well as joint instability. For these reasons the joints of elderly people are prone to damage. Care must be exercised in handling and positioning the joints of frail elderly people to ensure maximum joint protection. Because joints may stiffen after a period of inactivity it is essential to maintain mobility through active joint exercise or passive movements.

Progressive muscular atrophy leading to weakness has been demonstrated in old age but it is unclear whether this is a result of ageing itself or of the decline in physical activity experienced by most elderly people. There is evidence that muscles kept active through functional use and exercise show few structural changes with age because of the potential for increased recruitment of motor units. Again, evidence suggests that the rate of loss of strength depends on the peak value of strength attained during maturity and the level of continuing activity maintained. While there may be a relationship between declining strength and potassium deficiency, disuse is a major factor in muscle weakness. Disuse is complicated by the tendency to replace muscle cells with fibrous tissue, especially in conditions such as hemiplegia or multiple sclerosis. Muscular activity is, of course, affected by fatigue, the threshold decreasing with age. There is considerable evidence, however, that progressive exercise over time will improve oxygen uptake in muscles and thus endurance.

Although the capacity to work or exercise is dependent on the coordination of activities in many systems of the body a comment may be appropriate here. The capacity for moderate work does not decline with age but the limit to hard work is lowered considerably. The maintenance or redevelopment of endurance requires graded physical activity. Elderly people who are not otherwise hampered by certain pathological diseases may retain or regain an effective work capacity if they undertake graded exercise that stresses the body systems.

CARDIOVASCULAR SYSTEM

There is an increasing incidence of arteriosclerosis with age. Plaques develop from material deposited in the intima and are associated with changes in the media of the arterial wall. It is not an inevitable consequence of ageing but a progressive pathological problem that reaches significant proportions in elderly people.

The elasticity of the arteries, in particular the aorta, declines progressively with age. This may result in an increase in pulse and systolic pressure, but diastolic pressure remains relatively unchanged. This may account for the increased incidence of apparent hypertension in old age. Recent work has shown that systolic hypertension is associated with an increased incidence of cardiovascular and cerebrovascular morbidity. Therapeutic intervention to return the blood pressure to normal levels has been shown to be beneficial in the elderly population.

The state of the peripheral venous circulation is dependent, somewhat, on the tone and efficiency of the muscles of the limbs and trunk. Postural hypotension is a relatively common problem occurring when there is a too sudden change from the horizontal to the vertical position. Unfortunately, this problem may go undetected unless care is always taken to measure blood pressure in both lying and sitting or standing positions. Exercise and activity help to prevent peripheral stagnation. Many old people have adequate cardiovascular systems although there may be clearly demonstrated physiological changes.

The heart itself tends to decrease in weight and there is an increasing accumulation of lipofuscin in the myocardial fibres. Fibrotic lesions are common. While heart rhythm is essentially unaltered, cardiac output, oxygen consumption and maximum heart rate on exercise may decline with age. The system tends to be sensitive to sudden, extra loads but it retains the ability to hypertrophy in response to progressive increases in demand.

Healthy old people usually have normal red cell counts and are not anaemic, although their white cell counts tend to decrease. There may be a diminished clot reaction in the platelets and a rise in the erythrocyte sedimentation rate. Although whole blood viscosity may increase there is usually no change in plasma viscosity in the absence of disease.

RESPIRATORY SYSTEM

The mechanics of the respiratory system are impeded by a progressive increase in the calcification of the costal cartilages, decalcification of the ribs, and an increasing tendency to kyphosis. In the lungs, there is a progressive decrease in the thickness of the alveolar walls and the elastic recoil.

A fall in vital capacity levels concomitant with an increase in residual volume is common. On quiet breathing there is a decrease in the uniformity of ventilation which improves with increased respiratory rates.

Despite these physiological changes, elderly people tend to have an efficient respiratory system in the absence of disease. Activity and exercise stimulate deep breathing patterns and appropriate posture permits adequate lung expansion. There is considerable evidence that the lung function in elderly people continues to perform well under the stress of moderate exercise. Thus, bed rest or prolonged sitting are hazardous for elderly lungs.

ENDOCRINE SYSTEM

Atrophic and degenerative changes may occur in the ageing thyroid gland. Such changes are not often associated with reduced thyroid hormone production. There is decreased endocrine function in the gonads clearly seen in the climacteric or menopause of both women and men, but this decrease is not to be interpreted as a cessation of sexual function.

Diabetes mellitus is associated with ageing as is an increasing incidence of subclinical abnormalities in glucose tolerance tests. Diagnosis of diabetes may not be without its difficulties because of raised renal threshold level and, thus, a lower likelihood of glycosuria.

GASTROINTESTINAL SYSTEM

The teeth darken in colour and present changes in enamel, dentine formation, cement, pulp and gingival tissues all leading to a weakening of tooth structure. Loss of teeth is common in old age but whether or not this is normal is controversial. Adequate mouth and dental care is, obviously, essential if teeth are to be retained in a healthy and functional state. When teeth are lost they ought to be replaced with appropriate prosthetics to maintain mouth shape, facilitate chewing and promote cosmesis. Since dentures hiding in the drawer do none of these things it is imperative to ensure that dentures fit and are worn.

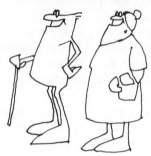

Saliva secretions are usually reduced but not sufficiently to produce a dry mouth. Taste and smell (see nervous system) decline progressively.

The incidence of achlorhydria due to gastric mucosal changes increases with age. Motor activity is thought to be delayed leading to a diminution of gastric contractions and delayed emptying.

The pancreas may show ageing changes such as duct hyperplasia which may contribute to alveolar degeneration and duct obstruction. Lipase production may be reduced leading to less effective fat absorption.

There is no evidence of increasing constipation as a physiological manifestation of ageing.

Ageing changes in the liver are significant, especially in relation to drug efficiency in elderly people. The liver tends to decrease in weight and the number of mitochondria per liver cell decreases. Liver glycogen and ascorbic acid levels tend to decrease while lipid level may increase. There is also a reduction in protein synthesis leading to higher blood levels of drugs which may result in adverse drug reactions. An altered, usually reduced, hepatic blood flow can affect the rate of metabolism of some drugs. Intrinsic hepatic clearance of drugs may decrease markedly in some cases.

Despite these changes, the gastrointestinal system as a whole presents a relatively efficient system throughout life in the absence of disease.

GENITOURINARY SYSTEM

In the absence of disease the kidneys of most elderly people function adequately throughout life despite a variety of physiological changes. There is usually a loss of weight and parenchymal mass while progressive hypertrophy in tubular and glomerulus tissues is common. A reduction in the number and size of nephrons may occur with an increase in interstitial connective tissue. A number of functions decreases: glomerular filtration rate and excretory and reabsorptive tubular capacities. Importantly, there is a progressive loss of the normal diurnal excretory pattern leading to nocturia. In younger adults, about two-thirds of the total daily urine output occurs during the day. With age this gradually changes to about half. Thus, nocturia is a normal feature of ageing.

Trabeculation of the bladder is present in the majority of old people. The most common bladder abnormality causing incontinence in old age, however, is the uninhibited neurogenic bladder.

While the incidence of incontinence increases with age it is essential to realise that incontinence is rarely due to ageing per se. Rather, incontinence is usually associated with a variety of causes, many of which may be corrected or ameliorated (see Ch. 7).

NERVOUS SYSTEM

As in many other systems of the body, it may be difficult to separate physiological ageing in the nervous system from pathological processes. Wisdom and adaptability may permit the elderly person to function adequately despite declining structures, thereby masking both the onset and the degree of change.

The brain tends to atrophy with age, especially in the anterior part of both hemispheres but also in the brain stem and the cerebellum. The vestibular system tends to enlarge. The loss of neurones is of significance because these cells are not replaced. There is some debate about the consequence of this neurone loss as a sign of ageing because of the brain's potential for recruitment of underutilised cells. The basal ganglia is also prone to degeneration with age, producing symptoms similar to the pathological parkinsonian syndromes.

The microscopic changes in the ageing brain include the presence of senile plaques and neuro-fibrillary tangles. It has been shown that these occur in small numbers in the brains of normal elderly people while in cases of Alzheimer's disease these are present in large numbers. The large increase in the number of plaques and tangles in Alzheimer's disease is a pathological change, the cause of which is not yet clear.

Nerve fibres, both white and grey, slowly atrophy. In the peripheral nerves there is an increasing incidence of thinning of myelin sheaths and damage to Schwann cells, in addition to a slowing in the velocity of nerve conduction.

The sensory system often demonstrates some changes with normal ageing, changes that may have a critical impact upon the effective performance of functional activities.

Reaction time, that is, the minimal time interval between the application of a stimulus and the beginning of a voluntary response, slows progressively. Many elderly people, therefore, need more time to integrate information and prepare a response. They may be able to cope if they shift from speed to accuracy in their functional performances. When rapid, sequential stimuli are presented the slowed reaction time usually creates a poor performance.

Reflexes such as the righting reflex may deteriorate, affecting the elderly person's ability to regain balance. Therapists who use reflex activity in facilitation therapy need to be aware that, in elderly people, new conditioned reflexes are induced with difficulty and appear neither stable or durable if they are formed.

Postural sway tends to increase with age. When this is associated with diminished righting reflexes and deterioration in other balance mechanisms, such as those of the inner ear and proprioception, loss of balance and subsequent falls may ensue.

Increasing *tremor* is not considered a physiological manifestation of ageing; rather, when present, it is probably pathological in nature.

Vibration sense is frequently impaired in old age. There are degenerative changes associated with age in the dorsal columns with consequent impairment of the proprioceptive system.

Thresholds for *temperature* recognition tend to increase for both hot and cold. This presents significant problems, especially in ambient temperature extremes when an increased death rate may occur. Temperature regulation, a feature of the autonomic system, may alter with age in some people. Responses to heat stress have a higher threshold while the reactions to the cold are less effective. Hypothermia is an important potential consequence of these changes. It should be noted that thermometer temperature taken by mouth has been shown to be an unreliable method of measuring body temperature in elderly people.

Kinaesthesia, the conscious sense of movement and position, tends to diminish with age because of changes in joint sensation, compression tension, muscle and tendon sensation as well as changes in the labyrinths and neck. This sensory deterioration has particular implications for walking and posture. Many elderly people must use visual clues, that is, watch their feet, to walk safely. When this is associated with poor night vision, walking in the dark is very hazardous. The wearing of bifocal lenses is dangerous for elderly people with diminished kinaesthesia because they attempt to watch their feet through the highly magnified lower section of the lens. Deficient kinaesthesia ought to be an important factor in care planning for very dependent elderly people. The impairment of this sensation may be a significant contributory factor in the grotesque sitting postures many institutionalised elderly people appear to adopt in the absence of effective chairs and alert staff.

Stereognosis, the ability to recognise form, progressively deteriorates with age. Stereognosis is really a synthesis of many sensations that help a person distinguish shape, size and composition — in other words, identify an object by touch alone. Many elderly people must use vision to supplement this deteriorating sense.

Pain is a significant problem in geriatric medicine. The mechanics of pain sensation are the subject of considerable controversy. Some writers suggest that the threshold for pain increases with age while others argue that it is the subjective response that actually changes. The disagreeable aspect of pain can be accentuated or depressed by mental or emotional states without any change in the physiological threshold.

Taste, especially to sour, bitter and sweet sensations, may deteriorate with age as there is a decline in the number of taste buds. The receptors of *smell* may also undergo changes reducing the ability to respond to odours. This deterioration in smell may prove a special problem because of the diminished ability to smell smoke and gas. *Flavour* sensations consist of a combination of taste and smell senses with smell predominating. Deterioration in the appreciation of flavour has important implications for nutrition, reinforcing the need to have meals presented in a visually interesting way to stimulate appetite, especially if the elderly person is not present when cooking, with its accompanying odours, takes place.

Vision is a very complex special sense with particular problems associated with normal ageing. The lens increases in size throughout life with a concomitant increase in rigidity. This results in a reduced power of *accommodation*. Visual *acuity*, the ability to distinguish objects against a background, tends to diminish. *Depth perception* becomes impaired progressively while *visual fields*, both peripheral and vertical, tend to contract. Visual *sensitivity*, or the ability to see in dim light, diminishes. There is an increasing inability to function in the dark. An 80-year-old person may need 300% more light than does a normal 20 year old. This does not mean that an elderly person should install high wattage light bulbs for reading or close work. It does mean, though, that careful planning must go into the placement of lights in relation to tasks.

Glare reactions are important considerations. Many elderly people are unable to tolerate glare and the recovery time from glare is usually increased substantially. Measures must be taken to protect an elderly person's eyes from glare as much as possible. *Colour vision* tends to deteriorate with age, especially the ability to discriminate between similar colours, tones and hues. *Critical*

flicker fusion is a significant problem for many elderly people, especially in relation to fluorescent lights and moving pictures on film or television. Normally, as the frequency of flashes increases, the ability to distinguish separate flashes decreases. Many elderly people have, however, a reduced capacity to cope with flickering lights.

This wide variety of visual functions that may deteriorate as a result of physiological changes in the many components of vision must be understood and appreciated by all people who contribute to the life of an elderly person. The implications of these changes for safe and effective function are significant. Unless environments are purpose planned to accommodate the more common vision changes many elderly people are disabled unnecessarily. Further, elderly people must be educated to become more aware of the limitations that may ensue. The role of diminished peripheral vision in the incidence of pedestrian accidents in people in the elderly age group may be significant.

Changes in the *auditory system* occur with age. Hearing impairment may be present in as many as 40% of people in their seventh decade. There is a progressive loss of higher sound frequencies in the initial stages progressing further until the lower frequency sounds are involved as well. As a result of these effects a person may have difficulty understanding speech and this difficulty may be compounded when background noise is present. The label of senility may be inappropriately applied to an elderly person as a consequence of problems with discrimination of speech which may make adequate communication impossible. The disability of deafness may be exaggerated by other effects of ageing such as impaired ability to concentrate, as listening

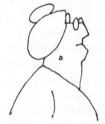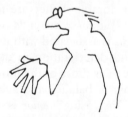

requires concentration. Impairment of vision reduces the ability to lip read and arthritic hands have difficulty in manipulating hearing aids. Impaired hearing is a common problem that attracts little sympathy but which may have unpleasant consequences for many people. It is essential, therefore, to approach such individuals with understanding while using correct communication techniques including facing the person with the light falling on the speaker and speaking with a firm voice but not shouting, preferably in an area free from background noise.

COGNITIVE CHANGES

Memory

It has long been known that there are cognitive changes associated with ageing. Unfortunately, these have been exaggerated generally by many people confusing pathological diseases such as Alzheimer's disease and multi-infarct dementia with normal ageing.

Memory may be affected by age, however, it seems that memory for things past is better preserved than memory for present events. Despite this, recent memory is not greatly disrupted by the ageing process. *Primary memory*, that is, the information that can be held for active processing at a given time, is essentially normal in old people provided that no reorganisation of that information is required. *Secondary memory* requires the transfer of information from primary memory into storage for removal at another time. It has been found that most elderly people perform less well on recall tests than do younger people. *Free recall*, for example, recalling a name, may become more difficult with age. However, if elderly persons are tested using a multiple choice format they generally perform as well as younger people. It would appear that information can be retrieved as effectively by elderly people when adequate clues are given.

There is considerable evidence to show that older people are quite capable of *learning* although they may take longer to do so. Elderly people have a large store of information acquired over time and the systems that maintain the store and make use of it tend to remain relatively intact. Learning, built on experience, is often easier for an older person. It was thought that the increased learning time was due to a slowing of the cognitive processes. It may, however, be that older people replace speed with accuracy, taking a little more time in an attempt to avoid errors.

Personality

While interest has been shown in the concept of changes in personality with age there is little evidence that such changes occur as a result of physiological ageing. With age there may be a decline in social standing and many may feel a loss of role, family and friends, all leading to a lack of purpose. On the other hand, many older people find old age a time for contentment.

Certain psychiatric disorders may be problems in later life. Depressive illness is perhaps the most common and may further impair alertness and cognitive ability to a degree that a diagnosis of dementing disease may be made. Anxiety, however, may be the presenting symptom of depression or, as is quite frequently the case, a series of somatic symptoms may dominate the picture. Remaining alert for the signs of depression is essential because the rate of suicide is high in the elderly population.

Confusional states, both acute and chronic, are a common problem in old age. Confusion, like any other symptom or sign, may have many causes. Defining the precipitating cause may be a significant clinical problem. It is essential to remember, however, that the majority of old people do not experience disabling levels of confusion or dementia and neither should be considered a normal feature of ageing.

REFERENCES

Blazer D, William C D 1980 Epidemiology of dysphoria and depression in an elderly population. American Journal of Psychiatry 137(4): 439–444

Bressler N M, Bressler S R, Fine S L 1988 Age related macular degeneration. Survival Ophthalmology 32: 375–413

Massoro E J 1987 Biology of ageing: current state of knowledge. Archives of Internal Medicine 1417: 166–169

5. Disability and disease presentation

John Hurley

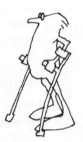

So far, this book has addressed the broad social context of normal ageing, and it is important to stress that the majority of people manage their lives independently or with moderate support until the end. This chapter should provide reassurance for many that disease and dependence are not inevitable consequences of ageing, and at the same time explain the significance of changes that may occur and the need for informed advice and appropriate action.

DIMINISHED FUNCTIONAL INDEPENDENCE

Although the proportion of elderly people who are significantly dependent is small, estimated at less than 20% of the over 65 population, there is a strong tendency for society to assume that this is the potential fate of all elderly people. Because of this, many functionally competent elderly people become anxious about the future. Of even more concern, families often attempt to coerce elderly people into dependency as they usurp decision-making responsibilities, often insidiously, though usually with the best intentions.

The 5% or so of elderly people who are in institutional continuing care are usually very dependent, physically or mentally or both. This may be due to fixed disease-based frailty and disability

but it may also result from dependency imposed by the institutional system. Unfortunately, identification of dependence in one activity often leads to assumptions of dependency in all activities. Because a person cannot walk, it does not follow that it is not possible to dress, bathe, laugh or converse.

A great deal of staff-paid time is expended on providing basic personal care services for these people. All evidence points to a growing demand for support programmes as the number of elderly people in the population grows. It would seem, therefore, that considerable work, that is research, planning, programming and, above all, education, must be undertaken if the system is not to be swamped by the demands of unnecessarily dependent elderly people.

Functional independence is the ability to perform tasks competently without the influence or assistance of other people. In normal daily life most people undertake a host of activities which may be classified as in Box 5.1.

To perform activities in any of these groups a person requires skills such as grasping, manipulating, walking, exploring, perceiving, thinking, learning, caring and sharing. Skill in relation to function implies a degree of competence that may be described as the smooth, purposeful and successful undertaking of an activity. Competence

Box 5.1	Functional activity groups
Cognition	Recreational
Communication	Self-care
Educational	Sexual
Home-making	Social
Judgemental	Vocational

includes the notions of coping and control. From birth, education, both formal and informal, is directed at gaining competence in the skills, both necessary and desirable, to live a life of purpose.

The majority of people develop a unique pattern of normal functional activities. This pattern usually emerges in response to the resources, talents and skills available. Each person in a democracy has the right to live in the manner of choice providing the resources are available and the modes are within the law. Often, a person's lifestyle is controlled more by the dictates of fashion or socially acceptable behaviours than essential personal desires. There is, however, still a place for the non-conformist, the eccentric. Freedom to choose how and when to function is an important element of independence.

The majority of mature people choose to share their lives with others, either permanently or temporarily in marriages, families and friendships. This sharing often involves interdependent, sometimes dependent, functioning. It is only the recluse who seeks a life of apparent complete independence.

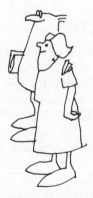

The desire for independent competency, inculcated in most people from babyhood, remains strong throughout life. However, the ability to function competently in the vast range of daily living skills may be thwarted by difficulties of a physical, psychological, social, economic or environmental nature.

The primary aims of geriatric care are the prevention of dependency, and the restoration or maintenance of functional competence. As far as possible every effort should be directed towards preventing problems; however, when they do occur it is incumbent upon the system to assist every person, regardless of age, to attain and maintain the highest level of functional skill within the limits imposed by disabilities.

On admission to any element of an extended care service, the elderly person must be assessed thoroughly to determine the range and extent of functional problems that may be present. Because each person is unique, a general regimen or schedule cannot be formulated in the hope that everyone will fit. Effective problem solving for each person can take place only if the problems are known. Further, it ought to be remembered that problems need to be viewed against the person's usual environment. Assessments undertaken in clinics or specially designed activities of daily living units must be somewhat inaccurate because it is impossible to simulate each person's unique normal environment. Further, such assessments may be unreliable because many people are poor witnesses and are unable to describe their home accurately and in detail. There is, then, no substitute for home assessment in planning for functional competence. The term 'home', as used here, includes both the private home and the institutional home.

The desire for independence requires the support of a suitable environment if success is to be achieved. There is little point in having a philosophical approach to independence when beds are too high, toilets are too far away, lighting is poor, directional cues are absent and floors are slippery. Careful planning ought to be undertaken to build or adapt living environments to suit the people who will use them. All aspects of the physical and organisational environments need to be considered.

Functional independence, its development and exercise, often involves a significant degree of risk. Elderly people cannot maintain or regain activities of daily living competence if they are cocooned or protected from all possible dangers. This does not mean that families or staff may ignore obviously hazardous situations. It does mean that alternatives, either direct or implied, must be explored. It is sad to realise that there is more concern about potential litigation resulting from a fractured femur than there is about the more disastrous consequences of a fractured mind or spirit. There is an urgent need for society to come to terms with this complex problem.

Many health care disciplines specialise in aspects of functional competence: for instance, physiotherapists in movement; occupational therapists in activity; and speech pathologists in communication. In the absence of skilled people from these professions, however, other people may contribute effectively if a practical, problem-solving approach is adopted.

Staff or families who do not have direct access to professional people who are experienced in dealing with problems of functional competence may obtain advice about such sources of help from a hospital, rehabilitation centre or health authority. In addition, there are a number of books and pamphlets that may be studied for guidance. Some of these are listed in the selective bibliography at the end of this book. The local health department's librarian may be a source of additional advice.

Training and practice may restore normal competence. This is, of course, the ideal situation. Where this is not possible there are other options such as teaching an alternative method of undertaking the activity by adapting aspects of it. For example, if independent dressing cannot be achieved because of an inability to manage buttons, hooks or zippers, they may be replaced successfully with Velcro fasteners. It may be necessary to provide aids or devices to facilitate independence in the task: for instance, a person may not be able to manage the degree of mobility required for using a bathtub normally but hand rails, a bath seat and a hand-held shower may permit effective bathing.

It must be stressed that aids should be kept to a minimum and tested thoroughly to ensure appropriateness. The elderly person, and the family or staff, ought to understand the nature of the device and how to use it effectively. There should be a clearly defined follow-up programme to provide occasional monitoring for maintenance and for evaluating use.

Of course, equipment that is on loan to a person should be returned to the equipment bank when no longer needed, another important function of a follow-up programme.

Many communities have established equipment display and testing centres where people, both public and professional, may obtain advice about the most suitable items available. A number of communities also have an organisation of skilled technical people who may be able to develop a special item of equipment to meet a particular need not available commercially. Recent advances in electronics and computers have expanded the range of assistive devices significantly. Unfortunately, expense is as yet a critical factor, but the future holds promise.

In domiciliary care it is essential to consider the functional needs of the family members who may be caring for a dependent elderly person. The caring family may need assistance with environmental planning, practical methods of managing their elderly relative and the use of equipment to facilitate the process. Often, an important aspect of family functional independence is the provision of assistance to permit some freedom from the caring task, for example, holiday breaks and regular planned admissions to a unit which can provide appropriate care on a short-term or shared care basis.

POOR MOBILITY

The consequences of limited mobility are wide ranging and may be seen readily on a visit to a hospital catering for geriatric patients. The inability to move freely where and when one chooses is the major cause of dependency in elderly people. For example, the inability to rise from a chair smoothly and safely may be the first step in a chain of circumstances that leads to the incontinence–depression–confusion syndrome often seen in nursing homes. The maintenance of the ability to move freely may prevent the occurrence of an accident that would mean disaster for an old person.

The control of impaired movement in elderly people requires an understanding of the many mechanisms that contribute to it. The physiological ageing process, itself, may be manifested by changes that contain the potential for disturbed movement. For example, research has indicated that there is progressive muscle atrophy in advanced age. Thus, old people decline in strength and vigour. If this fact is accepted in isolation, movement problems will be inevitable. Research, however, has found that most healthy muscles have the potential for recruiting previously inactive motor units if the muscles are exercised under some stress. Thus, a decline in strength and vigour may be partially corrected by exercise. Muscle atrophy is but one of many changes that may take place as a result of physiological ageing and which may have mobility consequences. People, especially elderly people, must be educated to understand these changes, to recognise the signs of onset and to prevent, as far as possible, the disabling consequences.

The pathological problems that have implications for mobility are legion. In fact, almost every illness due to disease or trauma may have a direct or indirect effect on mobility. A stroke, a fracture, and an arthritic disease are common pathological problems which disturb mobility effectiveness to some degree. Even those diseases resulting in blindness, deafness and respiratory distress may also produce mobility problems. Sometimes, the cause may be even more indirect. A skin disease such as psoriasis may not, in itself, cause a mobility disorder. However, the psychological effects may result in self-imposed isolation, with associated mobility disablement.

For elderly people, one of the greatest hazards for mobility is disuse resulting from bed rest or confinement in a chair. Immobility can have disastrous consequences which, with understanding and diligence, might have been avoided. When inactivity is essential it should be undertaken for the minimum time and be accompanied by vigorous efforts to maintain all movement components maximally. Careful research is essential to determine with accuracy the necessary frequency of range of movement exercises to prevent the development of position contractures. However, one full-range joint movement once a day with special attention to hips, knees and shoulders should be seen as a mandatory requirement for people who are dependent.

Psychological, social and economic problems may contribute to mobility disorders because they limit the person's ability to move. Depression, for example, may result in poor posture, inadequate nutrition and insufficient exercise. All of these are contributory factors in reduced mobility. Financial poverty may limit social mobility directly. It may also have consequences for adequate nutrition, heating and clothing, all of which may affect mobility.

Minor mobility problems are compounded for elderly people by adverse aspects of the environment. For example, an elderly person with some movement poverty such as stiffness, slight weakness and unsteadiness may be able to rise easily from a chair with a seat height of 50 cm (20 inches). However, when trying to stand from a chair of more usual height, 46 cm (17 inches), this elderly, person experiences difficulty. Unfortunately, high chairs are not readily available. Another elderly person may be disabled in mobility because the environment does not provide adequate cues. It may, for example, be very difficult for an elderly person to find the ward's toilet if the door is not clearly and appropriately distinguished from all other doors. The home environment may limit mobility because of steps or stairs, hazardous floor coverings, lack of convenience or too much furniture. When environments pose such limitations every effort ought to be expended upon correcting them in an appropriate way.

Dealing with mobility problems, either prevention or corrections, is the special province of the physiotherapist. In the absence of a skilled physiotherapist others can, and must, undertake the responsibility. Box 5.2 lists the skills of movement that are usually considered in assessment and management. If the problems appear to be beyond the available resources advice may be obtained from an appropriate hospital, rehabilitation centre or health authority.

Often elderly people with movement problems will require aids to promote safe and effective mobility. There are a wide variety of walking sticks, crutches and frames, each designed to

Box 5.2 Mobility skills

Bed:	*Transport:*
bridging	car
rolling	bus
moving up/down	
sitting up	*Walking:*
sitting maintenance	forwards
sitting over side	backwards
lying from sitting	turning
	carrying things
Chair:	managing doors
balance	smooth surfaces
posture	rough surfaces
posture correction	slopes
	steps, curbs
Transfers:	stairs
in bed	
bed to chair	*Level of competence:*
chair to bed	stability
chair to toilet	speed
chair to bath	endurance

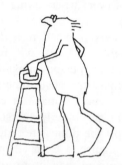

assist movement in a specific way. The choice of aid is dependent upon the needs of the elderly person and is subject to personal preferences. When a device is provided it must be suited to the individual requirements of the specific elderly person. For example, a tall person usually needs a higher walking frame than does a short person; a tall person with long arms, however, may need a shorter frame than does a person of the same height with short arms. Incorrectly adjusted sticks, crutches and frames are not effective and usually demand additional energy expenditure: energy is a resource few elderly people can afford to waste. The practice of sharing walking frames in long stay institutions to reduce clutter or expense is to be deplored.

The most essential aid to mobility is suitable footwear. Ill-fitting slippers and stockinged feet are very common contributory causes of falls in elderly people. Shoes should fit well, be in a good state of repair and provide adequate support. Painful feet force elderly people off their feet and into immobility far too frequently to be ignored. Thus, the podiatrist is a primary member of any extended care team.

Wheelchairs are becoming a common feature of the mobility scene for elderly people. If a wheelchair is used only to transport people within an institution, the quality of the chair, perhaps, is not of prime importance. There is one proviso, however: wheelchairs should have swingaway footrests so that transferring is facilitated. Fixed footrests prevent correct placement of the wheelchair with respect to chairs and beds, and increase the potential for trauma to the elderly person's legs.

A wheelchair used regularly to permit mobility, generally independent but sometimes assisted, must be prescribed specifically for the individual who is to use it. Wheelchairs, like people, come in various shapes, sizes and styles. A physiotherapist or an occupational therapist may be the most appropriate prescriber. If they are not directly available, advice should be sought from sources previously mentioned before a wheelchair is provided or purchased.

Wheelchairs must be maintained appropriately and kept in good condition as they are very expensive to replace and safety may be compromised, for example, by unfunctional brakes.

The user of a wheelchair must be taught to manage it efficiently. Self-propulsion by hands or feet needs instruction and practice. Power-driven wheelchairs usually require more intensive training before driving is mastered by elderly people. The people who push wheelchairs must also be taught to manage them correctly, especially on slopes and rough ground, over curbs, and up and down steps. It is always surprising that so few people have any idea about the simple manoeuvres that permit easy wheelchair management. Many people will need to be taught how to place the chair in and out of a car efficiently.

Independent mobility may not be possible for a small proportion of elderly people and varying degrees of assistance may need to be provided. The appropriate handling of people is a learned skill which must be understood and practised if

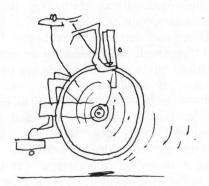

Table 5.1 Some diseases common in old age

System	Disease common in old age
Autonomic nervous	Hypothermia, postural hypotension
Blood chemistry	Anaemia, vitamin B_{12} deficiency myelodyplastic syndromes
Cardiovascular	Hypertension, ischaemic heart disease, peripheral vascular disease
Central nervous	Dementia, depression, stroke, Parkinson's disease
Ears	Deafness
Endocrine	Diabetes mellitus, gout, thyroid disease
Eyes	Cataract, macular degeneration, glaucoma
Gastrointestinal	Colonic carcinoma, constipation, diverticular disease, hiatus hernia
Genitourinary	Prostatic disease, renal impairment, incontinence, urinary tract infection
Musculoskeletal	Fractures, osteoarthritis, osteoporosis, polymyalgia rheumatica
Respiratory	Chest infection, pneumonia, obstructive airways disease, pulmonary tuberculosis
Skin	Pressure sores

efficiency and effectiveness are to be promoted and both the disabled person and the handler are to be protected from injury. The incidence of injuries to staff which occur during handling activities is testimony of the seriousness of this problem.

The occurence of injuries to elderly people is just as serious but, unfortunately, is less apparent. A study of shoulder disabilities in mishandled institutionalised elderly people compared with similarly disabled people who are handled effectively may indicate chronic joint damage as a result of being hauled by or under the arms. An energetic education programme for staff, families and the public should be a primary responsibility of those responsible for services for ageing or disabled people.

DISEASE PRESENTATION

The manifestation of disease in an elderly population is essentially similar to that of younger adults. There are, however, some fairly significant differences that need to be known by those caring for elderly people. Not only do certain clinical problems present differently but certain diseases, listed in Table 5.1, are more common in an elderly population.

In general terms, symptoms of disease demonstrated by elderly people are more non-specific, more insidious and sometimes atypical (see Table 5.2). The term 'going off' is frequently used by staff unable to identify a specific problem in an old person whose status is deteriorating.

A number of diseases can produce similar symptoms. For example, the onset of confusion

Table 5.2 Some atypical presentations of disease in elderly people

Problem	Atypical symptoms
Acute abdomen	
Acute myocardial infarction	
Chest infection	falls
Depression	
Hyperthyroidism	...ate ... ...ia, normal appetite, no thyroid enlargement
Hypothyroidism	Confusion, depression, aches and pains
Infection	Acute confusion, absent fever, white cell count not raised, reduced threshold for sweating
Parkinson's disease	Falls, rigidity without tremor

or incontinence, or both, can be due to illness not related to the central nervous system or genitourinary system. A disease process in an old person can, therefore, alter the function of several other organs in addition to the one originally involved. In the example given, pneumonia could be the cause of both the confusion and incontinence. Some diseases may be more virulent in old age, for example, acute appendicitis, whereas others may be more benign, such as breast cancer.

Multiple diseases are essentially the rule in old age. A number of factors tend to favour this situation. First, there is system interaction where the disease process in one system leads to problems in another, for example, falls caused by pneumonia. Secondly, many diseases have a long period of development, as is the case in vascular disease, which tends to appear later in life. Thirdly, there is an age-related increase in some diseases, such as carcinoma. Fourthly, there is a decline in immune function, leading to problems of infection and autoimmune diseases such as chronic thyroiditis. Finally, multiple problems often lead to multiple medications which may add iatrogenic diseases to the list.

A considerable amount of illness in elderly people is due to undiagnosed conditions such as dementia, urinary incontinence and a number of problems involving the locomotor system. This fact is sometimes regarded as the **'iceberg phenomenon of geriatric medicine'**.

Symptoms

A number of points about common symptoms need to be remembered when dealing with old people. Multiple abnormalities are evident; late detection of disease is common; and the four major disabilities of old age — immobility, instability, incontinence and confusion — may be present concurrently. The presence of one chronic disease may mask the development of another. The presence of a number of diseases, equally, can obscure the symptoms of a newly occurring illness. An example of such a situation would be chronic osteoarthritis with its general aches and pains delaying the diagnosis of polymyalgia rheumatica, which may present with similar symptoms.

Drugs may also produce problems of their own in older people. The incidence of adverse drug reactions increases with age and is a potent cause of hospital admission. Medications may precipitate various conditions, such as gout in the case of thiazide diuretics, and alter or modify symptoms and signs, such as non-steroidal anti-inflammatory drugs (NSAIDs) modifying pain. A review of drug therapy is mandatory in the initial assessment as wide-ranging problems, such as hypotension, electrolytic disturbance, confusion, depression and impairment of balance with resulting falls, may be produced.

As a consequence of illness being vague and ill-defined and because old people may present with complaints of inability to cope or reduced effectiveness, the elderly person may at first be reluctant to seek advice. Also, medical personnel may underestimate the symptoms, unwisely blaming the so-called process of ageing for the problem.

The problems of communicating with an elderly person can be formidable as a consequence of poor hearing, possibly impaired vision, and often poor concentration, all compounded by a change of environment if the person is first seen in a hospital setting (Table 5.3). Patience, tolerance and a sympathetic ear while giving the impression of having plenty of time may reap dividends. Too often, however, rush and bustle is the order of the day, with a poor history and inadequate diagnosis being the result.

Table 5.3 Common problems experienced in taking a history from elderly persons

Problem	Consequence
Anxiety	Inaccurate information
Chronic ill health	Fatigue, poor concentration
Deafness	Questions misunderstood
Depression	Lack of communication
Dysphasia	Communication difficulty
Fear of examiner	Reticence with information
Impaired recall	Inaccurate history
Impaired vision	Difficulty in reading
Strange environment	Possible confusion

Confusion

Confusion is a symptom that may be the final common pathway of presentation in a number of conditions. Confusional states are generally either acute or chronic. It is, thus, imperative to attempt to date the onset of the problem. It is remarkable how frequently this piece of information is missing in the elderly person's record and how ill informed staff may be on this point.

In general, acute onset of confusion is associated with a reversible cause such as an infection, metabolic abnormalities or heart disease. Chronic confusion, developing over months rather than days or weeks, more frequently may be associated with irreversible disease. This, however, should not be assumed to be the case and Alzheimer's disease should only be considered when other causes have been eliminated through thorough investigations. Some causes of chronic reversible confusion include hypothyroidism, hyperparathyroidism and normal pressure hydrocephalus.

Falls and immobility

The maintenance of upright posture is complex and age-related changes may predispose the individual to falls when an acute illness occurs. Falls that are not associated with trips or accidents may be an indication of serious underlying disease. The diseases that may present as falls or immobility are numerous and they include neurological and psychological problems. Some examples are parkinsonism, neuropathies, dementia and depression. Other problems include stroke, postural hypotension and locomotor-related difficulties. Falls without obvious accidental causes should be taken seriously and not dismissed as due to the ageing process.

Fatigue

General weakness or fatigue is a common presentation which may be the symptom of many diseases and is fairly typical of the non-specific complaints that elderly people report. Chronic infections of any type may produce such an effect and tuberculosis should be kept in mind, its incidence being higher in old people, in particular, among alcoholic old men. Other conditions to be considered include malignancy, other chronic inflammatory diseases and motor neurone disease, the latter being overlooked easily. The number of diseases that may be considered is formidable and could encompass more acute conditions such as polymyalgia rheumatica, biochemical abnormalities such as hyponatraemia, hypothyroidism and drug side-effects. Drugs with a sedative effect are particularly prone to produce the effect of weakness and lethargy.

Febrile response

Taking the person's temperature is a routine procedure in the normal course of investigating an illness. However, the febrile response in an elderly person may be reduced and if care is not exercised in recording the temperature a fever may be overlooked. The thermometer should be kept under the tongue for a period exceeding 3 minutes to improve the chance of recording an elevated temperature.

Compared with the younger population, old people have a higher temperature threshold before sweating occurs. Thus, a valuable sign may be missing in some old people suffering an infection. Where doubt exists, it is well worth taking the rectal temperature as this may show a fever to be present when the oral temperature has been normal. Usually, thirst goes hand in glove with fever, however, the ability of some elderly people to replace water loss is less effective and thus dehydration may occur quite rapidly.

Incontinence

Incontinence is a major problem in old age, although not due to the ageing process itself. Old age, however, may predispose the individual to becoming incontinent when an additional precipitating factor is brought into play. Incontinence is to be considered a symptom like any other and requires the cause to be determined. This symptom is one still tending to be hidden from the medical team because many people are reluctant, perhaps due to shame, to admit the problem. The multitude of causes need to be carefully considered with full and proper investigation being carried out to define the underlying condition. This condition will be dealt with in more detail in Chapter 7.

Signs

The conventional examination is usually undertaken with the person lying, probably in bed. This is effective for checking most systems but is inadequate when mobility and balance are of importance. Thus, for an examination to be complete it should include the person standing and walking if possible. Observing and examining the elderly person is very important as the history of symptoms may be less than clear.

Skin and general appearance

The clinical sign of pallor does not readily allow accurate diagnosis of anaemia in old age. Checking the skin for pallor is important, as is looking at the conjunctivae, tongue and nail beds.

Dryness of the skin with poor elasticity is usually normal and makes the diagnosis of dehydration by pinching the skin useless. A dry tongue also often goes with mouth breathing and may represent a false sign. Examination of the mouth may show a smooth tongue and angular stomatis suggestive of vitamin B complex deficiency, but these symptoms may also accompany poorly fitting dentures.

An unkempt appearance, especially if associated with a thin body, may indicate malnutrition, possibly associated with depression or dementia. An immobile facial expression may be related to depression, Parkinson's disease or hypothyroidism.

Locomotor system

The gait of the elderly individual is often abnormal and may give clues to the diagnosis: festination indicating possible Parkinson's disease; dragging of a foot or lower limb suggesting hemiparesis or foot drop; and a wide-based gait provoking thought of a cerebellar lesion. The presence of multiple bruises may indicate re-

peated falls while the examination of the system must include looking for evidence of arthritis in the joints. Not to be forgotten are the feet which are vulnerable to changes associated with the passing of the years. Proper care is important to maintain independent mobility so it is vital to look for corns, calluses and ischaemic lesions.

Cardiovascular system

The presence of peripheral oedema is not unusual in old people and a cause should be sought. Frequently, however, this oedema is of a dependent type secondary to sitting and inactivity. Prescription of a diuretic is not the first choice unless it is clearly indicated as, for example, in congestive cardiac failure which is also common in old age. Palpation of peripheral pulses is important as absence of pulses gives an indication of the state of the arterial tree. Auscultation of the carotid arteries and femoral arteries for bruits should also be routine as their presence indicates arterial disease.

Postural hypotension occurs with increasing frequency with age. All elderly people should have their blood pressure taken lying and standing. A number of conditions may precipitate postural hypotension, and among the more common are stroke, parkinsonism, prolonged bed rest and the use of a number of drugs including diuretics, phenothiazines, tricylic antidepressants and L-Dopa.

Hypertension is also prevalent in an elderly population but a number of blood pressure recordings need to be made before considering the diagnosis confirmed.

Respiratory system

Measurement of the respiration rate in an ill old person may reap considerable dividends, as the respiration rate may be a more reliable indicator of infection than the temperature. A rate of 25 breaths per minute or more may suggest such a problem. It should be remembered that pulmonary tuberculosis is more common in elderly populations and a high index of suspicion should be maintained.

Gastrointestinal system

Palpation of the abdomen needs to be carried out with care, feeling for abdominal masses while giving particular consideration to the bladder. A rectal examination is especially worthwhile as this may lead to a number of diagnoses common in old age, especially haemorrhoids, faecal impaction, prostatic hypertrophy or carcinoma and rectal cancer.

Central nervous system

Observation of the older person during the assessment process is particularly valuable from the neurological viewpoint. Various abnormalities of movement may be noted, particularly those of tardive dyskinesia and parkinsonism, which are not uncommon in this age group.

A number of changes occur which can be accepted as being within normal parameters in old people. These include a high incidence of absent ankle jerks and vibration sense, as well as some wasting of the small muscles of the hands. Failure to check intellectual capacity routinely using a validated mental function test may lead to incorrect impressions. Studies have shown that a 20% misdiagnosis in terms of absent or misleading description can occur when formal testing is not applied, especially in a hospital setting.

The special senses need to be tested and any impairment of hearing or sight noted, perhaps for further investigations.

Investigations

Care needs to be taken on interpreting laboratory results when investigating diseases in an elderly population. Anaemia is relatively common and pernicious anaemia increases with age, so taking notice of the haemoglobin concentration and mean corpuscular volume (MCV) as a matter of course is worthwhile as the MCV is elevated in vitamin B_{12} and folate deficiency. The total white cell count rises when infection occurs but in some infected old people the rise may be marginal or may not occur at all. However, a left shift in the white cell count is indicative of an inflammatory process taking place and, thus, paying attention to the blood film report is essential.

There is a reduction in kidney function in many elderly people with poor renal reserve. Further impairment produced by dehydration, hypotension or cardiac failure may cause elevation of the blood urea level. Electrolyte disturbances are commonplace, hypokalaemia and hyponatraemia being the most usual and very frequently associated with diuretic therapy. Both these conditions tend to produce similar symptoms, such as confusion, weakness and hypotension.

Elevated blood glucose levels are more common in the older than in the younger age group. In conjunction with this there is a tendency for the renal threshold for glucose to be higher in old people; thus, sugar in the urine may not be a reliable indicator of high blood glucose levels. A random blood sugar estimation is usually more effective.

X-rays and electrocardiography are useful diagnostic tools in the battery of tests available. The chest X-ray may be useful in diagnosing problems other than those involving the cardiovascular and respiratory systems; for example, hiatus hernia and osteoporosis may be incidental findings. In regard to the ECG, all abnormal findings are pathological because there are no abnormalities associated with age alone.

Conclusion

An elderly person may present disease in an atypical manner. Because there may be difficulty obtaining a proper history the examination must be meticulous and the interpretation of laboratory results needs to be made with care. Most essentially, multiple diseases occurring concurrently are common and each needs to be investigated carefully.

CONFUSION

Confusion is a word used to describe a group of symptoms due to cognitive dysfunction and often associated with distressed or disruptive behaviour. Confusion represents a common presenting problem in an elderly population and has similar diagnostic implications for the brain as shortness of breath has for the heart or lung. It demands, therefore, a no less careful analysis to elucidate its cause than does acute dyspnoea. It should be regarded as a symptom, the particular cause of which needs to be found.

Frequently, the causes of confusion are extracerebral and may result from a wide variety of conditions. Although psychological problems may produce symptoms of confusion in some circumstances, they are not usually a primary cause.

Acute confusion

Confusion may be divided into acute and chronic forms. As acute confusion tends to indicate underlying physical disease and, as most cases are reversible, it is essential to differentiate the two by taking a good history.

The first question to be asked, and documented in the record, is the time of onset of the confusion. Acute confusion develops rapidly and has a history dating back a matter of hours or days. Chronic confusion, on the other hand, usually presents with a story of insidious change developing over weeks or months. In the case of Alzheimer's disease the period of decline may cover several years.

The elderly brain is susceptible to acute confusional states due to age-related changes, both in the brain itself and in the body's homeostatic mechanisms. There is, for example, a reduction in the number of neurones, the extent of loss usually differing in various parts of the brain. Also, there is a reduction in some neurotransmitters including dopamine and acetylcholine. The latter changes may, in part, account for the sensitivity of old people to drug-induced confusion.

Acute confusion usually presents with a rapid onset of disorientation for time, place or person. In addition, hallucinations may be present, and the person may often be noisy and irrational, and usually experiences restless and disturbed sleep. The elderly person's degree of alertness may vary from drowsiness and apathy to hyperactivity. It is worth noting that the patient's mental state may fluctuate greatly during a 24 hour period,

from lucidity to apathy or agitiation. Attention may be impaired and the concentration span reduced, leading to an inability to complete even simple daily tasks. Taking a history from the elderly person may be impossible because of an inability to register the question and because of disorganised recent memory. Hence, it is vital to gather information from a close relative or friend.

The management of acute confusion depends on an accurate diagnosis which depends largely on a precise and detailed history. This involves all team members gleaning as much information as possible from relatives, friends, neighbours and supporting services. The history should contain information on the duration of confusion, speed of onset and any changes, either physical or social, immediately prior to onset. An accurate drug history should also be taken including information on 'over the counter' medication which may be misused. The most effective method is to obtain all medication for perusal and to identify those drugs most recently commenced. Part of the drug evaluation should include alcohol intake, a factor often overlooked (Box 5.3).

Box 5.3 Drugs frequently associated with the onset of confusional states in elderly people

Alcohol	Benzodiazepine
Anaesthetics	Cardiovascular
Analgesics	Beta-blockers
	Digoxin
Anticonvulsants	Diuretics
Antidepressants	Hypnotics
Antihistamines	Hypoglycaemics
Cimetedine	
	Hypotensive agents
Anti-Parkinson	Non-steroidal anti-
Anticholinergics	inflammatory drugs
L-Dopa	
Antispasmodics	Phenothiazines
Barbiturates	Steroids

The list of those conditions most likely to produce acute confusion is remarkable in its breadth (Box 5.4) and extends a considerable challenge to the team members dealing with this problem. It is their job to identify and treat the underlying

Box 5.4 Common causes of acute confusional states

Cardiovascular
Cardiac failure
Dysrythmia
Complete heart block
Transient tachycardia
Hypotension
Myocardial infarction

Cerebral
Cerebral tumour
Cerebrovascular
   accident
Infarct (occipital lobe)
Embolus
Haemorrhage
Epilepsy (temporal
   lobe)
Subdural haematoma
Transient ischaemic
   attack
Vertebrobasilar
   insufficiency

Chest
Carcinoma of bronchus
Hypoxia — acute or
   chronic infection
Pneumothorax

Deficiency states
Vitamin B$_{12}$
Folate
Iron
Multiple vitamin
Potassium
Sodium

Depression

Endocrine
Diabetes mellitus
Hypoglycaemia
   (chlorpropamide)
Hyperglycaemia
Hypoparathyroidism
Thyroid
Myxoedema
Thyrotoxicosis

Infection
Bacterial endocarditis
Cellulitis
Pneumonia
Urinary tract infection

Necrosis
Pressure sores
Gangrene

Toxic
Alcohol
Carcinoma
Liver failure

Uraemia
Dehydration
Chronic renal failure

Miscellaneous
Change of scene
Urine retention,
   chronic or acute
Constipation with
   impaction

disorder and to control the confusion in such a manner as to alleviate distress and harm to the elderly person.

A thorough examination is mandatory. This is particularly necessary if the historical data are limited. A very careful measurement of the elderly person's temperature is required so as not to miss minor febrile responses and hypothermia. It is also imperative to overcome the reluctance to carry out a rectal examination as a number of causes of confusion may be discovered through this procedure. Part of the assessment includes the mental status examination. A formal test, using one of a number of standard validated short questionnaires, is helpful, especially as it may also be used to monitor improvement over the period of illness. Particular regard should be paid to the possibility of depression presenting with features suggesting confusion.

Appropriate laboratory investigations may be of benefit. Although there is no fixed battery of tests that needs to be carried out certain tests may be helpful. A full blood count may show a raised white cell level or a left shift indicating an infection. Urea and electrolyte levels may point to dehydration, or abnormal potassium or sodium levels as a cause of the problem. A random blood glucose level may pick up a new case of diabetes, or hypoglycaemia in an established case, and thyroid status is worth evaluating as both underactive and overactive thyroid function may present atypically. A chest X-ray and electrocardiograph may also be of assistance as silent or pain-free myocardial infarction is a relatively common feature in old age. In addition, more detailed testing may be required when the clinical picture indicates the need.

Measures to minimise confusion should be taken while the underlying disease is being treated. Sedative agents may be used in restless elderly people, the doses and duration of courses of drug therapy being kept to a minimum. It is preferable to use sedatives with a shorter duration of action to prevent accumulation of the drugs; such drugs include thioridazine, haloperidol, chlormethiazole and chloral hydrate. If a major tranquiliser is required by injection small doses of haloperidol may be useful. It should be kept in mind constantly that sedatives and tranquilisers may cause confusion in their own right or make existing confusion worse. Certainly, physical restraints should be avoided as they usually increase distress. The approach taken by staff, especially nursing staff, to an agitated elderly person is an extremely important factor in management and is dealt with in Chapter 16.

Chronic confusion

Characteristically, chronic confusion develops gradually over a period of weeks or months, even years. It tends to be linked with the term dementia which, in its turn, is frequently associated in the mind of many people with irreversible disease. It may be easier to think of chronic confusion as being a symptom that requires a cause to be found, some causes being reversible and some not. It is of great importance not to equate prolonged confusion with irreversible disease before a definite cause for the confusion has been established. A list of some causes of chronic confusion are shown in Box 5.5, and it should be noted that many of these can be put in the reversible category.

Box 5.5 Some causes of chronic confusion

Alcohol	Multiple sclerosis
Alzheimer's disease	Myxoedema
Depression	Neurosyphilis
Drugs	Normal pressure hydrocephalus
Hungtington's chorea	
Hyperparathyroidism	Parkinson's disease
Intracranial tumour	Pick's disease
Multiple infarct dementia	Subdural haematoma
	Vitamin B$_{12}$ deficiency

The history is, again, important and may suggest the presence of conditions with a reversible aetiology. An onset that is rapid, within a few months, and the presence of quick deterioration tend to indicate a disease process that is treatable. The past history is also particularly relevant. For example, previously treated thyrotoxicosis is suggestive of myxoedema being the current precipitating factor. The drug history is once again highly relevant, the drug groups with anticholinergic characteristics being particularly notorious for contributing to confusion.

Careful examination is again very important. Signs of depression should be looked for; evidence of thyroid disease should be sought, and normal pressure hydrocephalus with its associated ataxic gait plus incontinence should be remembered. The mental status should be evaluated by a standard, validated questionnaire. A series of 'I don't know' responses as answers to questions may suggest the presence of depression.

Laboratory investigations should be as for acute confusion but additional tests may be valuable. The erythrocyte sedimentation rate may give a clue to the presence of cranial arteritis or neoplastic disease. Vitamin B$_{12}$ levels may be low in the absence of signs, and screening tests for syphilis need to be considered. Endocrine causes should be eliminated, thyroid function tests being of special importance. Checking serum calcium levels is often useful, a result above normal necessitating the measurement of parathyroid hormone levels which would be elevated in the case of hyperparathyroidism. CT scans are helpful when the cause is not clear, and where intracranial lesions with normal pressure hydrocephalus are possible. Lumbar puncture is generally retained for the identification of possible infections.

Management should begin with the treatment of reversible causes. When the condition is irreversible, therapy may be aimed at stabilising the situation and preventing deterioration (as is the case in multi-infarct dementia where the use of daily aspirin may be effective). The majority of cases will, however, be due to Alzheimer's disease, for which attempts to modify behaviour through various support programmes and medication are all that is available at present (See Ch. 10). It is clearly important not to miss any treatable condition.

CHRONIC PAIN

Physiology of pain

Any painful stimulus will provoke a response within the central nervous system which involves three main areas — the autonomic system, the limbic–hypothalamic area and the myoneural reflexes. The autonomic system produces physical expression through dry mouth, tachycardia and changes in blood flow: the most severe form of this being reflex sympathetic dystrophy with its associated pain, swelling and hot trophic skin. The limbic system is related to the emotional response to pain so behavioural factors such as emotional lability, sleep disturbance, depression and hostility may be evident. The myoneural response is based on protective muscle reflexes that may result in muscle tension, trigger spots and, in extreme cases, disuse atrophy.

The reaction to a painful stimulus is complicated further by other factors such as the intensity of the stimulus and the type of stimulus applied. The individual's personality, past pain experience, and cultural background may influence the interpretation of pain. Also the presence of external stresses may have a considerable impact. Clearly, pain is a very complex matter.

Age and pain

Pain is a common problem experienced by elderly people. It has been suggested that over 60% of visits to medical practitioners occur because of pain. As older people are afflicted more frequently with disease it could be assumed that pain would be a common presenting symptom, but balanced against this is the impression that either elderly people may not perceive pain to the same degree as younger age groups or that they tolerate pain better. Some research indicates that the pain threshold increases with age whereas others suggest that this is not so, older people just complain less. Whichever is the case, complaints of pain from elderly people should not be taken lightly.

Chronic pain in old age

Chronic disease is common in old age and it would appear that problems of chronic pain also, especially neurological pain, increase with age. There is little doubt that the quality of life is significantly reduced in the presence of chronic pain. In many instances pain interferes with sleep. High ratings of depression and anxiety may be present and significant restriction of daily activities occurs. The use of tricyclic antidepressants may benefit the elderly person greatly by alleviating the anxiety and depression, and allowing the elderly person to cope more effectively with pain.

It is important to understand that treatment may be difficult because of the inevitable multiple abnormalities present in old age, but suffering in this group of people could be reduced with proper pain management. Factors to consider are:

- That the prevalence of pain increases
- That diagnosis is important
- That psychological support is required
- That individualised drug regimens are necessary
- That therapy other than drugs is often effective.

Approach to chronic pain

Chronic pain has usually been present for longer than one month and has not responded to conventional therapy. This means that an organic and emotional component are present and will need to be considered in the therapeutic regimen. Pain is a symptom, not a diagnosis. It is essential, therefore, to obtain an accurate history. The assistance of relatives and friends may be helpful to achieve a clear picture. The elderly person should be questioned carefully regarding the pain, especially being asked to point to the site of the pain. This may help to prevent errors in terminology. A thorough and detailed examination should be carried out even though this may be difficult, perhaps because of mobility difficulties and possible reluctance to cooperate. The use of appropriate laboratory and other investigations may be needed to make or confirm the diagnosis. It needs to be stressed that the first step in treatment of patients with chronic pain is accurate identification of the problem.

An explanation of the causes of the pain needs to be given to the elderly person along with an indication of the therapeutic plan that is to be followed. Where an emotional component is involved this should also be addressed while reassuring the individual that assistance with the physical aspect of the pain will be continued. A positive approach needs to be maintained with the emphasis on rehabilitation rather than a more passive illness-like attitude focused on pain problems alone. The elderly person needs to develop a sense of sharing the responsibility for pain control.

Some specific pain problems

An accurate diagnosis helps proper pain control: for example, general pains and stiffness may be attributed to arthritis which responds to NSAIDs. Should pain, however, be due to polymyalgia rheumatica, dramatic recovery occurs with the use of steroids. Similarly, an acutely inflamed joint due to gout is better controlled in the long term when specific therapy with allopurinol is used to prevent further episodes.

Neoplastic diseases increase with age and unfortunately may present at a stage when the disease cannot be controlled at all despite various interventions. In this situation, care needs to be taken not to attribute all symptoms to the cancer but to evaluate each symptom individually and treat accordingly. When the symptom, particularly pain, is due to cancer, then it will persist and requires control in its own right. The therapeutic approach still is to diagnose the cause of the pain and begin specific treatment in an attempt to avoid analgesics; for example, abdominal pain due to constipation. If analgesia is necessary then it should be given regularly. Continuous pain cannot be treated on an as required basis. The dose of analgesic should be the smallest that controls the pain.

Analgesics are not the only type of intervention that is possible for pain due to neoplastic disease. Others include:

- Specific radiotherapy
- Local nerve blocks
- NSAIDs for secondary bone pain
- Psychotropic medication
- Transcutaneous electrical nerve stimulation (TENS)

Finally, emotional support is vital and should not be overlooked during the battle to control pain.

The use of opiate drugs is commonplace in controlling cancer-related pain. One of the greatest problems may be a too timid approach to the dose used. Respiratory depression is one of the anxieties often expressed in relation to these drugs but is rarely a major problem. By treating each person as an individual there should be few difficulties. Starting with low-dose oral morphine every 4 hours and increasing every 24 hours or more frequently, if necessary, pain can be relieved quickly and safely. The starting dose for old people is probably best set at 2.5 mg every 4 hours, initially used orally. Morphine, however, is only commenced should pain control not be possible with simple analgesics such as paracetamol. Morphine may also be given by continuous subcutaneous injection (using a syringe driver), intravenous infusion or by the intrathecal route in specific situations.

Various arthritic and rheumatic conditions are common in an elderly population. NSAIDs help to relieve discomfort by reducing pain and swelling in the affected tissues. Thus, the use of this group of drugs is often the first choice in controlling pain. The choice between the various drugs is empirical but a simple twice daily regimen is often the most convenient for an elderly person. The NSAIDs do have side-effects which need to be known, in particular, intestinal mucosal damage leading to upper gastrointestinal bleeding. Other problems involve depression of renal function which is reversible with the cessation of the drug. Consequently, these drugs need to be used with caution. Measures other than drugs to control arthritic pain should not be overlooked. These include heat, exercises, especially hydrotherapy and swimming to maintain mobility, the use of sticks and splints as necessary to support joints, and appropriate aids in the home. Surgery of various kinds, especially joint replacement, is effective in relieving pain in selected cases.

Neurological pain is decidedly more prevalent in the older generation. *Post-herpetic neuralgia*, as a complication of infection with herpes zoster virus, increases dramatically with age to the point where it may be as high as 70% in people aged 80 years and over. As the pain occurs secondary to a central lesion involving the spinal cord, the standard analgesics produce a less than satisfactory response. The best results are obtained through the use of tricyclic antidepressants such as amitriptyline, 25–50 mg at night. These may act centrally by inhibiting the re-uptake of amines such as serotonin and noradrenaline which are involved in many processes including pain perception. The concomitant use of carbamazepine (Tegretol) may help to control the shooting type of pain. The use of TENS may also be of assistance.

The TENS unit is believed to act by closing the pain gate in the spinal cord. The gate theory suggests that the input of pain via C fibres (small nerve fibres) could be inhibited or blocked by A fibre stimulation (large nerve fibres). If C fibre stimulation is greater than A fibre stimulation, then the gate is open and pain is felt. If A fibre stimulation is greater, then the gate is closed and pain is diminished or abolished. TENS therapy has been shown to stimulate A fibres, and has been demonstrated as being effective in a wide range of syndromes including low-back pain as well as post-herpetic neuralgia.

Trigeminal neuralgia is a disease also more common in old age most usually affecting the maxillary or mandibular divisions. With the onset of the problem, light touching of the affected area triggers a severe shooting pain. The treatment of choice is carbamazepine, 100 mg three times daily, increasing as necessary to a maximum dose of 1600 mg. Should the condition fail to respond then a variety of nerve blocks are available.

It is important to remember that there are other approaches to pain which should be considered. Physiotherapists may play a key role with gentle manipulation, stretching exercises, massage and ultrasound in addition to the use of heat and cold as required. Relaxation therapy can be of considerable benefit and these techniques can be carried through into the home. Hydrotherapy may be a very useful modality. Other therapeutic adjuncts such as acupuncture and trigger point injections may be used.

Summary

The treatment of chronic pain may be a complex matter involving physiological, sociological and emotional factors. Thus, a number of professionals may be included in the clinical team. It is the growing awareness of the complexity of this issue which has led to the development of pain clinics. Those involved with chronic pain issues in old people need to keep in mind the importance of:

- Accurate diagnosis
- A proper management plan
- Psychological support
- Referral to a specialist pain clinic as soon as practicable if control is difficult.

Finally, the tendency of many elderly people to make less fuss regarding their pain should not lead to the magnitude of the problem being underestimated with the consequent risk of improper diagnosis and inadequate treatment.

REFERENCES

Barton R, Hurst L 1966 Unnecessary use of tranquilizers in elderly patients. British Journal of Psychiatry 112: 989

Bermau P, Hogan D B, Fox R A 1987 The atypical presentation of infection in old age. Age and Ageing 16: 201–207

Caradoc Davies T H 1984 Non steroidal anti inflammatory drugs: arthritis and gastro intestinal bleeding in elderly patients. Age and Ageing 13: 295

Cheiltin M D 1989 The spectrum of cardiovascular disease in the elderly. International Journal of Cardiology 22: 283–288

Clive D M, Stoff J S 1984 Renal syndromes associated with non steroidal anti inflammatory drugs. New England Journal of Medicine 310: 563

Collier D S T, Pain J A 1985 NSAIDs and peptic ulceration. GUT 26: 359–363

Crowe M J, Forsling M L, Rolls B J, Phillips P A, Ledingham J G C, Smith R F 1987 Altered water excretion in healthy elderly men. Age and Ageing 16: 285–293

Davis P B, Robins L A 1989 History taking in the elderly with and without cognitive impairment. Journal of the American Geriatrics Society 37: 249–255

De La Monte S M, Hutchins G M, Moore G W 1988 Influence of age on metastatic behaviour of breast carcinoma. Human Pathology 19: 529–534

Downton J H, Andrews K, Puxty J A H 1987 Silent pyrexia in the elderly. Age and Ageing 16: 41–44

Edelstein J E 1988 Foot care for the ageing. Physical Therapy 68: 1882–1886

Fulton J D, Pebbles S E, Smith G D, Davie J W 1989 Unrecognized viscus perforation in the elderly. Age and Ageing 18: 403–406

Gjorup T, Hendriksen C, Luwd E, Stromgard E 1987 Is growing old a disease?: study of the attitudes of elderly people to physical symptoms. Journal of Chronic Disease 40: 1095–1098

Hamblin T J 1987 Myelodysplasia. British Journal of Hospital Medicine 38: 558–561

Heath D A, Wright A D, Barnes A D, Oates G D, Dorricott N J 1980 Surgical treatment of primary hyperparathyroidism in the elderly. British Medical Journal 280: 1406–1408

Homer A C, Honovar M, Lantos P L, Hastie I R, Kellett J M, Millard P H 1988 Diagnosing dementia: do we get it right. British Medical Journal 297: 894–896

Hutton J T 1981 Senility reconsidered. Journal of the American Medical Association 245: 1025–1026

Iredale J P, Symons A J, Briggs R S J 1986 Audit of the assessment of mental impairment. Journal of Royal College of Physicians 20: 268–270

Janko M, Trontelj J 1980 TENS: micro-neurographic and perceptual study. Pain 9: 219–230

Larson E B, Kukull W A, Buchner D, Reifler B V 1987 Adverse drug reactions associated with global cognitive impairment in elderly persons. Annals of Internal Medicine 107: 169–173

Lau W Y, Fan S T, Yiu T G, Chu K W, Lee J M 1985 Acute appendicitis in the elderly. Surgery, Gynecology and Obstetrics 161: 157–160

McAlpine C H, Martin B J, Lennox I M, Roberts M A 1986 Pyrexia in infection in the elderly. Age and Ageing 15: 230–234

Melzack R, Wall P 1965 Pain mechanisms: a new therapy. Science 150: 971–979

Melzack R 1975 Prolonged relief of pain by brief intense transcutaneous somatic stimulation. Pain 1: 357–373

Melzack R 1977 Trigger and acupuncture points for pain. Pain 3: 3–24

Meyer J S, Rogers R L, McClintic K, Mortel K F, Lofti J 1989 Randomised clinical trial of daily aspirin therapy in multi-infarct dementia: a pilot study. Journal of the American Geriatrics Society 37: 549–555

Nathan P, Wall P 1974 Treatment of post herpetic neuralgia by a prolonged electrical stimulation. British Medical Journal 3: 645–647

Nordenstram G R, Brandberg C A, Oden A S, Svanborg-Eden C M, Svanborg A 1986 Bacteria and mortality in an elderly population. New England Journal of Medicine 314: 1152–1156

Reynold C F, Hoch C C, Kupfer D J, Buysse D J, Houck P R, Stack J A, Campbell D 1988 Bedside differentiation of depressive pseudo dementia from dementia. American Journal of Psychiatry 145: 1099–1103

Rosenblatt R M, Reich J, Dehring D 1984 Tricyclic antidepressants in the treatment of depression and chronic pain. Anesthesia and Analgesia 63: 1025–1032

Smerlon M 1984 Anticonvulsant drugs and chronic pain. Neuropharmacology 7: 51–82

Smith J S, Kiloh L G 1981 The investigation of dementia: results of 200 consecutive admissions. Lancet 1: 824–827

Tucker M A, Andrew M F, Ogle S J, Davison J G 1989 Age associated change in pain threshold measured by transcutaneous neuronal electrical stimulation. Age and Ageing 18: 241–246

6. Common problems of ageing

John Hurley

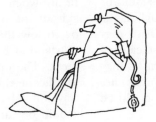

This chapter covers a number of common problems resulting from physiological change, which in turn can result in serious consequences unless measures are taken to improve functioning and safeguard against accidents.

FALLS

Falls are a common accompaniment of old age. They may have a devastating effect on an elderly person, both as a result of the consequent trauma and, perhaps more significantly, the ensuing loss of confidence. Recurrent falls may result in the older person being afraid to leave the immediate home environment. The all too common problems of isolation and immobility may well follow. This is unfortunate because many causes of falls are correctable.

Many research projects have been undertaken into the causes, incidence and effects of falling in elderly populations. Generally, this research has shown a fairly consistent pattern of information:

- Some 30% of elderly people fall each year.
- Elderly women are more at risk, falling twice as frequently as men.
- A significant number of elderly people fall recurrently.

- The number of falls sustained by an elderly person tends to increase with age.
- Drugs, especially hypnotics and sedatives, are often associated with falls.
- Most falls occur at times of greatest activity.
- The majority of falls occur indoors — in the person's home, in residential accommodation or in hospital.
- People who live alone are particularly at risk.
- There is a significant incidence of pre-existing abnormality or disease.

Environmental factors

Research has indicated that the majority of falls occur indoors. It is, therefore, essential to begin a preventive campaign with a careful study of the environment in which an elderly person normally functions. Since most elderly people live at home a review of the home environment should be a basic feature of routine health care. Institutional accommodations, including hospitals, are also common sites for falls, so the same, detailed environmental analysis should be undertaken regularly in those places. Because one-third to one-half of all falls are due to accidental trips and slips it is reasonable to begin an environmental assessment with the floor.

The type of floor covering plays a major role. Slippery surfaces should be eliminated. Frequently, the polishes used have antislip properties while retaining a very high gloss. This gloss, however, may be perceived as being slippery and cause hesitancy in walking. High gloss also produces hazardous glare with which many elderly eyes cannot cope. Thus, shining floors should be eliminated. A further complication, though, is the all too common use of loose mats. These may slip when stepped on or may catch a toe causing the person to trip. The removal of such mats may prevent an accident. Loose floor boards are another potential cause of a fall. They should be repaired promptly.

It needs to be remembered that the decision to undertake environmental modifications belongs to the elderly person and, where appropriate, the family. Carefully tendered education and advice may be rejected, the elderly person preferring to continue with long held habits. One can but continue to counsel.

Inadequate lighting is a frequently overlooked cause of accidental falls. Vision, generally, deteriorates with age so the majority of elderly people require an increased intensity of illumination to see adequately. The simple process of changing a low wattage light bulb for one of higher intensity may make all the difference to mobility safety. Larger watt bulbs, however, may not be an appropriate solution for lighting for close work or reading. Here, the closeness of the light source to the work is significant. A 60 watt bulb in a gooseneck lamp 800 mm from a book may be much more effective than a 100 watt bulb at ceiling height. Additional considerations include the presence of a bedside light to promote safety when getting out of bed at night; the planned use of night lighting to facilitate safety when going to the toilet; and the elimination of wide variations in light and dark within an area of mobility.

Steps and stairs are potential hazards for most elderly people. The edge of the step must be clearly distinguishable from the surrounds. A strip of white or brightly coloured paint on the step edge is an essential safety feature. Hand rails may also be important but care must be taken to ensure their correct placement. Many a fall occurs because a hand rail stops short of the top or bottom step and, thus, presents false information. Consideration may be given to replacing steps with ramps.

Attention should be paid to the furniture used by the elderly person. The height of the bed is especially important. Feet should touch the floor firmly when the elderly person is sitting on the side of the bed. The bed, however, should not be so low that the elderly person must struggle to stand. Chairs also demand a similar assessment. The organisation of furniture may have a significant effect on mobility safety. Clear pathways must be arranged and trailing electric cords should be carefully positioned.

The bathroom and toilet are frequently the sites of mishaps. The provision of aids may be necessary to make these safe environments. Such aids include rails, bath seats and non-slip mats or strips.

Footwear is an important environmental consideration in the assessment of the potential for falling. The common practice of wearing slippers that are ill-fitting and have slippery soles should be discouraged. Of course, walking in stockinged feet is most hazardous.

Disease factors

Accidental falls may be countered with commonsense advice. Other falls, though, may be associated with illness. Where a clear history of an accidental fall, such as a definite trip or slip, cannot be demonstrated a careful history and examination is required to ascertain the cause. Box 6.1 indicates the great range of diseases which have been implicated as significant causes of falls.

Cardiovascular causes of falls are numerous. The elderly person may report feeling breathless and giddy after walking a short distance prior to falling. This may be the result of an inadequate cardiac output caused by silent myocardial infarction, cardiomyopathies or aortic stenosis. Falls may be the result of dysrhythmias of which the elderly person may or may not be aware. Some elderly people may report a history of palpitations prior to a fall but often this symptom is not presented clearly. When tachycardia or bradycardia are suspected, 24 hour ambulatory electro-

Box 6.1 Disorders commonly associated with falls

Cardiovascular
Syncope
  Vasovagal attacks
  Cough syncope
  Micturition syncope
  Defaecation syncope
Paroxysmal arrhythmias
  Supraventricular tachycardia
  Atrial fibrillation
  Ventricular tachycardia or
    ectopics
  Bradycardia
  Heart block
Carotid sinus sensitivity
Myocardial infarct
Pulmonary embolus
Aortic stenosis

Metabolic and endocrine
Hypoglycaemia
Hypokalaemia
Addison's disease
Septicaemia
Toxaemia

Miscellaneous
Anaemia
Subclavian steal syndrome
Malnutrition

Locomotor
Unstable joints
Osteoarthritis
  Rheumatoid arthritis
  Neuropathic joints
Myopathies and muscle weakness
  Osteomalacia
Thyrotoxicosis
  Neoplastic disease
  Cushing's syndrome
  Polymyalgia rheumatica
Miscellaneous
  Fractures
  Dislocations
  Painful feet

Postural hypotension
Drugs
Hot baths
Prolonged bed rest
Dehydration
Sympathectomy
Automatic neuropathy
Hypokalaemia
Peripheral vascular insufficiency

Neurological
Cerebellar lesions
Parkinsonism
Transient ischaemic attacks
Epilepsy
Proprioception impairment
  B_{12} deficiency
  Tabes disorders
  Cerebrovascular accident
  Vertebrobasilar insufficiency
  Meniere's disease
  Cervical spondylosis
  Shy-Drager syndrome

Iatrogenic
Sedatives
Hypnotics
Hypotensive agents
Diuretics
Antidepressants

Psychological
Depression
Dementia
Anxiety states

cardiograph monitoring is an appropriate way of identifying the dysrhythmia. A precise diagnosis is necessary to permit correct medication.

A thorough examination of the lower limbs is mandatory for the elderly person who falls. Assessment of joint mobility and muscle strength as well as a full neurological examination may highlight problems. Scrutiny of the feet may reveal deformities such as hallux valgus, callosities, ingrowing toe nails and other painful conditions which lead to an abnormal gait and consequent falls.

Myxoedema may be associated with ataxia, giddiness, and an unsteady gait pattern. This may be compounded, in some instances, by arthralgia. Hypoglycaemia should always be considered when elderly people with diabetes mellitus present with a history of falls associated with episodes of confusion.

Neurological lesions are another group of conditions often associated with falls. One of the most frequently encountered is Parkinson's disease. The classical case is usually clear but the person presenting with increased tone and little in the way of tremor may be overlooked. Giddiness precipitated by head movement may indicate vertebrobasilar insufficiency or an inner ear problem.

Falls may happen during a transient ischaemic attack. These may occur over a period of months with spontaneous recovery following each episode, and these are associated with the effects of vascular disease creating platelet and fibrin micro-emboli. Transient ischaemic attacks may culminate in a major cerebrovascular accident. Epilepsy also has a well known association with cerebrovascular disease and should not be forgotten when tracing the cause of a fall.

Iatrogenic causes of falls must be considered when reviewing an elderly person. Drugs are a too common cause of falls. The most common offenders are sedatives and hypnotics but the list may include hypoglycaemics, hypotensive agents and antidepressants. Diuretics are often associated with falls, especially in the morning, when they force an elderly person to rush to the toilet.

An elderly person's mental status should be assessed carefully. There may be a lack of concentration or forethought which frequently results in accidents. This is particularly hazardous if it occurs in conjunction with nocturnal wandering. A depressed elderly person is often apathetic, slow and lacking in alertness. An anxious elderly person may grab at objects for support without regard for stability. Both situations may result in falls.

Investigations

It is helpful to have a reliable witness to the event when attempting to build an accurate history of the fall.

Considerable care should be taken to determine the elderly person's medication, both physician- and self-prescribed. Compliance with prescription instructions must be assessed.

The measurement of blood pressure, both lying and standing, should be part of the routine medical examination of all elderly people to determine the presence, or not, of postural hypotension.

Other investigations that may be pursued usefully are measurements of the haemoglobin concentration and erythrocyte sedimentation rate. The latter, if high, may suggest disease such as polymyalgia rheumatica, rheumatoid arthritis or underlying carcinoma. The estimation of urea and electrolyte levels plus random blood sugar testing may pick up hypoglycaemia or hyperglycaemia. Electrolyte disturbances may, in particular, indicate hypokalaemia or hyponatraemia, both inducing hypotension and muscle weakness. Further investigations that may be helpful in establishing an accurate diagnosis include a thyroid function test and measurement of serum Vitamin B_{12} levels, looking for both increased and decreased thyroid activity and Vitamin B_{12} deficiency.

Cardiac conditions may be responsible for falls. An ECG may be useful but it is important to remember that the dysrhythmias responsible for falls are transitory and may be missed by routine testing. The 'Holter' monitor ECG, which tests cardiac function over a period, may be of benefit in this situation.

Apart from invasive techniques such as angiography, most of the investigations may be carried out in the general medical practitioner's surgery, outpatient department or day hospital.

Management

Falls are a major problem for many elderly people because the consequences may be disastrous. Prevention is, obviously, the most appropriate course of action. The management programme depends on the diagnosis but may consist of treatment of the reversible medical problems, the correction of hazards within the elderly person's environment and education.

Research has indicated that there is an increased mortality, within the year following a fall, for elderly people who fall compared with matched controls. The association of falls to illness, often apparently symptomless, has been demonstrated clearly. Thus, particular care should be taken to elicit, accurately, the cause of any fall. Treatment of the consequent trauma without due regard to the cause is a disservice to the elderly person who falls.

The importance of accurate diagnosis has been recognised in a number of centre's by the development of falls clinics. These clinics are staffed by multidisciplinary teams, including a geriatrician, cardiologist, neurologist, physiotherapist and psychologist. Relatives or friends are also important members of the clinic team, both for their potential contribution to the diagnosis and for their later role in educating the elderly person.

HYPERTENSION

Ageing is associated with progressive rigidity of the aorta and peripheral arteries. The elasticity of the aorta declines but the calibre increases. In association with these changes there is an increase in the velocity of the pulse wave. These changes result from alterations in the media of the aorta, that is, changes in the amount or nature of the collagen plus fibrosis and calcification leading to rigidity and elevation of systolic pressure.

The underlying cause of hypertension in the majority of persons, including elderly people, is increased peripheral vascular resistance. A measure of 160/90 mmHg or above is indicative of hypertension in elderly people, just as it is in younger adults. The diagnosis, however, should not be made on the basis of one reading since anxiety, among other factors, may produce an elevated recording. Also, blood pressure varies throughout the day. Consequently, a series of readings should be taken before any action is contemplated. At least three recordings should be made, at varying times, to verify the reading.

A thorough examination to determine any complications of hypertension such as retinopathy or heart disease should follow the initial detection of an elevated blood pressure. The presence of such complications will, of course, influence treatment.

It is well known that many middle-aged people, men in particular, are at risk of hypertension. The consequences of this state include strokes, dissecting aneurysms and cardiac disease. These risks are reduced substantially when the hypertension is corrected by hypotensive agents.

The transition of similar assumptions to elderly people has been controversial. Arguments used to be advanced to suggest that potent hypotensive agents were unnecessary and may, in fact, seriously impair the quality of life experienced by many elderly people.

Epidemiological studies have, however, shown that isolated systolic hypertension in older individuals is associated with an increased risk of cardiovascular death. This may be in the order of twice the rate for people who are normotensive. In a similar manner, the incidence of stroke is twice that occurring in elderly people without systolic hypertension. Further, various studies into the effects of treatment of hypertension have shown that the incidence of stroke may be reduced by some 40%. The European Working Party on High Blood Pressure in the Elderly (in consultation with the World Health Organization) indicated that this was also the case in people over the age of 60 years, further suggesting that the probable benefits, in terms of reduction of stroke, may be even greater in the older age group. The European Working Party also showed a decrease in cardiovascular deaths as well as a reduction in severe cardiac failure. Thus, it appears that therapeutic intervention in the event of hypertension is worthwhile.

Despite much effort there is very little data available related to very old people, those aged 80 and over. Some epidemiological studies conducted in Finland suggest that the association of raised blood pressure with increasing cardiovascular problems may not apply to this age group. In fact, the risk of death may actually diminish. This throws open the debate about commencing, or even continuing, active therapy for hypertension in the over 80 age group.

Treatment

Treatment of hypertension should begin with non-pharmacological regimens. Weight reduction to an ideal body weight should be attempted. Exercise programmes, beginning very gently and progressively increasing in intensity according to tolerance, have been found to produce a reduction in blood pressure. Such activity should be encouraged. Consumers of alcohol should be encouraged to moderate the level. Similarly, more prudent use of dietary salt may be beneficial. Approaches such as these may be sufficient to bring mild hypertension under control.

The pharmacological treatment of hypertension in elderly people must be undertaken with caution to avoid a rapid drop in blood pressure and the possibility of provoking a stroke. Regular manometry in lying and standing is mandatory. The first line of treatment may be a thiazide diuretic which is effective in the majority of people. Thiazides, however, are not without their problems. The consequent development of hypokalaemia is not uncommon and may require careful monitoring, especially if digoxin is used concurrently. Other difficulties such as an aggravation of symptoms may be encountered in elderly people with associated diabetes, gout or prostatism, all quite common in old age. The use of thiazide diuretics as an automatic first choice is now debatable.

Beta-blockers may be used cautiously although they are best reserved for specific cases rather than general use in an aged population. The hepatic metabolism of propranolol is poor. Less of the dose is removed on the first pass of the drug through an elderly person's liver than is usual in a younger adult. This results in a higher than anticipated blood level for the same dose. Consequent side-effects include bradycardia and hypotension, while cardiac failure may be precipitated if the hypertension is associated with ischaemic heart disease. Atenolol may be used, especially since it is water soluble and, thus, excreted through the kidneys. Again, though, smaller than usual doses are recommended for elderly people. The presence of chest disease or peripheral vascular disease may exclude people from this therapy because both may worsen with the use of beta-blockers.

It is essential to note that clonidine should be prescribed with great care. When clonidine is stopped after a period of successful therapy there may be rebound hypertension. The danger of this phenomenon is more likely in elderly people with impaired memory where the potential for compliance problems exists.

Methyldopa has been shown to be an effective agent but is less commonly used because of associated problems such as depression and sedation.

A newer group of drugs, *vasodilators*, have been found to be more effective, especially for older people with systolic hypertension. Prazosin is one of these drugs but it needs to be introduced in small doses because it is known to produce severe postural hypotension initially in some elderly people. Angiotensin-converting enzyme (ACE) inhibitors have been shown to be both effective and safe for elderly people with hypertension. These drugs, for example, captopril, are well tolerated and do not interfere with lipid or carbohydrate metabolism, nor are they likely to cause hypokalaemia or hyperuricaemia. However, the ever present danger of hypotensive episodes must be considered and commencing treatment with smaller doses, increased in small amounts over a longer period, is recommended.

Calcium-channel blockers are also effective in reducing blood pressure by vasodilation. There are a number of agents in this group of drugs including nifedipine, verapamil and diltiazem. They vary in their characteristics. For example, nifedipine is a very potent peripheral vasodilator with little inotropic and chronotropic effects. Verapamil, on the other hand, is a much less effective dilator. These agents have the added advantage of being effective for angina and can be used where ischaemic heart disease coexists with hypertension. Further, they do not interfere with lung function or upset biochemical parameters. Because they may improve cerebral circulation their use in hypertension with associated ischaemic cerebral disease may be less hazardous.

In summary, recent work has shown that the treatment of hypertension in people over 60 years of age can produce benefits although there is still controversy regarding treatment for those aged 80 or more years. Recent advances in therapy with the introduction of ACE inhibitors and calcium-channel blockers means that elderly people with hypertension may be treated more safely.

POSTURAL HYPOTENSION

Normal postural compensation

When a person changes position from lying or sitting to standing gravity shifts the blood from the upper body to the legs and lower abdomen. Normally, this state instantaneously triggers several reflexes which fire compensatory adjustments to prevent a sudden fall of arterial blood pressure. The action of pressor reflexes induces constriction of the peripheral arteries and arterioles. Aortic and carotid reflexes accelerate heart action, while muscle activity accompanied by increased respiration stimulates venous return. Usually, as a person moves to the upright position there is a transitory drop in blood pressure followed almost immediately by a compensatory rise. Most people are unaware of these rapid shifts in pressure on position changes.

Age and postural compensation

People with postural hypotension have an altered response to the effects of gravity on the circulation as they change to an upright posture. The blood pressure initially stabilises at a slightly lower than usual level but the failure of the compensatory mechanisms leads to a precipitous fall in pressure.

Postural hypotension is a condition that occurs with increasing frequency in old age. The prevalence may be as high as 20% in an elderly population. Unfortunately, hypotension is often overlooked.

There are many factors that may be responsible for the presence of hypotension in elderly people. Reduced blood volume associated with sodium and water depletion may occur with the prolonged use of diuretics. The increased rigidity of the arteriovenous walls prevents rapid constrictions of the vessels and, thus, is a factor in producing slowed circulatory adaptation. Autonomic dysfunction, probably the major cause, is due to an age-related decline in the physiological mechanisms, especially those which promote compensation. In addition, the incidence of pathological processes which affect the autonomic systems increases with age. Perhaps,

though, the most common causes of the problem are those related to drugs. Box 6.2 summarises some of the conditions that may have postural hypotension as an associated problem.

Symptoms

Pathological hypotension is considered present when the systolic blood pressure drops 20 mmHg or more as the person moves from lying to standing. This drop may be detected through palpation of the radial pulse and is seen as a clear reduction in volume or even a disappearance of the pulse. Frequently, hypotension presents as dizziness or a faint, often associated with a fall. Recovery is usually rapid when the person returns to lying. Early symptoms, though, may not be as profound as these. Apathy and lack of interest in activity may be the clue to the diagnosis, particularly when the elderly person does not progress as the in-bed assessment indicated. A person recovering from a stroke is especially prone to present in this way.

It is necessary to note that postural hypotension may be symptomless. Asymptomatic hypotension of 100 mmHg systolic and 60 mmHg diastolic may be consistent with good health in some elderly people. This may be due to the fact that cerebral perfusion is being maintained despite the drop in blood pressure.

Diagnosis

Blood pressure should be measured with the elderly person in both lying or sitting and standing postures. The examination of an elderly person should not rely on recumbent manometry because the potential effects of hypotension may be missed. Because postural hypotension is often noticed first in a restorative care programme, occupational therapists and physiotherapists, especially, should be encouraged to palpate the radial pulse and note any reduction in volume when bringing the elderly person into an upright position. Blood pressure measurement also should be part of the assessment skills of such therapists.

It is important to measure postural blood pressure on first rising in the morning and half

---

Box 6.2 Some causes of postural hypotension

Lesions of CNS	*Drugs*
Diabetic autoneuropathy	Diuretics
Acute polyneuropathy	Phenothiazines
Transverse myelitis	Tricyclic antidepressants
Parkinsonism	Benzodiazipines
Cerebrovascular disease	Levo dopa
Alcoholism	Alcohol
Shy-Drager syndrome	Hypotensive agents
Tabes dorsalis	

Other causes	
Prolonged bed rest	Myocardial disease
Bilateral varicose veins	Cardiac infarct
Bilateral sympathectomy	Cardiac dysrhythmias
Addison's disease	Vasodilation
Fall in plasma volume	Hot bath
Dehydration	Exercise
Haemorrhage	

an hour after meals as these are the times when maximal drop is likely to occur. Ideally, the blood pressure should be taken after the elderly person has been lying flat for at least 5 minutes, then immediately after standing, and then again after at least 2 minutes of standing.

Treatment

The treatment of postural hypotension should be directed toward the precipitating factor. A careful history and examination ought to be carried out, including a thorough review of the drug consumption. Drugs that may induce postural hypotension need to be identified, reduced in quantity, or even withdrawn. In conjunction with this, antigravity support in the form of graduated elastic stockings may be worn to support the blood supply of the legs. The elderly person needs to be advised against quick changes in posture, particularly on rising from bed in the morning, when the problem may be more acute. A rapid exit from a warm bath should also be discouraged. Where the problem does not respond to these simple measures the elderly person's tolerance may be improved by maintaining at least a semi-upright position. A tilting chair or raised bedhead may prove useful.

Drug therapy plays an important role in the control of hypotension. When necessary, water and electrolyte replacements may be administered. The most effective drug at present is fludrocortisone acetate, 0.1 mg daily. During this treatment excessive fluid retention may need to be managed. Hypokalaemia should be guarded against as it may reduce the efficiency of treatment. Other drugs that may be used include inhibitors of prostaglandin synthesis, especially those that reduce prostaglandin-induced vasodilation, Indocid being particularly effective. Clonidine may be helpful for those elderly people with severe autonomic neuropathy and reduced sympathetic outflow as it promotes venocontraction and venous return to the heart.

Most elderly people respond well to simple practical measures and the withdrawal of offending medications.

CONSTIPATION

Although constipation is probably no more common in an elderly population than in any other age group, it certainly figures prominently as a complaint and may have considerably more severe effects in an older person. The definitions of constipation are as varied as the people experiencing the complaint. To some, it may be reduced frequency of bowel action while to others it may be that the stool has hardened in consistency. The most common definition, however, would appear to be straining to defaecate. The symptom of constipation, however, should not be shrugged off as just being associated with age because it may well be indicative of underlying disease.

The function of the colon is complex, influenced both by systemic and local factors. There are three types of muscular activity in the colon. First, rhythmic segmentation waves that mix the contents; secondly, regularly occurring, coordinated peristaltic waves that are responsible for some forward movement; and thirdly, mass movements, occurring once or twice a day, that move the stool further and faster than any other action. Mass movements are generally related to meals, most usually occurring soon after ingestion. It is known that the parasympathetic system promotes propulsion of the stool while the sympathetic system increases segmentation preventing forward movement.

Causes of constipation

Constipation may be caused by or associated with lesions of the gastrointestinal tract (Box 6.3). Intestinal carcinoma may present as constipation resulting ultimately in obstruction. Haemorrhoids and fistula in ano may be extremely painful and result in fear of defaecation and suppression of normal action with consequent constipation. Severe chronic constipation can be, at times, associated with idiopathic megacolon.

Metabolic disorders and drugs may also be responsible for the development of constipation. The drugs most likely to cause such problems are those with anticholinergic effects such as tricyclic antidepressants and some drugs used for

Box 6.3 Some causes of constipation in old age

Gastrointestinal
Anal fissure
Diverticular disease
Haemorrhoids
Megacolon
Pseudo-obstruction
Tumour
Volvulus

Drugs
Laxative abuse
See Box 6.4

Psychiatric
Dementia
Depression

Metabolic
Hypokalaemia
Hypercalcaemia
Phaeochromocytoma
Uraemia
Porphyria

Neurological
Spinal cord lesions
  Paraplegia
  Cauda equina
    compression
  Tabes dorsalis
Cerebral lesions
  Cerebral vascular
    disease
  Parkinsonism

Endocrine
Hypothyroidism
Diabetes mellitus

General conditions
Immobility
Dehydration

Box 6.4 Examples of drugs that may cause constipation

Analgesics
Codeine
Morphine
Pethidine

Antacids
Aluminium compounds

Anticholinergics
Benzhexol
Benztropine
Orphenadrine
Procyclidine
Hyoscine hydrobromide
Propantheline bromide

Antidepressants
Tricyclic antidepressants
  Amitriptyline
  Doxepin
  Imipramine
  Nortriptyline
Monoamine oxidase
  inhibitors
  Iproniazid
  Isocarboxazid
  Phenelzine
  Tranylcypromine

Antihistamines
Cyproheptadine
Azatadine
Promethazine

*Calcium-channel
  blockers*
Diltiazem
Nifedepine
Verapamil

Disopyramide

Diuretics

H₂ antagonists
Cimetidine
Ranitidine

Iron tablets

Phenothiazines
Fluphenazine
Chlorpromazine
Promazine

Vincristine

Parkinson's disease. Other drugs producing similar difficulties are analgesics with a codeine base and antacids containing aluminium salts (Box 6.4).

Hypercalcaemia may also produce constipation and should be considered as a possible, if not common, cause.

Hypothyroidism and depression are two insidious and not uncommon causes of constipation. Both conditions do not necessarily present in typical fashion in old age so an elderly person with persisting symptoms should be considered as a possible candidate for one condition or the other.

Management

The management of constipation should include the elimination of possible underlying disease as the first manoeuvre. This should consist of taking a history and examination, including rectal examination, when the elderly person first presents with complaints. The history may give a clue to the aetiology while a rectal examination may produce evidence of haemorrhoids, fistula or carcinoma. Further investigations in the form of proctoscopy and colonic endoscopy or barium enema may be indicated when there is a history of bleeding. Laboratory tests and other studies may be required in some instances, especially when hypothyroidism or a carcinoma is suspected.

In the majority of cases, no serious condition will be evident. In this situation, simple preventive measures should be undertaken. First, an adequate fluid intake is essential. Some elderly people take reduced quantities of fluids, particularly those people trying to avoid frequency and problems of urinary incontinence. In other situations, the elderly person may be immobile and have to rely on others to assist. In these situations particularly, as well as in general, an elderly person should aim at an intake of 2 L of fluid per day. The diet should contain an adequate quantity of fibre which tends to bind water in the intestine thus reducing the reabsorption of water from the large intestine. The faecal content is, therefore, bulky and soft. It would appear that the fundamental requirement is a diet rich in fibre and the first dietary change should be a switch to wholemeal bread as well as sufficient bran and cereal to provide 10 g of fibre per day. A high fibre diet has been encouraged in many geriatric institutions to reduce the problems of constipation and the ad hoc use of purgatives.

Laxatives may be self-administered by some elderly people, often over long periods, while suppositories and purgatives are often used in an inappropriate manner in institutions. A rational policy for the use of such substances should be developed and implemented. Bulk purgatives other than bran are probably not indicated for elderly people. Faecal softeners having few side-effects may be beneficial and may be used alone initially or in combination with an irritant purgative. Dioctyl sodium sulphosuccinate is probably preferable to the lubricant aperient paraffin be-

cause of the problems associated with the latter in impaired absorption of fat soluble vitamins and lipid pneumonia (see Boxes 6.5 and 6.6).

Irritant purgatives are many in number but, in practice, are reduced to senna and bisacodyl. Senna is effective and is usually taken by mouth at night. Bisacodyl is effective by mouth and in the form of a suppository.

Osmotic laxatives may also be used. Lactulose (Duphalac) is a synthetic disaccharide which is split into fructose and galactose by colonic bacteria. This results in water being drawn into the gut, the bacterial flora changing, and gas being produced. It should be noted that this is an expensive agent, often slow in onset, and not always effective. Magnesium and sodium salts act by drawing water into the lumen by osmosis. However, they may produce cramps and electrolyte disturbances and are probably best avoided. Certainly, magnesium salts should not be used for elderly people with renal impairment as hypermagnesaemia may ensue.

When softening and irritant purgatives have not been effective, then enemas may be used. There is no longer an indication for large volume enemas as they are no more effective than the small volume variety and are more likely to produce unpleasant effects. In cases of severe impaction, treatment should continue until the build-up of scybala is known to be cleared.

Constipation is a problem which may be prevented by an adequate diet of fibre and fluid intake in association with exercise and activity. People with recent onset of symptoms should be checked for possible underlying disease before embarking on regular treatment with faecal softeners alone or in conjunction with irritant purgatives. All laxatives, however, like other drugs, produce side-effects. Consequently, care should be taken when deciding on their use.

The problem of *impaction* needs to be considered from a different perspective. When it exists, efforts to remove it from above by laxatives are ineffective and may worsen abdominal pain. Enemas and suppositories alone may dislodge the impaction but it is usual for manual removal to be required. Once partial removal has occurred suppositories or enemas may be used. Phosphate enemas should be avoided as they cause

---

Box 6.5 A classification of laxatives with some examples

Bulking agents	*Stimulant (irritant) agents*
Bran	Bisacodyl
Ispaghula	Phenolphthalein
Psyllium hydrophilic mucilloid	Senna
Sterculia gum	Ricinoleic acid (castor oil)
Osmotic agents	*Softening (secretory) agents*
Lactulose	Ricinoleic acid
Magnesium salts	Dioctyl sodium sulphosuccinate
Lubricant agents	
Liquid paraffin (mineral oil)	

Box 6.6 Some adverse effects of laxatives

Abdominal discomfort or pain

Chronic abuse syndromes

Diarrhoea

Effect on absorption of drugs

Electrolyte disturbance

Flatulence (bran)

Fluid depletion

Lipid pneumonia (mineral oils)

Malabsorption (mineral oils)

Skin reactions (phenolphthalein)

hyperphosphataemia in those elderly people with renal impairment and, more recently, associated

problems with rectal necrosis have been observed.

REFERENCES

Agate G 1979 Effects of indomethacin on postural hypotension in Parkinsonism. British Medical Journal 2: 1466–1468

Becker G L 1974 The case against mineral oil. Journal of Digestive Diseases 19: 344–348

Brocklehurst J C, Kirkland J L, Martin J, Ashford J 1983 Constipation in long stay elderly patients: its treatment by lactulose, poloxalkol, dihydroxy anthroquinolone and phosphate enemas. Gerontology 29: 181–184

Clark A N G, Scott J S 1976 Wheat bran in dyschezia in the aged. Age and Ageing 5: 149–154

Collins K J, Exton Smith A N, James M H 1980 Functional changes in the autonomic nervous responses with ageing. Age and Ageing 9: 17–24

Cummings S R, Nevitt M C, Kidd S 1988 Forgetting falls: the limited accuracy of recall of falls in the elderly. Journal of the American Geriatrics Society 36: 613–616

Eastwood M A 1973 Effects of dietary supplement of wheat bran and cellulose on faeces and bowel function. British Medical Journal 4: 392–394

Forette F, Handfield-Jones R, Henry-Amar M, Fouchard M, Boucharcourt P, Hervey M P, Henry J F, Bilaud-Meoguifh E, Alexandre J M 1988 Rationale for ACE inhibitors in the elderly: treatment of arterial hypertension with enalapril. Gerontology 33 suppl 1: 9–16

Frohlich E D 1988 Hypertension in the elderly. Current Problems in Cardiology 13: 313–367

Giles T D, Massie B M 1988 Role of calcium antagonists as initial pharmacologic monotherapy for systemic hypertension inpatients over 60 years of age. American Journal of Cardiology 61(16): 13H–17H

Grimley Evans J 1987 Blood pressure and stroke in an elderly English population. Journal of Epidemiology and Community Health 14: 275–282

Hazell J W P 1979 Vestibular problems of balance. Age and Ageing 8: 258–260

Imms F J, Edholm O G 1979 The assessment of gait and mobility in the elderly. Age and Ageing 8: 181–185

Jansen P A F, Schulte B P M, Meyboom R H B, Grimnay F W J 1986 Anti hypertensive treatment as a possible cause of stroke in the elderly. Age and Ageing 15: 129–138

Kannel W B, Wolf P A, McGee D L, Dawber T R, McNamara P, Castelli W P 1981 Framingham Study: systolic blood pressure: arterial rigidity and risk of stroke. Journal of the American Medical Association 245: 1225–1229

Lakatta E G 1989 Mechanisms of hypertension in the elderly. Journal of the American Geriatrics Society 37: 780–790

Langer R D, Ganiats T G, Barret-Connor E 1989 Paradoxical survival of elderly men with high blood pressure. British Medical Journal 298: 1356–1359

Lewis A, Lipsitz M D 1989 Orthostatic hypotension in the elderly. New England Journal of Medicine 321: 952–957

McRae A D, Bulpitt C J 1989 Assessment of postural hypotension in the elderly. Age and Ageing 18: 110–112

Mattila K, Haavis M, Rajala S, Heikinheimo R 1988 Blood pressure and five year survival in the very old. British Medical Journal 296: 887–889

Morris J C, Rubin E H, Morris E J, Mandel S A 1987 Senile dementia of the Alzheimers type: an important risk factor for serious falls. Journal of Gerontology 42: 412–417

Prudham D, Grimley Evans J 1981 Factors associated with falls in the elderly: a community study. Age and Ageing 10: 141–146

Radado J A, Rubenstein L Z, Robbins A S, Heng M K, Schulman B L, Josephson K R 1989 The value of Holter monitoring in evaluating the elderly patient with falls. Journal of the American Geriatrics Society 37: 430–434

Robinson B J, Johnson R H, Lambie D G, Palmer K T 1985 Autonomic responses to glucose ingestion in elderly subjects with orthostatic hypotension. Age and Ageing 14: 168–173

Sixt F, Landhal S 1987 Postural disturbances in a 75 year old population: prevalence and functional consequences. Age and Ageing 16: 393–398

Smith R G 1980 A study of bulking agents in elderly patients. Age and Ageing 9: 267–271

Sweeney J L, Hewett P, Riddell P, Hoffman D C 1986 Rectal gangrene: a complication of phosphate enemas. Medical Journal of Australia 144: 374–375

Tinetti M E, Speechley M 1989 Prevention of falls among the elderly. New England Journal of Medicine 320: 1055–1059

Vetter N J, Ford D 1989 Anxiety and depression scores in elderly fallers. International Journal of Geriatric Psychiatry 4: 159–168

Whitehead W E, Drinkwater D, Cheskin L J, Hellar B R, Schuster M M, 1989 Constipation in the elderly living at home. Journal of the American Geriatrics Society 37 5: 423 429

Wolf-Klein G P, Silverstone F A, Basavaraja N, Foley C J, Pascarv A, Pi-Huai M 1988 Prevention of falls in the elderly population. Archives of Physical Medicine and Rehabilitation 69: 689–691

Wollner L, McCarthy S T, Soper N D W, Macy D J 1979 Failure of cerebral auto regulation as a cause of brain dysfunction in the elderly. British Medical Journal 1: 1117–1118

Wyke B 1979 Cervical articular contribution to posture and gait: their relation to senile disequilibrium. Age and Ageing 8: 251–258

7. Incontinence

Cynthea Wellings

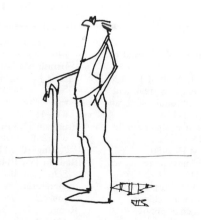

This chapter addresses the widespread nature of incontinence, and the realisation that much more can be done to identify the remediable causes, to institute more effective modes of management, and to improve the quality of life for those in whom the condition is irreversible.

Incontinence is a common clinical problem and, although it is experienced by people of all ages, it appears to be more prevalent in elderly populations. This is probably due to the following factors:

- The higher incidence of multipathological disease
- Increased use of medication
- Altered environmental situations, e.g. change of place of abode
- Greater overall exposure to health care services making identification of the problem more likely.

URINARY INCONTINENCE

Involuntary loss of urine is very distressing, and may have a devastating affect on a person's life: '*I am . . . eighty eight years old. For the past three years I have gone through 'hell' being unable to hold my urine until I get to the bathroom. I have been confined to my home . . . I can't go to church anymore and that really hurts*'. (Gartley 1986).

There appears to be no correlation between the amount of urine lost and the depth of distress experienced by the individual. A totally, incontinent person may perceive their leakage to be of minor importance, while another person who leaks infrequently may be overwhelmed by the problem. It is very important that health care personnel acknowledge the psychological impact of incontinence, regardless of the amount or frequency of the urine loss.

Involuntary urine loss is a major cause for concern for all health care workers because incontinence:

- Can cause much personal suffering
- May signal a major underlying health problem
- Can be the precipitating factor in admission to institutional care
- Can be improved, and in many cases, cured.

Most importantly, incontinence should never be ignored on the mistaken assumption that it is a normal feature of ageing.

Prevalence

A landmark study performed by Thomas et al (1980) showed that 17% of people in Britain over the age of 65 experience urinary incontinence. This and other surveys on the prevalence of urinary incontinence conducted in both the hospital and the home environment indicate that this is a significant health problem. Experience suggests

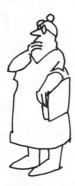

that incontinence is a major reason for nursing home admission. Certainly, the most dense concentrations of elderly incontinent people live in nursing homes where it may affect as many as 60% of residents (Howe & Preston 1985).

Normal micturition

Micturition is controlled by three structures — brain, spinal cord and peripheral nervous system — although the exact neural mechanisms are not fully understood. The desire to void is produced in the cerebral cortex as a result of impulses initially caused by increased tension in the bladder. The stretch receptors in the bladder pass impulses along the sensory pathways to the sacral micturition centre (S1–S3). This information is relayed to the cortical centre which prevents or suppresses reflex emptying until voluntary voiding is appropriate. When the time and place is right, the muscles of the pelvic floor relax allowing the neck of the bladder to descend. Bladder contraction and simultaneous relaxation, or drawing up, of the sphincters then occurs allowing the urine to pass along the urethra. Coordination of all this activity takes place in the pontine micturition centre of the brain.

Neuropharmacology of micturition

During the phase of storage of urine the bladder muscle (detrusor) is relaxed. The beta-sympathetic receptors, acting on the detrusor muscle, are probably responsible for maintaining muscle tone and thus produce a net relaxing effect with an increase in bladder capacity. At the same time, the alpha-sympathetic receptors acting at the bladder neck and proximal urethra (internal sphincter) produce an increase in pressure, thus ensuring continence.

During the phase of voiding, the activity of the parasympathetic (cholinergic) receptors causes the detrusor muscle to contract. At the same time the sympathetic activity is inhibited so that the internal sphincter relaxes and micturition occurs.

The external sphincter consists of striated muscle of the pelvic floor, enervated by the cholinergic pudendal nerve. During micturition there is cortical inhibition of this sphincter. The internal sphincter, consisting of involuntary smooth muscle, is the more important of the two in maintaining continence.

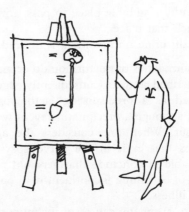

The cholinergic parasympathetic nerve system is responsible for bladder contraction and thus voiding, whereas the alpha fibres of the sympathetic system cause contraction of the internal sphincter and maintain continence.

Normal age-related changes of the genitourinary system

- Decreased urine flow rate with possible spraying and post-micturition dribble.

- Decreased bladder sensation resulting in delayed awareness of a full bladder.
- A slight decrease in bladder capacity may be present in some people.
- Decreased tone in voluntary muscle manifesting as weakness of the external sphincter and pelvic floor.
- The prostate may be increased in size and sponginess on digital examination, associated with a benign hyperplasia.
- Female labia may become smooth, shiny and pale and may retract to within or near the vagina due to a relaxed perineum.
- The urethra becomes sensitive to any decrease in oestrogen levels; fibrous tissue increases and urethral pressure decreases.
- Nocturnal diuresis occurs due to changes in circadian rhythm (Thompson et al 1989, Brocklehurst 1984).

It is important to remember that other age-related changes may impact on the ability to maintain continence. It is essential that a person is able to:

- Identify a suitable place to pass urine
- Reach that place
- Retain urine until voiding is desired.

Abnormalities of micturition do occur with age as described above. Consequently, age may be regarded as a predisposing factor for incontinence, although a precipitating event would need to occur. When one considers the age-related changes that exist in the nervous system it is reasonable to conclude that very old people are at risk of becoming incontinent with only a fairly minor illness.

There are many causes of incontinence in old age (Box 7.1), and within the general list of causes some are worthy of special mention.

Dementia is a major cause of incontinence being particularly common in the very old. Confusion in identifying a toilet may be compounded by lesions which affect the micturition centre in the frontal lobe of the brain and its connections. This can produce a dysinhibited bladder and subsequent wetness.

Parkinson's disease affects 1% of people over 60 years and approximately 30% of these people will

---

Box 7.1   Some causes of incontinence in old age

Central nervous system
Autonomic neuropathy
   Underactive bladder
Chronic brain failure
Epilepsy
Multiple sclerosis
Parkinson's disease
Spinal cord lesion
Cerebrovascular
   accident

Endocrine system
Diabetes mellitus
Hypothyroidism*
Hyperthyroidism*

Locomotor system
Osteoarthritis
Rheumatoid arthritis

Psychiatric
Acute confusion
Dementia
Depression

Genitourinary system
Atrophic vaginitis
Idiopathic unstable
   bladder
Intrinsic bladder
   disease
Stones
Tumour
Prostatic disease
   Benign hyperplasia
   Carcinoma
Retention with overflow
Stress incontinence
Underactive detrusor
Urinary tract infection

Gastrointestinal system
Constipation,
   impaction
Rectovaginal fistula

Medication
Diuretics
Hypnotics

* Uncommon causes

---

develop dementia (Thompson et al 1989). Once again, the problem may result in a dysinhibited bladder and incontinence. This may be further compounded by mobility problems, hindering speedy access to the toilet.

Diabetes can cause an underactive bladder which results in painless retention of urine, overflow incontinence, urinary tract infection and occasionally *Candida* infection. This type of incontinence can be relatively difficult to treat as it is often a longstanding problem.

Cardiovascular problems including hypertension are also common correlates in incontinent people. This may, in part, be due to the side-effects of medication, such as polyuria caused by diuretics.

Arthritis is also an extremely common condition found in elderly incontinent people.

It is possible that incontinence in this age group may be multifactorial in origin; consequently, a comprehensive psychosocial assessment plus medical history and thorough clinical evaluation are required. Whatever the cause of incontinence it should not be regarded as a normal process of ageing. It is a symptom, the cause of which needs to be determined and treated, especially as many reversible causes exist.

Types of incontinence

There are four major categories of incontinence resulting in bladder dysfunction (Abrams et al 1987).

1. Urge incontinence is an involuntary loss of urine (usually 50 mL or more) associated with a strong desire to void. In this case, there is inability to inhibit voiding after the sensation of bladder fullness is perceived.

2. Stress incontinence is the involuntary loss of urine (usually less than 50 mL) which occurs when detrusor activity is absent and the bladder pressure exceeds the maximum urethral pressure.

3. Reflex incontinence occurs in neurogenic disorders. A detrusor contraction and/or involuntary urethral relaxation occurs without the individual experiencing the sensations of needing to void.

4. Overflow incontinence occurs when there is an overdistension of the bladder causing involuntary loss of urine. This may or may not be associated with a detrusor contraction.

Diagnosis

As in any other assessment process the exact cause of the problem is sought. Each specialty brings its individual skills to assist in understanding the nature of the problem. The nurse will be particularly concerned about the impact that incontinence is having on the life of the individual and what steps need to be taken to minimise these effects. The doctor will be primarily concerned with the aetiology of the incontinence. Hilton & Stanton (1981) produced a useful algorithm which summarises an approach to the medical management (Box 7.2).

An assessment includes establishing a medical diagnosis to define the cause of the problem, and determining whether the incontinence relates directly to bladder function or is secondary to another disease process. The past and current medical history may provide important clues. Previous genitourinary surgery and parity are especially significant. Bladder function assessments need to be tailored to suit the needs of each individual. Few elderly people will have access to urodynamic investigation and thorough pelvic floor appraisal. A careful abdominal examination may provide valuable information: distension or tenderness may suggest retention; a palpable bladder indicates a volume of urine greater than 500 mL; prostate abnormalities may be detected; or faecal impaction may be contributing to the problem. An examination of the vagina and vulva, if the elderly person permits, may reveal gynaecological abnormalities such as discharge, cystocele or atrophy. The male genitalia may be examined for phimosis and discharge and the skin of the lower trunk and legs assessed for excoriation. Finally, a rectal examination will provide information about prostate size, sphincter tone and faecal impaction.

An assessment of mobility is mandatory when incontinence is a problem. Stiff hips and knees and even pain may prevent an elderly person from rising from a low chair or bed. This is particularly significant if the person has urge incontinence. An inaccessible toilet is a common problem, especially at night. Such inaccessibility may be due to distance, or unfamiliarity with surroundings caused by admission to institutional care such as a hospital or nursing home. Problems with eyesight or managing clothes caused by dyspraxia or paralysis may further hinder toilet access. Finally, incorrect height of toilet and lack of hand rails could be the final handicap in remaining continent.

A mental state assessment may be appropriate if problems related to confusion or poor memory are involved. The elderly person's social history may reveal contributory factors such as the death of the spouse or a recent hospitalisation which may have precipitated depression. The degree of insight the elderly person has or could develop to facilitate an understanding of his/her problem is invaluable information. An appraisal of the person's level of motivation and possible commitment to correct any unhealthy lifestyle habits that

Box 7.2 Summary of approach to the *medical* management of incontinence (adapted from Hilton & Stanton 1981)

Step 1: Initial assessment

History
  Social
  General
  Genitourinary
  Drug

Examination
  Central nervous
  Abdominal
  Abdominal standing
  Rectal, vaginal

Investigations
  Blood chemistry
  Midstream urine
  Residual urine (if retention suspected)

Follow-up
  Continence chart

Step 2: Therapeutic intervention — correction of identified problems

Problem	Action
Constipation, impaction	Aperients, enemas, education
Gynaecological abnormality	Gynaecological opinion
Medication-induced incontinence	Withdrawal of drugs
Stress incontinence (cough)	Pelvic floor exercises
Urinary tract infection	Appropriate antibiotics after cause is sought
Urge incontinence alone	Trial of medication/bladder training
Palpable bladder/voiding problems	Urology opinion

Steps 3: No response to intervention

Review assessment, further investigation preferably in conjunction with a urologist/geriatrician

- Cystometrogram
- Cystoscopy
- Surgical intervention may be required

Step 4: Intractable incontinence

- Counselling and family support
- Appropriate aids and equipment
- Catheterisation in specific cases

may be contributing to the incontinence is also mandatory if management is to be realistic.

The medication history is very important (see Ch. 12). The following drugs especially should be reviewed in the presence of incontinence:

- Diuretics, which increase urine output, perhaps beyond the elderly persons ability to cope
- Sedatives, which may slow reactions or decrease comprehension
- Tricyclic antidepressants, which may lead to retention
- Cholinergics, which may produce frequency
- Lithium, which may cause polydypsia and polyuria

- Cold medications, which may cause increased outlet resistance
- Prazosin, which may reduce urethral resistance.

In recent years great interest has been shown in drugs that may affect the urinary system as many of these are prescribed for elderly people. These drugs usually produce few problems but when used concurrently they may cause considerable difficulties. In reviewing the medication history it is advisable to be aware of some of the offending drugs and their mode of action (Table 7.1)

Box 7.3 lists those items which should be considered in urological assessment. Many

Table 7.1 Drugs used for other disorders that may affect the urinary system

Drugs	Mechanism	Improve	Aggravate/cause	Comments
Sedatives Antihistamines Antidepressants Antipsychotics Tranquillizers Hypnotics Alcohol	Decrease awareness of bladder sensations (including external sphincter) (NB This effect unlikely if sedation does not occur)	Nil	Urge (mainly)	Could aggravate any incontinence. Common belief but few case reports. Antipsychotics also have prazosin type action (Kiruluta & Andrews 1983)
Cardiovascular 1. Prazosin Phenoxybenzamine Labetalol Methyldopa Guanethidine Reserpine	Relax urethra and internal sphincter	Overflow (prazosin may assist complete bladder emptying Romanowski et al 1988)	Stress, ? Complex (i.e. stress and urge)	Handful of reports but consistent, worth special attention (Kiruluta & Andrews 1983)
2. Calcium-channel blockers	Decrease bladder contractions	Urge	Overflow	No reports of incontinence found
Anticholinergics Antihistamines Antidepressants Anti-Parkinson's Antispasmodics Disopyramide	Decrease bladder contractions	Urge	Overflow	Commonly stated but few case reports of incontinence found
Diuretics including caffeine	Increase urine output	Nil	Urge (mainly)	Could aggravate any incontinence. Loop diuretics or excess caffeine more likely than thiazides. 'No' reports (? too obvious)
Lithium	Increases urine output (polyuria)	Nil	Urge (probably others too)	Lithium uncommonly used for elderly patients but a predictable side-effect
Muscle relaxants Baclofen Dantrolene	Relax skeletal muscle (? external sphincter)	Nil	1 case report ? cause of incontinence	Single report (baclofen) (Williams & Pannill 1982)
Miscellaneous Bromocriptine	Three-fold action 1. Contracts detrusor 2. Relaxes urethra and internal sphincter 3. Anticholinergic action (Caine 1984)	Urge — poor results as a treatment (Delaere et al 1978, Cardozo & Stanton 1980)	Overflow (Lees & Kohout 1978, Cardozo & Stanton 1980, Gopinathan & Caine 1980, Sandyk & Gillman 1983)	Well documented
Metoclopramide	Unclear (Hasen 1984)	Nil	? Overflow	Single report of association with incontinence (Kumar 1984)
Clonazepam	Unclear	Nil	Unclear	Single report of association with incontinence (Romanowski et al 1988)

Compiled in association with Stuart Baker, Director of Drug Information Services, Office of Psychiatric Services, Health Department Victoria.

Box 7.3 Items to be considered in a urological assessment

Duration of incontinence	Flow rate
Mode of onset — sudden, gradual	Dysuria present
	Inhibition time
Degree of wetness	Haematuria present
Nocturia present, amount	History of urinary tract infections
Enuresis present, amount	Hesitancy present
Frequency over 24 hours	Stress incontinence present
Urgency	Type and amount of aids used
Sensation of complete emptying	

---

practitioners have developed these into a chart for easy reference and analysis. Such a chart, however, is only of value if the information is used in a meaningful way for care planning and for future comparative studies.

There are a number of specific diagnostic tests that may be appropriate in the assessment of incontinence:

• Routine urine analysis to test for the presence of protein, nitrates, glucose, blood, etc.
• Midstream urine test to screen urine for specific bacterial infections
• Residual urine measure to assess the emptying ability of the bladder
• Blood chemistry to evaluate renal function
• Cystometrogram to measure bladder function
• Flow rate to determine the speed of urine flow during micturition
• Perineometer to measure the strength of the pelvic floor muscles
• Intravenous urography to assess renal function.

Routine analysis of the urine may detect abnormalities such as glycosuria which could precipitate incontinence through the large volume of urine produced. The presence of haematuria may indicate the possibility of tumour or bladder calculi.

Bacteriuria is common in old age and has a particularly high prevalence in people aged 70 or more; such bacteriuria is often asymptomatic. Asymptomatic bacteriuria is not believed to reduce life expectancy and thus treatment is not required. The elderly person with cognitive impairment may not be capable of giving a clear history of symptoms and, consequently, a course of antibiotics is warranted. It is important to remember that a cause needs to be sought for urinary infections that are notoriously likely to recur when treated. For example, poor fluid intake or high residual urine may be the underlying cause of the problem.

Residual urine measurement is performed immediately following voiding. The normal residual urine volume is less than 50 mL. Ultrasound can also be used to assess residual urine of more than 50 mL. High residual urine volume indicates outflow obstruction, an underactive bladder associated with neurological problems or drug–induced retention.

Urine flow rate measurement is non-invasive and simple to perform. This requires the person (usually male), to void while the rate of flow is measured by a flowmeter. For an accurate result 200 mL or more is desired. The normal urine flow rate range is approximately 15–45 mL/sec. A urine flow rate of less than 10 mL/sec is highly suggestive of outflow obstruction or poor detrusor muscle contraction.

Urodynamic or cystometric studies are helpful in accurately identifying the cause of bladder pathology by measuring detrusor function. A catheter with a pressure transducer attached is placed in the bladder and fluid, or less commonly gas, is introduced. For extra accuracy a second catheter can be inserted into the rectum to - measure abdominal pressure. Bladder contractions are provoked by distension of the bladder. Diagnosis can be made from the reaction the bladder makes to this , challenge. It is impractical and inappropriate to use such an invasive technique in all cases and, consequently, only relatively few elderly incontinent people are investigated in this manner.

Urethral pressure measurements may be used for women to help diagnose genuine stress incontinence. The measurement is performed by withdrawing a pressure transducer slowly along the urethra while recording the pressures. A pressure profile is thus produced. There is some debate on the value of this test because an overlap exists between lower values in normal women and those with stress incontinence.

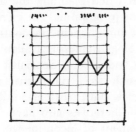

Bladder charts

Charts are valuable tools that may be used to create a clear picture of bladder function. The chart serves two functions: first, it may provide essential diagnostic information and, secondly, it is useful for monitoring progress during the management phase. Whenever possible, the person with the problem is in the best position to complete the bladder chart accurately, and should be encouraged to do so. This also helps to involve the person in his/her own care. The chart, therefore, should be in a format that may be managed by the individual elderly person. For instance, it

may need to be enlarged for a person with poor eyesight.

The chart should be simple and easily completed. Information to be recorded should include:

- Frequency — the number of episodes of micturition in each 24 hour period
- Volume of urine passed each time of voiding
- Incidence of micturition and number of incontinent episodes
- Degree of severity of each episode, that is, damp, wet or saturated.

This information should be collected over a 3–5 day period. The days need not be consecutive if the elderly person is medically stable (see Fig. 7.1).

Management

The goal of incontinence management is to assist the elderly person to reach and maintain his/her

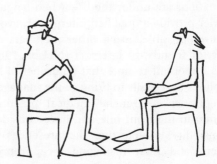

optimum level of continence. This may mean correction of the problem or it may mean learning to live effectively despite the presence of incontinence. Dryness should not be viewed as the only measure of success. Avoidance of accidents, elimination of odour, reduction in physical and mental stress, reduced financial outlays and increased social interactions are often essential prerequisites of a successful management programme.

An incontinence programme consists of four elements:

- Defining the pathological problems precisely

Day 1			
Time	Damp Wet Soaked	Dry	Measured amount passed

Fig. 7.1 Example of a continence chart.

- Assessing the impact the problem has on the individual elderly person and, if appropriate, the carer(s)
- Developing and implementing a realistic care plan
- Evaluating the plan to ensure that it is effective.

Effective management requires efficient teamwork. The elderly person and the carer(s) must be involved as fully as possible in the development and implementation of the care plan. This may not be easy if the person is anxious, embarrassed or even depressed. Experience has shown that the best results occur when the elderly person, and his/her carer(s), when appropriate, play the leading role in the management programme. To facilitate this it is necessary to: provide for confidentiality and personal privacy, while promoting dignity to the greatest possible degree; involve the elderly person and carer in all decisions taken, especially allowing the freedom to refuse any procedure or therapy; provide complete and accurate information; and ensure explanations are understood — when language is a barrier provide a qualified interpreter, avoiding, whenever possible, using other members of the family, or friends, to interpret (Nelson 1988).

It is important to note that a number of health disciplines have skills to bring to the management of incontinence. General medical practitioners are often in the front line and have considerable responsibility in detecting the presence of the problem and then managing it appropriately. Elderly people, particularly women, need to be informed that incontinence is not a normal feature of ageing and therefore proper investigation is required as with any other symptom. The medical practitioner should be vigilant and prepared to elicit information by including appropriate questions in any general examination.

Domiciliary nurses are often the first to become aware of an incontinence problem. When this is the case a rigorous nursing assessment should be carried out with sensitivity. With the permission of the person concerned or, when appropriate, the carer, the problem should then be discussed with the medical practitioner and relevant health care workers. The aim is to effect maximum communication between all relevant professionals, and most importantly, with the individual with the problem.

The views of a number of specialists may be called upon when planning the assessment and management programme. An increasing number of specialist nurses, including continence, urology and gerontology nurses, is available to work with individuals and carers. Specialist medical practitioners, such as geriatricians, urologists and gynaecologists, have particular skills in this area. Many physiotherapists also have special skills in the management of incontinence. This includes increasing an elderly person's general mobility and, mainly in females, strengthening the muscles of the pelvic floor.

Finally, it is important to remember that health care workers need to be sensitive to the considerable emotional and social stresses associated with incontinence, not just for the individual but the carer(s) also. As Wykle (1989) stated, 'There are times when the old person being cared for is actually healthier than their caregiver'.

Management planning

The management plan will, of course, depend on the findings of the assessment and the decision of the individual. It is not possible to propose a

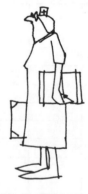

standard care plan because each elderly person will have unique needs. If the individual is living in the community it is important to consider and value the care giver in the management process. For example, extra laundry can be an enormous burden; good management therefore, must look realistically at the wider effect of the problem and intervene accordingly. This may mean recommending the provision of large body worn pads initially to minimise the effect of the problem while the assessment plan is commenced.

Incontinence caused by acute confusion resulting from recent pathology (often a urinary tract or chest infection), will need urgent treatment and in such cases the incontinence will not be viewed as the immediate and urgent problem. Further, it should not be forgotten that depression and the person's living conditions may be the cause of incontinence. In such a situation a social worker could assist in resolving the social problems.

Success in continence management should never be confused with the achievement of dryness. For many elderly people it is unrealistic to become continent. The focus should be on assisting the person to reach and maintain his/her optimum level of continence.

There are certain approaches to the management of incontinence which are commonly used with elderly people. These include:

- Bladder training programmes
- Lifestyle changes
- Medications
- Environmental modifications
- Pelvic floor exercises
- Surgery
- Aids and clothing.

Bladder training programmes are very popular as a form of continence management. Indeed, many nursing homes use timed voiding, usually 2 hourly, as their main method of management. There are a number of other bladder training regimens which may be considered depending on the needs of the person. Urgency, or urge incontinence may be assisted with training which progressively extends the intervals between voiding by conscious deferral of micturition. This form of bladder training needs a highly motivated and well orientated elderly person who has a good understanding of bladder function, especially the role of the pelvic floor muscles.

Incontinence due to diuretics or mild neuropathy, which may occur in the presence of diabetes, may be assisted by habit training. The toileting time is adjusted and fixed to pre-empt incontinent episodes and thus avoid them. Habit training demands precision and a good understanding of the individual's patterns of micturition if it is to be successful. Finally, prompted voiding is a useful tool aimed at reminding the person to go to the toilet when mild confusion is present. A continence chart may be used occasionally to monitor the success of the toileting regimen (see Fig. 7.1).

Lifestyle changes include altering habits that may be deleterious to the person's health and as a result be causing the incontinence. The health professional has an important role in educating people to lessen the impact of, and where possible, to prevent incontinence occurring. For instance, poor diet could lead to constipation which in turn may lead to urinary as well as faecal incontinence; inadequate fluid intake (a common phenomena seen in incontinent elderly people) can cause serious ill health, infections and incontinence.

Medications may be used to treat certain types of incontinence. Urge incontinence is commonly treated with anticholinergic agents (e.g. propantheline and the tricyclic antidepressant, imipramine). These act against the parasympathetic cholinergic nerve fibres that cause bladder contractions. This results in a decrease in the frequency and strength of unstable contractions and an increase in bladder capacity (see Table 7.2). It is important to ensure bladder outlet obstruction, infection and neuropathy are not present before prescribing such drugs. Also, anticholinergic medication can have significant side-effects in the elderly such as postural hypotension which may lead to falls.

Atrophic vaginitis and stress incontinence may be relieved with oestrogen cream, which acts by increasing the periurethral blood flow, strengthening periurethral tissue and reducing inflammation. However, many older women do not want, or are unable, to administer vaginal creams themselves and may need nursing assistance. Alpha-adrenergic agonists (e.g. imipramine, ephidrine and phenylpropanolomine) stimulate alpha-adrenergic fibres causing an increase in urethral smooth muscle contraction. This improves urethral sphincter tone which helps to prevent

Table 7.2 Drugs used to treat incontinence

Drugs	Mechanisms	Improve	Aggravate/cause	Comments
Anticholinergics Flavoxate Dicyclomine Oxybutynin Belladonna Penthienate Propantheline	Decrease bladder contractions (relaxes detrusor)	Urge	Overflow	
Antidepressants Imipramine Amitriptyline	Decrease bladder contractions Contract urethra and internal sphincter	Urge Stress Complex (i.e. stress and urge)	Overflow	
Adrenergics Ephedrine Pseudoephedrine Phenylpropano-lamine Mazindol	Contract urethra and internal sphincter — increases urethral resistance	Stress	? Retention	Adrenergics and oestrogens may be used together to manage stress incontinence
Oestrogens Various (topical or oral)	Increase urethral resistance (women)	Stress	? Retention	See above
Cholinergics Bethanechol	Contract detrusor	Overflow	Urge, stress, complex (i.e. stress and urge)	
Calcium-channel blockers Terodiline Nifedipine	Decrease bladder contractions	Urge	Overflow	

Compiled in association with Stuart Baker, Director of Drug Information Services, Office of Psychiatric Services, Health Department Victoria.

leaking. Alpha-blocking agents (e.g. prazosin) should be reviewed as they reduce urethral tone and may aggravate stress incontinence.

There are other medications not currently available in Australia which have a role in continence management. For example, tests in Europe show terodoline to be of value (Macfarlane & Tolley 1984).

Environmental modifications are commonly used to minimise incontinence. If the toilet is not readily accessible a commode or chemical toilet located in a convenient but appropriate place may be provided. A general assessment of the situation by an occupational therapist will reveal the types of adaptations necessary to assist in promoting continence.

Pelvic floor exercises, aimed at strengthening the voluntary, periurethral and pelvic floor muscles are important in the management of incontinence in the elderly. The contraction of these muscles exerts a closing force on the urethra. It has generally been the case that these techniques have been promoted for women with stress incontinence, but they may be useful for men, particularly after a prostatectomy. However, in most cases this treatment will require a well motivated and committed elderly person if it is to be successful over a long period. A physiotherapist with additional qualifications in continence management is invaluable in teaching such regimens.

Surgery for incontinence is relatively uncommon in the elderly. It is most frequently used for the treatment of prostatic and, to a lesser extent, gynaecological problems. The transurethral resection of the prostate is the most widely accepted treatment for urethral obstruction. Fortunately, many advances in surgical technique have occurred which make prostatectomy a relatively safe and much less uncomfortable procedure than previously. However, there still remains an associated morbidity and mortality. Expandable tubular stents of stainless steel mesh have been used in men with recurrent strictures and can also be very effective in managing obstructions in older people who are not suitable for surgery. Stones in the bladder and tumours, both benign and malignant, can precipitate incontinence and are best managed by a surgeon.

Aids and clothing are useful adjuncts to other management programmes. There is a wide range of equipment available and independent living centres or disabled living foundations have excellent ranges of such aids and appliances on display and can offer sound advice. The aim of an aid is to assist the person to maintain social continence. This means it should not be obvious that the person has a bladder problem; the aid should totally disguise the incontinence, leaving the person confident and dignified.

The most common aids used are pads and pants. Such systems are effective for 24 hour use if pad changes occur frequently and good skin hygiene is maintained. Disposal of the pad may

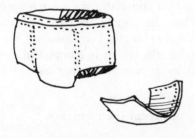

cause a problem as there are clear environmental as well as hygiene problems involved. It is best to consult the local council for advice on disposal. Condom drainage has a limited use as it is not suitable for all men. Contraindications include a retracted penis or a confusional state. The correct size of condom is essential to ensure adequate function.

Hydrophobic materials which drain urine through them while remaining dry have made a significant impact on the comfort of an individ-

ual. The material is made into sheets upon which the person rests. Should the individual become wet the urine is rapidly absorbed by the sheet and the person should be able to continue sleeping, undisturbed. These sheets can be difficult to dry due to their absorbent nature, but they are generally hard wearing and appear quite popular, especially in extended care facilities.

Urinals are also popular and very useful. There are various types available and most men tend to prefer those with a low, wide neck which make insertion of the penis easy.

Indwelling catheters have diminished in popularity over the last decade. Indeed, long-term catheterisation is seen as a last resort but may be necessary for selected people. Indwelling catheters lead to bladder infection and frequently are bypassed by urine causing subsequent incontinence which results in the individual being wet as well as being catheterised. Inserting a catheter to control incontinence without first determining its cause is poor continence management.

Judicious and discreet adaptations to clothing can assist a person to remain continent. Clearly, a person with urge incontinence is more likely to remain continent if he or she can quickly reach the toilet. Track suit pants are very useful as they are easy to pull down. In addition, gussetless pants may be helpful for women who wear longer skirts.

The cost of incontinence

It is very important to assess the cost of the problem both in social terms as well as financial. Withdrawal from social life and a feeling of shame may be the most significant costs experienced by the elderly incontinent person. In addition, many people are forced to spend considerable sums on protective pads and other aids. The cost, especially in physical terms, of constant laundering, and coping with wet bed linen, can be very taxing. Stress on family life is a major price paid by many caring families. These areas need to be fully explored during assessment to highlight the importance which must be placed on doing something to correct the problem. 'It's your age', is a pathetically inadequate response on the part of a health care worker in the light of the overwhelming problems associated with incontinence.

Evaluation

Management of a health problem usually requires some form of adjustment to an individual's lifestyle. The extent of such an adjustment will depend on the type of therapy and the person's ability to adapt. Clearly, not all programmes will work. It is, therefore, essential to appraise outcomes within reasonable time frames. For instance, once the treatment is established and appears to be appropriate, ongoing evaluation may be required, initially at 3 monthly, then 6 monthly and finally yearly intervals. Unsatisfactory progress will require modifications and review of the assessment and management plan.

Because an elderly incontinent person may be a high-risk candidate for nursing home admission it is essential to monitor progress carefully and on a continuing basis to prevent relapse and avoidable dependency.

FAECAL INCONTINENCE

Few substantial surveys have been undertaken to determine the prevalence of faecal incontinence. British research has suggested that one adult in every 200 experiences the problem with the incidence rising to 50% in some psychogeriatric facilities. While the transit time from ingestion of food to defaecation does lengthen with age there is no evidence to suggest that age-related changes contribute to faecal incontinence. Inappropriate use of purgatives, a common practice in past decades, may predispose the current elderly population to bowel problems. Faecal incontinence frequently occurs in combination with urinary incontinence.

Faecal incontinence is one of the worst human conditions. It is humiliating and embarrassing for both the elderly individual and the family. It is often repugnant and unpleasant for the carers. The extreme social stigma associated with the problem makes it a real affliction whether the elderly person is at home or in an institution. Every

effort must, therefore, be made to correct the problem or to overcome its devastating consequences.

Control of defaecation

The maintenance of bowel control is complex and relies on a number of factors including an intact nervous system. Because of this complexity, the following description includes only essential details (Smith 1983).

1. The puborectalis muscle forms a sling around the lower end of the rectum, producing a 90° angle in the rectum. This results in the anterior wall of the rectum being in apposition with the posterior wall in the horizontal plane. This forms a valve which is maintained by intra-abdominal pressure.
2. The internal and external sphincters are constantly in a state of tonic contraction.
3. The external sphincter, which is part of the pelvic floor musculature, may account for 15% of the closing pressure.
4. The anal canal is so arranged that it acts as a flutter valve.
5. Central control from the cortex can suppress the urge to defaecate which occurs when a mass of faeces enters the rectum and by distension stimulates the stretch receptors.
6. When the urge to defaecate is inhibited, the external sphincter contracts and the anorectal angle, which is diminished during defaecation, is returned to normal.

Causes of faecal incontinence

Faecal incontinence may be due to localised disease of the rectum, systemic problems such as neurological disorders and, on rare occasions, psychological dysfunction. In addition, faecal incontinence may be present in terminal disease due to carcinogenic pathology as well as constipation (see Box 7.4).

The most common cause of reversible faecal incontinence in older people is faecal impaction resulting from constipation. Such a cause may easily be overlooked in an assessment. Faecal impaction is accompanied by the frequent passage

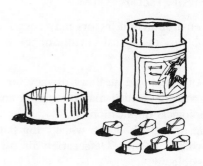

Box 7.4   Some causes of faecal incontinence in old age

Gastrointestinal system	*Central nervous system*
Carcinoma colon	Dementia
Carcinoma rectum	Diabetic neuropathy
Crohn's disease	Multiple sclerosis
Diverticulitis	
Fissure in ano	
Fistulae	
Gastroenteritis (acute)	*Drugs*
Impacted faeces	Purgatives
Incompetent anal	Iron preparations
sphincter	Antibiotics
Ischaemic colitis	
Surgically damaged	
sphincter	
Ulcerative colitis	

of small amounts of faeces and mucus. This is produced as a result of irritation by the hard faecal mass in the colon and rectum. A hard faecal mass may be felt on rectal examination; however, this will not be the case if the impaction occurs at a higher level. Further, it is possible for incontinence to occur with a soft mass of faeces in the rectum.

Anal fissure is an example of a localised painful condition which can cause faecal incontinence. It is well managed by surgery as are other problems such as anal fistula and carcinomata of the colon or rectum. All of these conditions may present with faecal incontinence.

Certain gastrointestinal diseases can lead to incontinence. For example, diverticulitis, ischaemic colitis and gastroenteritis may cause symptoms of abdominal pain, severe diarrhoea and incontinence. Also, laxity of the anal sphincter and rectal prolapse may allow faeces to escape, in which case local surgical intervention will be required.

Certain drugs can cause diarrhoea and faecal incontinence. These include purgatives, antibiotics, iron preparations and certain antacids, particularly those containing magnesium salts. Long-term purgative abuse may be responsible for a condition called megacolon which is characterised by chronic constipation, distension of the abdomen and overflow incontinence.

The central nervous system is fundamental in controlling defaecation, by both voluntary control and the coordinating effects of the autonomic system. Any major disturbance of these systems may lead to faecal incontinence. In normal circumstances, voluntary initiation of bowel action is controlled by the cerebral cortex which allows the person to choose the appropriate time and place for elimination.

Faecal incontinence associated with dementia may be due to an inappropriate awareness of ones surroundings and social niceties. In some cases, it may also be caused by the loss of inhibition of the reflex emptying of the rectum. However, faecal incontinence does not occur in all people with dementia and therefore rigorous assessment to exclude a reversible cause is essential.

Incontinence may also develop in some people with diabetes mellitus. This is probably due to a disruption of the coordinating role of the autonomic system through the development of diabetic neuropathy. In the case of multiple sclerosis, there may be widespread damage throughout the central nervous system leading to incontinence. Such people are relatively difficult to treat.

Rarely, psychological problems such as personality disorder or even depression may cause an older person to have faecal incontinence. Although treatment in such cases may be difficult, it is extremely important to refer such individuals for appropriate psychiatric assessment and, when necessary, counselling.

Terminally ill people commonly experience bowel problems. Indeed, as many as 75–80% of people seen by terminal care teams in hospitals and the community are found to be very constipated (Doyle 1987), which may cause faecal soiling.

Contributory factors

Certain environmental factors may contribute to the problem of faecal incontinence. These include:

- Lack of visual and auditory privacy for toilet activities which may have profound psychological implications
- Trying to use a bed pan while lying flat in bed which can make defaecation almost impossible
- A lifetime habit of defaecating which may not fit into an institutional routine
- Diminished mobility which could hamper or prevent access to the toilet or interfere with comfortable posture for defaecation.

Management

Because such a profound impact can be made on the life of the elderly person and his/her carer(s), the development of a management programme for all people who experience faecal incontinence (regardless of whether the problem is amenable to treatment) is essential. Clearly, any alleviation of such devastating symptoms, will be of benefit to the person, even if such management is only a body worn pad which discreetly contains the faeces. Development of the management programme will depend on the particular circumstances revealed by the assessment. It is important to note that a thorough medical examination is required to exclude the presence of disease. Once again, faecal incontinence should never be accepted as an inevitable correlate of old age and/or dementia. It should, however, be remembered that faecal incontinence is rare and care should be taken to assess thoroughly a resident living in an institution or the community.

A general assessment of a person experiencing faecal incontinence includes:

- A history of the problem itself and the impact it is having on the individual, on relatives or other carers, particularly if the main problem is dementia
- A medical appraisal to exclude disease

- Assessment of mental and psychological status (possible presence of confusion or depression)
- Physical examination (including abdominal and rectal).

Further tests that may be required are stool culture, proctoscopy and sigmoidoscopy. Invasive procedures must be performed by skilled medical practitioners. In selected instances, a more extensive review may include colonoscopy and barium enema.

Once a thorough assessment has been made a rational approach to management can be planned. Once again it is essential that the person concerned is involved as far as possible in planning care and is fully informed and supported during the process.

As there are many causes of faecal incontinence only the most common will be discussed.

Constipation is the most common cause of faecal incontinence characterised by spurious diarrhoea. When faecal impaction is a problem, it will be necessary to empty the rectum. This can be achieved by using small volume enemas daily until there is no return and evidence of the impaction has ceased. Regular bowel actions need to be maintained there after, through sensible diet, which includes appropriate amounts of fibre, exercise and occasionally aperients. For some people, such as those with megacolon, a suppository may be necessary. It is also useful to utilise the gastrocolic reflex by recommending toilet use after a hot cup of tea or after a meal, usually, breakfast.

The prevalence of Crohn's disease peaks in the 60 to 70 years age group. Fistula formation, left iliac fossa pain, malaise and diarrhoea resulting in incontinence may result. Sulphasalazine and prednisolone are useful medications and surgery may be required. Diverticular disease is also common in the elderly having a prevalence approaching 70% in people over 80 years of age. Acute attacks may precipitate incontinence requiring antibiotics and intravenous therapy. Long-term management includes education about the need for a high fibre diet and antispasmodics. Ischaemic colitis generally affecting the splenic flexure and left side of the colon is less common and, in mild cases usually presenting with diarrhoea, blood loss and colicky pain, may heal spontaneously. However, when the problem is severe, it may well become an acute surgical emergency. Diagnosis is made through X-ray and colonoscopy. Ulcerative colitis has a bimodal distribution with its second peak in the seventh decade. Acute exacerbations may cause symptoms of severe diarrhoea and incontinence requiring intravenous therapy for rehydration plus either oral prednisolone or intravenous hydrocortisone. Prednisolone enemas and sulphasalazine suppositories are frequently required to control the diarrhoea.

Other diseases of the bowel, such as carcinoma, haemorrhoids, rectal prolapse or incompetent anal sphincter may be treated by surgical intervention.

Clearly, education of the individual and, where appropriate, carer(s) will form an integral part of most management programmes. Such education may include adjustment to diet including recommending an increased amount of fresh fruit, vegetables and cereals, adjustment to fluid intake (usually an increased amount) and adjustment to timing of meals.

A bowel retraining programme may be appropriate with an evacuation schedule established, consistent with preferences and habits. Carefully controlled use of laxatives and stool softeners may assist with the timing of defaecation. Pelvic floor exercises can assist the elderly person to achieve control by strengthening the muscles to facilitate sphincter closure.

Appropriate continence aids such as pads and pants should be selected and worn constantly if the time of defaecation is unpredictable. This will reduce the likelihood of embarrassing accidents. This personal protection needs to be fully disposable as odour may cause anxiety both in the home and in the institutional setting. Certain products have recently been produced which dissolve odours by use of an enzyme. They are readily available in pump spray canisters and are of enormous value for the incontinent person no matter where they live.

In the event of a faecal incontinence episode the elderly person should be assisted to wash, rinse and dry the area and to change clothing if necessary. At all times, the elderly person should be treated with dignity and respect. Because faecal incontinence can be stressful for the carers of the incontinent person it is essential that the management programme provides the carer(s), whether family or paid staff, with opportunities to obtain relief and support from the problems associated with such care.

REFERENCES

Abrams P, Blaivas J G, Stanton L, Anderson J 1987 The standardisation of terminology related to lower urinary tract function. International Continence Society Standardisation Committee, Glasgow

Brocklehurst J C 1984 Ageing, bladder function and incontinence, In: Brocklehurst J C (ed) Urology and the elderly. Churchill Livingstone, Edinburgh

Caine M 1984 Bromocriptine and urinary incontinence. Lancet i: 228

Cardozo L D, Stanton S L 1980 A comparison between bromocriptine and indomethacin in the treatment of detrusor instability. Journal of Urology 123: 399–401

Delaere K P J, Debruyne F M J, Moonen W A 1978 Has bromocriptine a place in the treatment of the unstable baldder? British Journal of Urology 50: 169–171

Doyle D 1987 Domiciliary terminal care. Churchill Livingstone, Edinburgh

Gartley C B 1986 Managing incontinence. Souvenir Press, London

Gopinathan G, Caine D B 1980 Incontinence of urine with long term bromocriptine therapy. Annals of Neurology 8: 204

Hadley E C 1986 Bladder training and related therapies for urinary incontinence in older people. Journal of American Geriatrics Association 256: 372–378

Hasen J 1984 Urinary incontinence associated with metoclopramide. Journal of the American Medical Association 252: 3251

Hilton P, Stanton S L 1981 Algorithmic method for assessing urinary incontinence in elderly women. British Medical Journal 282: 940–942

Howe A L, Preston A N 1985 A comparative analysis of nursing home populations in Australia. National Research Institute in Gerontology and Geriatric Medicine, Occasional Paper in Gerontology No. 10, Melbourne University, p 75

Kiruluta H G, Andrews K 1983 Urinary incontinence secondary to drugs. Urology 22: 88–90

Kumar B B 1984 Urinary incontinence associated with metoclopramide. Journal of the American Medical Association 251: 1553

Lees A J, Kohout L J 1978 Bromocriptine in Parkinsonism. Archives of Neurology 35: 503–505

Macfarlane J R, Tolley D A 1984 The effect of Terodiline on patients with detrusor instability. Scandinavian Journal of Urology and Nephrology (Supplement) 87: 51–54

Nelson M L 1988 Advocacy in nursing. Nursing Outlook 36.3: 136–141

Romanowski G L, Shimp L A, Balson A B, Cahn M I 1988 Urinary incontinence in the elderly. Drug Intelligence and Clinical Pharmacy 22: 525–530

Sandyk R, Gillman M A 1983 Urinary incontinence in patients on long-term bromocriptine. Lancet ii: 1260–1261

Smith R G 1983 Faecal incontinence. Journal of the American Geriatrics Society 31 : 694–697

Thomas T M, Plymat K R, Blannin J, Meade T W 1980 Prevalence of urinary incontinence. British Medical Journal 281: 1243–1245

Thompson J M, McFarland G K, Hirsh J E, Tucker S M, Bowers A C 1989 Mosby's manual of clinical nursing, 2nd edn. C V Mosby Co, St Louis

Williams M E, Pannill F C 1982 Urinary incontinence in the elderly. Annals of Internal Medicine 97: 895–907

Wykle M 1989 Extract. In: Andreopoulos S, Hogness J R (eds) Health care for an aging society. Churchill Livingstone, New York, p 155

8. Calamity of ageing — stroke

Doreen Bauer and John Hurley

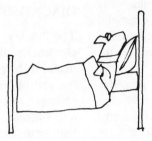

Strokes are a formidable problem in today's society: they account for 20% of deaths in persons over the age 80 years and produce a considerable number of chronically disabled persons. Although the incidence of stroke rises considerably after the age of 60 years, the overall incidence of stroke in the general population has declined slowly over the past three decades. More recent evidence, though, suggests that this reduction has ceased and the incidence of stroke has plateaued. The survival rate and quality of life seem to be better in those aged under 75 years when compared with a more elderly age group. With an increasing elderly population the management of stroke is going to be an important challenge to those who work in the field of geriatric medicine.

CLINICAL MANIFESTATIONS

The clinical manifestation of cerebrovascular disease is varied and may be divided into four categories:

1. Transient ischaemic attack (TIA)
2. Reversible ischaemic neurological deficit or (RIND)
3. Stroke in evolution
4. Completed stroke.

A transient ischaemic attack is a focal neurological event with complete recovery occurring within 24 hours. A reversible ischaemic neurological deficit, while similar in many respects, requires more than 24 hours for complete recovery. Stroke in evolution is a term to describe a neurological event that progresses over a period of hours and ends in a completed stroke. Recovery may occur, fully or partially, after the maximal effects have developed and the situation stabilises.

The *pathological basis* of a stroke may be an embolism, a thrombosis or a haemorrhage. Emboli, which are generally extracranial, mainly arise from the atrium associated with atrial fibrillation, from atheromatous plaques in the internal carotid or vertebral arteries, and from damaged aortic or mitral valves. Cerebral thrombosis is the result of the formation of a clot within the cerebral vessels, while cerebral haemorrhage is associated with a rupture of a vessel, an aneurysm or an arteriovenous malformation. To try to distinguish between the various pathological processes on the basis of clinical signs alone is very difficult.

The brain is supplied by three main arteries — anterior, middle and posterior cerebral arteries — of which the most commonly involved in producing symptoms is the middle. Damage to this artery frequently results in a cortical infarct and the development of hemiplegia. When blockage of the main trunk occurs, then dysphagia (dominant hemisphere) or dyspraxia (non-dominant hemisphere) plus homonymous hemianopia and conjugate eye deviation accompany the hemiplegia. However, when individual branches of the middle cerebral artery are involved, then only part of this picture develops. For example, thrombosis of the left inferior branch may result in no loss of power, but a visual field defect with a speech defect of the Wernicke type.

The middle cerebral artery also provides narrow, perforating branches to the internal capsule where the nerve fibres from the motor and sensory areas of the cortex pass, while closely packed together, on their way to the spinal cord. Damage in this area may also lead to hemiplegia by interrupting the nerve impulses from the cortex to the limbs. These capsular infarcts have a much better prognosis because cognitive skills remain intact and alternative blood supplies are good, aiding recovery.

The anterior cerebral artery mainly supplies the paramedian frontal lobe and the caudate nucleus. A thrombosis of this artery results in contralateral weakness of the leg, mainly affecting the foot, combined with sensory loss in the same limb. Slowness in mentation, speech perseveration and urinary incontinence are often associated with this lesion.

Interruption of blood flow to the posterior cerebral artery results in damage to the occipital lobes and inferior part of the temporal lobes. The consequences of this lesion are the development of hemianopia with other signs, depending on the areas damaged, such as altered memory, agraphia and dyspraxias. There is, however, little or no paralysis.

Several other vascular lesions may occur involving the medulla, pons and midbrain, resulting in paralysis and severe incapacity. These lesions are generally less common and are beyond the scope of this chapter.

Clearly, strokes vary in their severity depending on the site of the lesion and the magnitude of damaged brain tissue. It is important, therefore, to be aware of this fact when discussing the likely outcome with relatives. A blockage of the main trunk of the middle cerebral artery producing a hemiplegia will have a catastrophic effect with little chance of recovery to independence, whereas a hemiplegia due to a small capsular infarct generally resolves, with independence in daily activities being quite likely.

DIAGNOSIS

The history of the event is a very important element in the diagnosis so witnesses are very useful in helping to describe the clinical picture. An abrupt onset suggests an embolism or haemorrhage as the cause. A rapid recovery is also suggestive of embolism. Unilateral headache with tender temporal arteries may suggest cranial arteritis, while a story of convulsion prior to the neurological deficit occurring may indicate Todd's paralysis.

The possibility of a non-vascular cause should be considered and excluded if possible. Problems that may fall into this category include:

- Subdural haematoma
- Cerebral tumours — benign, primary or secondary malignant
- Cerebral abscess
- Meningitis
- Todd's paralysis (post epilepsy)
- Giant cell or cranial arteritis
- Syphilis.

General examination

General observation of the elderly person may suggest a precipitating cause. The presence of petechiae suggests the possibility of multiple emboli due to bacterial endocarditis or a haemorrhagic diathesis, while evidence of periorbital bleeding suggests that trauma may be a factor.

The *cardiovascular system* should be examined with care. Routine measurement of blood pressure is essential since hypertension is the most common risk factor for cerebrovascular disease. Auscultation of the carotid arteries is mandatory as a bruit heard at the bifurcation of the carotid artery is highly suggestive of vascular disease being the basis of the stroke. It needs to be remembered, however, that some bruits are not accompanied by cerebral lesions while the absence of bruits is not uncommon in the presence of carotid artery disease. Valvular lesions may lead to emboli as may subacute bacterial endocarditis, the appropriate murmurs being heard on auscultation. Cardiac dysrhythmias may be responsible for emboli secondary to atrial fibrillation while bradycardia may suggest a Stokes-Adams attack.

The *respiratory system* may be the site of carcinoma which may produce signs suggesting a secondary cerebral deposit as the cause. In addition, the possibility of pulmonary emboli or atelectasis as complications of the stroke itself should be considered when abnormal signs are discovered in the lungs.

The *gastrointestinal system* should not be forgotten in the hunt for indications of the cause of a stroke. An abdominal mass may indicate a tumour, while enlargement of the spleen in combination with a plethoric appearance would suggest polycythaemia. It is always necessary to palpate the bladder because of the frequency of urine retention in association with cerebrovascular accidents.

Specific neurological examination

The level of consciousness should be noted with particular reference to the elderly person's ability to maintain an open airway. A prolonged duration of unconsciousness is usually a poor prognostic sign.

The cranial nerves need to be examined, with special reference to swallowing, speech and sight. Depending on the site of the lesion, nystagmus, dysarthria and ataxia may be the dominating signs.

Swallowing difficulty (dysphagia) frequently occurs after a stroke and may result in the accumulation of secretions in the mouth with dribbling and choking. During feeding, care must be taken to avoid inhalation of solids and fluids.

Speech is a complex mechanism which is frequently impaired by a stroke. The two major speech centres are supplied by the left middle cerebral artery. Blockage of the superior branch leads to Broca's aphasia. This is characterised by sparse, effortful speech with poor pronunciation of syllables, but with preserved comprehension of the spoken word. This defect is usually described as an expressive dysphasia. A thrombosis in the inferior division results in Wernicke's aphasia, which produces fluent speech with well pronounced syllables but a tendency to use wrong or non-existent words, thus making little sense. Further, comprehension and repetition of speech are poor. This problem is described as receptive dysphasia. A lesion blocking the main middle cerebral artery prior to its division results in damage to both areas, leading to both receptive and expressive dysphasias.

As *sight* may be impaired in several ways a thorough examination is required. The main deficiency to look for is homonymous hemianopia, testing for which is best accomplished by assessing the ability to follow finger movements. When cooperation is not possible, a threatening movement, such as an apparent attempt to strike the person from the side, should elicit a blink response. When this reaction is absent, a hemianopia should be suspected. During the eye examination other signs may be found including nystagmus or third, fourth and sixth nerve palsies indicating lesions in the brain stem.

Motor function

The assessment of motor function is important. The degree of impairment may be determined by observing the person attempting voluntary movements. Gross abnormalities will be detected readily while minor degrees of control loss will require more careful testing.

Reflex consequences

All normal voluntary movements performed by a person are a response to sensory stimuli that act upon the central nervous system. These sensory stimuli are received by the brain via receptor nerves of which there are two groups:

- Exteroceptors, such as vision, touch and hearing, which carry messages from the external environment.

- Proprioceptors, such as sensory nerves in the muscles, joints and ears, which carry messages from within the body about its position.

These sensory messages are integrated in the sensory and motor cortex of the brain and result in the production of a coordinated motor or movement response. Each person with hemiplegia following a cerebrovascular lesion presents a unique picture depending on the degree and distribution of the effects of the lesion. In spite of the great variety of symptoms, there are certain sensory and motor disturbances in reflex activity which are similar in many people with hemiplegia.

Perhaps the most common area of disturbance is that of muscle tone, resulting in what may be termed paralysis. At all times, voluntary muscles are maintained in a state of mild contraction ready to respond to the call to move. This state of mild contraction is called normal muscle tone. It is present, to some extent, in all voluntary muscles but it is more marked in the muscles that hold the body upright against gravity. In the lower limbs, trunk and neck, the antigravity muscles are the extensors. In the upper limbs the antigravity muscles are those which, in prehistory, used to lift the body weight. These are the scapula retractors, shoulder depressors, and shoulder, elbow, wrist and finger flexors.

Muscle tone is entirely reflex in character and is maintained by reflexes. These reflexes are located in the spinal cord but are controlled by the brain. A stroke reduces or abolishes the cortical control of the brain over the spinal reflexes, resulting in the change from normal tone. Immediately after the onset of the hemiplegia there is usually a state of flaccidity or hypotonicity. This decreased tone may last for a few days. Occasionally, the flaccidity persists for months but this is quite rare. A flaccid limb feels heavy and abnormally relaxed when being moved. There is no active adjustment of muscles to changes of posture, no active control of movement and no ability to arrest a movement or hold the position against gravity when not supported.

Flaccidity usually gives way to spasticity or hypertonicity. This is increased muscle tone resulting from the cortical brain's failure to exert control over the primitive reflexes. Spasticity is felt as undue resistance to a movement performed passively.

Spasticity is not confined to any one muscle or muscle group but occurs most commonly in patterns. These patterns are so characteristic or stereotyped as to be able to be recognised at a glance in a person with hemiplegia.

Spasticity usually occurs in the antigravity muscles. In the arm there is usually retraction and depression of the scapula and humerus, internal rotation of the shoulder, flexion of the elbow, flexion and ulnar deviation of the wrist, and finger flexion and adduction. The spastic pattern in the leg produces rotation backwards and upward hiking of the pelvis, external rotation of the hip, extension of the hip and knee, extension with inversion of the ankle and plantar flexion of the toes.

It is essential to remember that the level of spasticity is not static but is constantly changing. Postural positioning has a definite effect on the release of reflex activity and, to a large extent, governs the degree of tone. For example, turning the head to the left will increase the normal flexor tone in the right arm and leg. The position of the head is important in assessing or controlling tone in the limbs. The effect is called a tonic neck reflex, an example of the very complicated reflex actions present in both the normal and the abnormal body.

Spasticity can be increased and the chance of normal movement decreased in many ways. Stimulation of the ball of the foot will increase extensor spasm in the leg. It is the extensor spasm which prevents normal function in the leg. It is often suggested that a footboard is essential for the prevention of foot drop. Unfortunately, a footboard creates pressure on the ball of the foot, increasing the spasm and so forcing the foot into the dropped position. Another common way of increasing extensor spasm in the leg is encountered when the person tries to get out of a too high bed. Sliding onto the forefoot will increase the extensor spasm and any chance of a consequent normal step is negated. The person with hemiplegia must put the heel down before weight-bearing.

Flexion spasm in the arm can be increased by efforts to perform movements unless particular postures are adopted. Many health workers do not understand this and attempt to judge a person's recovery by testing the ability to squeeze the hand. When nothing happens but an increase in spasm through the whole arm there is disappointment. Recovery after a stroke almost always occurs in the direction of proximal to distal. That is, recovery in the shoulder precedes recovery in the hand; recovery in the hip occurs before recovery in the foot. Early testing of finger and foot function is depressing as well as a waste of effort.

Spastic muscles are unable to function because of the increased tone and function can only be restored when the spasticity has been controlled. Strengthening exercises for apparently weak muscles following a stroke are inappropriate. In fact, the effort required by the person with spasticity to perform the exercise may only succeed in increasing the spasm. Giving a person with spastic hemiplegia a ball to squeeze, for example, may contribute significantly to the failure to restore functional movement in the hemiplegic arm.

Changes in muscle tone are perhaps the most apparent reflex disturbance following a stroke. Changes in normal postural reflex mechanisms, which are the basis of normal voluntary and skilled movements, are also common following a stroke. The normal postural reflex mechanisms consist of a great number of automatic motor responses that are acquired and gradually developed during the first three years of life. There are two groups of automatic postural reflexes that are of particular importance when considering stroke.

First, *righting reactions* are automatic movements which serve to maintain and restore the normal position of the head in space and in its normal relationship to the body. The developmental patterns of these righting reflexes are seen in the earliest activities of rolling over, kneeling, sitting and standing. They develop in the growing infant, are gradually modified and disappear towards the end of the fifth year. The motor patterns or movements of adult life are possible because of the developmental patterns established by these reflexes. A stroke usually destroys the normal movement patterns on the affected side.

The restoration of normal movement requires the re-establishment of these patterns.

Secondly, *equilibrium reactions* are automatic movements which maintain and restore balance during activity, especially when in danger of falling. For example, if pushed, a person will step back without thinking. These postural adjustments to change in the centre of gravity are continuous while a person moves. Even the smallest change in equilibrium needs to be countered by muscle action. For example, when reaching forward there is compensatory muscle work in the trunk and legs to ensure the maintenance of balance.

A person with hemiplegia following a stroke will have lost these equilibrium reactions on the affected side. Any attempt to move toward the affected side is hazardous because it does not have the necessary protective mechanisms. Redevelopment of these most basic reflex responses is a basic aim of rehabilitation training.

Investigations

Investigation through laboratory tests is an essential part of the diagnostic approach to strokes and may be of great assistance in arriving at a diagnosis.

Haematology

The haemoglobin level is normal in most cases. A low haemoglobin level may indicate neoplastic disease or chronic renal disease; the former may be associated with a cerebral deposit while the latter may indicate widespread vascular disease. An elevated haemoglobin level should indicate further investigation for the presence of polycythaemia which is associated with an increased likelihood of thrombosis and lacunar infarcts.

The white cell count may be elevated in cases of infection including subacute bacterial endocarditis which may produce cerebral emboli, and in leukaemia with its associated problems of haemorrhage.

The erythrocyte sedimentation rate may be greatly elevated, in which case cranial arteritis must be suspected as extension of the arteritis may cause intracranial thrombosis. Neoplastic diseases may also cause this elevation and thus the possibility of cerebral secondaries may need to be considered.

Biochemistry

Urea and electrolyte levels are indicative of renal function and the state of hydration. Correction of dehydration is important for effective blood flow, so essential when the cerebral blood supply is compromised.

Random blood sugar tests, 2 hours postprandially, may be helpful in the diagnosis of diabetes, a condition which is associated with arterial disease and, thus, cerebrovascular disease.

Hypoglycaemia may masquerade as a stroke, the signs and symptoms disappearing after the blood sugar level has returned to normal.

Cerebrospinal fluid (CSF)

A lumbar puncture is usually not necessary except when there is doubt about the cause of the stroke or when subarachnoid haemorrhage or meningitis is suspected. After having ascertained that papilloedema is not present, CSF may be obtained.

Blood-stained CSF is indicative of haemorrhage. An increase in white cells suggests meningitis or possibly leukaemia involving the meninges.

Electrocardiography

An ECG provides evidence of myocardial infarction which may have precipitated a stroke secondary to a drop in blood pressure. It also produces information of pre-existing and prolonged hypertension.

Scanning procedures

Scanning procedures may be used to provide additional and more specific information.

CT scanning is a non-invasive technique and is appropriate to use for elderly people. It is able to differentiate a cerebral infarct from cerebral haemorrhage as well as to identify tumours.

Ultrasonography is now a reasonably effective method of determining the patency of the carotid artery and, as it is non-invasive, has an important place in the investigation of TIAs and carotid bruits, supplanting angiography as the first line of investigation in this group of conditions. Studies have shown that people with neck bruits have a higher risk of stroke than is the case in the general population. However, where the bruit is not associated with symptoms such as TIAs, the risk is not high enough to justify carotid endarterectomy.

Echocardiography is only required to identify a cardiac source of embolism when there is clinical evidence of such a source being possible, for example, when atrial fibrillation is present.

Angiography

Digital subtraction angiography is another method that may be used in determining the extent of the damage in the carotid arteries. The investigation, which is invasive, previously used a venous route, but arterial injection is more effective and has become safer as a result of improved techniques.

Angiography is used to visualise the extracranial and intracranial blood vessels through the use of radio-opaque material. Because it is not without risk it should be used for specific reasons only. People with TIAs may be considered as candidates in view of the potentially good results that may be obtained through surgery on the carotid artery.

THERAPEUTIC APPROACH TO STROKE

Acute management

The acute stage of stroke management involves the maintenance of:

- The airway (ventilation)
- Fluid/electrolyte balance
- Urinary output
- Skin integrity
- Motivation.

With care, the person will pass through the acute phase without avoidable disabilities, allowing the rehabilitation phase to take place at the earliest opportunity. It is particularly necessary to avoid contractures and pressure sores. All joints should be put through a full range of movement, either active or passive, each day and a careful positioning and turning programme implemented.

Positioning

Although initially the hemiplegic side may be flaccid or lacking in tone it should be remembered that an increase in tone, or spasticity, may develop. This spasticity may be minimised by diligent positioning. This is particularly important in the very early stages. Positioning requires the use of the antispasm or recovery patterns at all times. An understanding of the spastic pattern is necessary to fully appreciate the recovery pattern (Table 8.1).

Table 8.1 Spasm and antispasm patterns of importance when planning a positioning programme

Region	Spastic Pattern	Antispasm pattern
Spine	Head and trunk bent toward hemiplegic side	Head and trunk in neutral alignment
Shoulder	Retracted, depressed and inwardly rotated	Scapula brought forward and raised arm rotated outward
Elbow	Flexed	Extended
Wrist	Flexed and ulnar deviation	Extended and radial deviation
Fingers	Flexed and adducted	Extended and abducted
Pelvis	Pulled up and backward	Forward and dropped down
Hip	Extended and externally rotated	Flexed and internally rotated
Knee	Extended	Flexed
Foot	Plantar flexed	Neutral

To minimise the effects of reflex activity careful attention should be paid to positioning. Because a person with acute hemiplegia cannot be in a total antispasm position at all times it is appropriate to use components. Lying on the back is a position that is often chosen but it should be used with care as it is the position that produces maximum spasm.

Lying on the back

Upper limb. The arm and shoulder are placed on a pillow and are thus lifted forward. In addition, the arm is turned outward with the elbow, wrist and fingers extended. Note that nothing is placed in the hand.

Lower limb. A thin pillow or pad is placed under the hip and thigh, keeping the pelvis forward and knee slightly bent. Note that nothing is placed against the sole of the foot.

Lying on non-affected side

Upper limb. The arm is brought forward from the scapula with full extension of elbow, wrist and fingers across a supporting pillow.

Lower limb. The pelvis is rolled forward and the leg is bent and supported by a pillow for comfort.

It should be noted that if there are too many pillows under the head the neck will be bent toward the hemiplegic side, thus increasing the spasm.

Lying on the hemiplegic side

Upper limb. The arm should be brought forward from the scapula with full extension of the elbow, wrist and fingers.

Lower limb. The pelvis should be pulled forward slightly with the hip and knee in some flexion. A pillow should be placed under the top leg for comfort.

Postural movements

As soon as possible the elderly person should learn to move in bed. Bridging, rolling and sitting are important functions both for the elderly person's independence and for reducing the physical demands on carers.

Bridging is useful for assisting with bedpan use as well as for relieving pressure on the buttocks. The elderly person lies supine with both knees bent — crook lying. The pelvis is lifted while pushing down on both feet. This manoeuvre should be practised as an exercise until it can be undertaken easily.

This manoeuvre may also be used for moving across the bed. The feet are moved first, a few inches across the bed in the direction the elderly person wishes to move. After the pelvis is raised it is lowered in line with the feet. The chest and head may then be brought into line with the pelvis. The process is repeated until the elderly person is in the desired position.

Rolling may be quite a traumatic experience unless it is performed carefully. It must be remembered that because the hemiplegic limb may be flaccid and lacking in sensation the elderly person may not be able to protect it. Since the arm, particularly, has a tendency to become trapped, dragged or pulled, the carers must be very cautious to avoid damage. Before attempting to roll the elderly person should move across the bed, away from the direction of the roll. After assuming the crook lying position the elderly person should hold the hemiplegic arm stretched out in front. The carer should stand on the appropriate side to be in front at the end of the roll. Assistance may be given at the posterior shoulder and hip while the elderly person rolls, first moving the head, then the chest, legs and pelvis.

Too often the elderly person with hemiplegia is seen *sitting*, falling toward the affected side, the arm hanging, the leg carelessly slipped forward while the person looks toward the unaffected side. Just at a glance, one can see that this is an abnormal posture which is just as uncomfortable and demoralising as it looks. The elderly person should be positioned upright with the trunk in a good vertical alignment. A thin pillow or pad may be needed to support the affected hip. The hemiplegic arm should be placed on a pillow positioned to maintain level shoulders, the scapula pulled forward and the arm and fingers in extension. The chair should be positioned so that the elderly person is encouraged to turn the head toward the affected side.

Selection of a suitable chair is very important. If it is too wide the elderly person will slip to one side. If it is too high the feet cannot maintain the correct, flat on the floor, knees bent, position. If

the upholstery is smooth plastic the elderly person may slip forward.

Rehabilitation phase

Therapeutic programmes are usually designed to facilitate recovery through managing the environment, which may be defined as the surroundings in which a person functions. The environment encompasses all the contents of those surroundings — physical, emotional and social.

People function as an integral part of the environment, acting and reacting according to input received from the environment. If input is absent or distorted a person's reactions will also be absent or distorted. For example, an elderly person with homonymous hemianopia following a stroke does not react to the environment on the side of the visual deficit; an elderly person with perceptual disorders often reacts incorrectly or inappropriately to the visual stimuli received from the environment.

The hospital environment

Illness or disability may result in an altered perception of the environment and thus produce altered reactions. One of the reactions often seen in elderly people after a stroke is that of thinking the disabilities are due to being in hospital and that on return to home all will be well again. This unrealistic attitude is a result of the elderly person's altered perception of self and the environment.

The physical environment is assumed to set the stage and perhaps define the person's role in human relationships and activities. Therefore, a specific environment may evoke a range of expected behaviours. A hospital environment will cause a person to become a patient who should be unwell, in bed and dependent.

All aspects of the environment need to be considered carefully in relation to the elderly person who has had a stroke. The first aspect needing attention is the placement of the bed in the hospital ward. Not only should it allow for freedom to transfer and for carers to assist the patient, it should also be positioned for visual input and social interaction.

A common consequence of the stroke is left hemiparesis with neglect on the same side. There is decreased awareness of the environment on the left and the elderly person often avoids looking toward the affected side. This is often coupled with poor spatial orientation, impaired body image and hemianopia. As much as possible, the elderly person needs to be encouraged to become aware of the affected side. Efforts should be made to draw attention to the affected side by approaching the elderly person from that side and encouraging relatives and friends to do likewise. Ideally, placement in the ward should be such that the elderly person is forced to look to the affected side to focus on areas of activity. The bedside chest and the visitors's chair should be

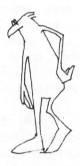

on the affected side to encourage the elderly person to look that way for needed items or social contact. During later stages of rehabilitation, however, it may be necessary to change the placement to facilitate safe moving to the stronger side.

The elderly person should be placed in an area that enables convenient access to toilets, dining room and day room. This becomes even more important when the elderly person becomes mobile but does not have sufficient endurance to walk more than a short distance.

The second aspect of the environment which should be considered carefully is the type and placement of the furniture. No space is more important in the early rehabilitation phase than the elderly person's bedroom, especially if it forms the centre of the elderly person's life. For many elderly people the bedroom, for a time, will become the reception area for visitors, a dining room, a television room, library, perhaps even bathroom and toilet.

The most common pieces of furniture in the bedroom are, of course, the bed, the locker, chair and overbed table. These items of furniture constitute the elderly person's immediate environment and their placement either enhances or detracts from the ability to function adequately. Some features of furniture that are important to consider are: correct height, appropriate support and comfort. The chair should be placed on the stronger side, positioned at an angle to facilitate transfer from bed to chair. The chair itself should be sturdy, with arms of an appropriate height to assist an upright posture, wide enough to allow the arms to rest without having to lean sideways, and of the correct height for the person, enabling the feet to be placed flat on the floor.

The bed should be of the correct height to facilitate transfers and should have a firm mattress to enable easy mobility in bed. An 'overbed triangle' or rope ladder may be useful aids for in-bed mobility. The bedside locker and overbed table should be positioned so the elderly person is able to reach items. There can be little more that is as frustrating as being able to see a cup of tea or a favourite book and being unable to reach them.

The areas used for social interaction, other than the bedroom, should be considered carefully. These places, in hospital, include the dining room and day room. As with the bedroom the furniture should be functional and promote independence and it must be placed to promote function. The day room should promote social interaction and activity. If chairs are placed around the walls with nothing in the middle of the room, opportunity for social interaction with others may be lost. Placing chairs in conversation groups around a table that contains magazines or books and is easy to reach gives the idea of comfort and conviviality and promotes social interaction. Having a comfortable area to go to other than the bedroom also gives the elderly person a reason to become mobile. In the rehabilitation ward there should also be an area for individual and group activity.

The dining room should be spacious enough to allow for free access around tables that have sturdy, comfortable chairs with arms. Aids that may be required for independence in eating should be available for use and, if needed, placed within easy reach.

In the hospital, where there is a need to share ward accommodation, it is helpful to provide private places for the elderly person to be alone, alone with family, clergy or, from time to time, staff. Too often, the need for personal privacy is neglected in hospital.

Of major importance is consideration of the general ward environment. This includes such areas as the floors, lighting, windows and corridors. The dilemma of finding a floor surface that is not slippery and does not produce glare is a constant one for designers. For the person with hemiplegia, a non-slip floor can make the difference between dependence with transfers and walking and being completely independent. If the flooring in the hospital is slippery and shiny, or even appears to be so because of a high gloss, the use of non-skid bath mats may be helpful, especially if placed in front of the chair or by the bedside. The mat may provide a secure, non-slip surface for the elderly person to stand on, allowing time to gain balance before walking. Lighting should be indirect and diffuse, reducing the glare factor while giving a good even light. Again, this is very important for those elderly people who have visual field defects or perceptual problems. Having a room or a corridor that is well and evenly lit reduces the distortions in vision that may occur if lighting is poor.

The emotional or psychological environment must promote the idea of personal independence despite disability. Once the elderly person has passed through the acute phase of the illness resulting from the stroke and has become medically stable, he/she should not be considered a 'sick' person. Every encouragement must be given to undertaking activities as independently as possible and to participating in a normal day. The elderly person should be encouraged to get up and dress in day clothes, go to the dining room for meals and the day room for activities. Normal leisure activities should be re-introduced as quickly as possible, even if competence is not what it was. If the pre-stroke leisure activities are no longer possible, the elderly person should be encouraged and helped to develop new interests.

An atmosphere of kindness, caring concern and unlimited time must be attempted. It may seem very difficult in a busy hospital to present this attitude but the attempt must be made and made in such a way that the elderly person has the feeling that staff have all the time in the world to spend helping, talking through worries about the future, the family or the disabilities.

'Ability not disability' should be the motto for the rehabilitation ward and everything that can be done to develop an environment that promotes this should have a high priority.

The home environment

While the environment in the ward or institutional setting is important in the rehabilitation process, so too is the home environment at the time of discharge. A careful assessment of the home environment should be undertaken by appropriate personnel and the family members who will assist the elderly person at home (see Ch. 15).

Steps in the household should be examined with a view to fixing hand rails or providing ramps. The ability to cope in the toilet and bathroom is very important and, because each will have its own idiosyncracies, care should be taken to assess thoroughly. In the toilet, appropriately placed hand rails, the use of a raised toilet seat and non-slip matting may be of great benefit as may be the use of a commode by the bed at night in preventing incontinence and improving the elderly person's morale by independent toiletry. The bath may also be a hazard. Here again, skill and ingenuity may be needed to improve the elderly person's ability to function. Bath seats and transfer boards may be useful as are hand-held showers, hand rails, and non-slip mats. Where a shower is available a shower chair may be helpful. The shower floor should be flush with the surrounding surface to avoid the need to step over a ledge.

The kitchen area is important and again there is a wide variety of aids available to assist function: tap turners, tea pourers, bread spreading boards, cutlery plates, mugs and other devices for use by a one-handed person may be appropriate.

Aids and assistive devices should only be provided if they are necessary, if they have been thoroughly tested, if the elderly person is trained to use them and, above all, if the elderly person wants them.

Motor skill learning

Relearning motor skills, such as standing, walking, dressing, eating and so on, is a vital aspect of the rehabilitation programme. Currently, a variety of theoretical approaches are used by therapists, all beyond the scope of this book for detailed descriptions. Further, considerable research to evaluate these approaches is being undertaken, especially as they apply to elderly people. Whatever the theoretical approach chosen, the primary goal of the rehabilitation process must be to get the elderly person home, functioning as effectively and safely as possible in the shortest time possible. All team members must keep this goal in focus at all times and not become side-tracked by prolonged efforts to restore movements or functions to normal.

There is considerable evidence that motor learning is best achieved when a person practises the whole skill, incorporating specific refinements where and as possible. For example, to relearn walking the elderly person needs to walk with purpose, to the toilet, to the dining room, in the garden, using whatever aids or assistance makes the activity possible, effective and safe. There is little evidence that practice of the various parts of walking — weight shifting, step placement, control of hip, knee and ankle and so on — in parallel bars or other artificial environments, makes a great deal of difference to the eventual outcome, other than perhaps delaying progress.

The process of recovery may continue for some time; thus, the rehabilitation programme may continue after the person has left the inpatient hospital service. This may be carried out in an outpatient rehabilitation service or day hospital. Alternatively, the family may cope adequately carrying on a regimen developed by the team. It is essential that the team remembers that it includes the elderly person and the family who should have considerable input into the development of realistic functional goals. However, it

must be accepted that continuing formal rehabilitation on an indefinite basis, especially when there is little evidence of further progress, cannot be supported.

The role and function of a self-help group or stroke club cannot be underestimated in assisting people who have had a stroke, and their families, come to terms with the limitations of therapeutic intervention and prolonged rehabilitation.

Communication

When communication skills have been altered by the stroke the speech pathologist is a vital asset to the rehabilitation team and should be involved as early as possible. Restoration of effective communication channels is of the greatest importance and the speech pathologist will be able to suggest the best approach given the specific form of disability. There is considerable evidence that lack of communication is the most frightening and frustrating feature of a stroke. Finding a way to communicate is, therefore, a priority goal.

Rehabilitation programmes aimed at restoration of speech and other communication skills may be designed by the speech pathologist and carried out in therapy sessions or by the elderly person and family practising at home under the guidance of the speech pathologist. As in other rehabilitation programmes, communication skill learning should be goal directed and not prolonged beyond reasonable progress.

Motivation of the person after a stroke

Motivation in the context of stroke rehabilitation is a complex process. It may be defined as the elderly person's willingness to mobilise all physical and psychological resources to cope with the disability.

People are judged to be motivated if they engage in behaviour that contributes to their recovery. In this situation, the goals of the elderly person and the other rehabilitation team members concur. The elderly person is easy to treat because of a willingness to cooperate with procedures and tests; an eagerness to attend therapy sessions and work diligently; a desire to maintain relationships with family and friends and keep up with current events.

If the goals of the elderly person and the rest of the team diverge the elderly person may be labelled unmotivated or poorly motivated. In fact, the elderly person may be highly motivated, consciously or subconsciously, in a different direction. For example, the elderly person may be motivated to be dependent, to remain in hospital because it represents an improved living situation or because it offers relief from making difficult decisions.

Cerebrovascular accidents represent a massive assault on the person. Deficits occur in motor skills, sensation, vision, perception and intellectual abilities. Frequently, personality changes result. The emotional reactions which often follow a cerebrovascular accident can be thought of as normal reactions to these abrupt and often devastating changes to a person's lifestyle.

It is little wonder that reactions include acute depression, hyperanxiety, anger, withdrawal and defeat. Until adjustments to the changes occur, these reactions adversely affect motivation.

Action can be taken in a therapeutic way to correct feelings of anxiety and depression through the use of drugs and other means which may have a considerable effect on the rehabilitation process. However, anger that is often associated with aggressive behaviour may be very difficult to manage. Tact, tolerance and understanding may, in time, lead to improvement.

The anxieties and frustrations that impair the forces involved in motivation may be helped by careful explanations of the symptoms and possible ways of compensating for the disabilities. Rehabilitation goals may have to be revised in the light of the elderly person's reaction. A lack of encouragement and effort by carers to promote independence may result in an elderly person becoming unnecessarily dependent. Any excessive pressure, however, may confirm the sense of failure which leads to giving up and refusing to try.

To help the elderly person succeed to the highest levels possible requires constant encouragement and great sensitivity on the part of the rehabilitation team, especially the elderly person's relatives.

SURGERY IN STROKES

Surgery on the carotid artery or the surgical anastomosis of the extra- and intracranial arteries is unhelpful or even harmful in the acute phase of a stroke. However, surgical intervention is most likely to be considered when prevention of an initially mild episode becoming a major event is considered possible. This is the usual attitude adopted towards TIAs and RINDs from which there is complete recovery. Surgical treatment of carotid stenosis, often associated with TIAs, is now undertaken in selected cases. Surgical intervention for localised intracranial artery disease is, at present, unproven.

PREVENTION

When considering measures or programmes of disease prevention the first step is the identification of the risk factors. There is, for example, an almost exponential increase in the incidence and mortality of stroke with age. Age, though, does not stand alone so it is necessary to focus attention on those factors that also contribute and which may be ameliorated through therapeutic intervention. These include:

- Diabetes mellitus
- Heart disease
- Hypertension
- Polycythaemia
- Transient ischaemic attacks
- Cigarette smoking
- Hypocholesterolaemia
- Obesity

Many studies have confirmed the role of hypertension and have also provided compelling evidence that controlling blood pressure reduces the chances of cerebral disease occurring.

Diabetes mellitus and its association with arterial disease and stroke is well documented. Unfortunately, efforts directed at more effective control of blood pressure levels in the presence of diabetes mellitus have not been shown to reduce the risk. Despite this, it is suggested that good control is maintained.

The risk of a completed stroke following TIAs is greatest within the first year of the initial incident, the expected stroke incidence in that period being 17%. Carotid artery surgery may improve the prognosis in selected cases. The use of antiplatelet drugs following the TIA is also of benefit.

Obesity and its association with stroke is equivocal, although it is a proven risk factor for hypertension and diabetes. Despite the lack of evidence of a clear relationship for obesity with stroke the maintenance of weight within the expected range for height and age should be encouraged.

As in the case of elevated blood lipid levels the evidence for a direct link between smoking and stroke is not consistent. However, there is little doubt of the relationship between smoking and heart disease and peripheral vascular disease so smoking should be discouraged.

PROGNOSIS

The overall mortality rate within the first month is approximately 20% for the first stroke. Of those people who survive the first month, some 50% make a good recovery to normal or near normal function.

There is not a good outlook for a return to independent function in people over the age of 75 years, mainly because of the increased prevalence of associated disabilities.

The rate of recurrence after the first stroke is about 10% per year and people who have survived a stroke are more likely than age-matched controls to die.

Many people are left with considerable disability after a stroke and require considerable support from the family and the community to remain at home. Otherwise, residential care may be an essential option.

9. Sensory change — vision and hearing

Jennifer Gibbons

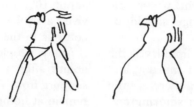

The previous chapter dealt with the calamity of 'stroke'; however, the slow and often insidious development of sensory loss, particularly dual loss of vision and hearing, is no less a calamity for those so affected. It is important to bear in mind the compounding effect of impairment in both of these vital senses, and the implications for an older person striving to function independently day by day. Individuals may find the problems so daunting that they become resigned to withdrawal from normal patterns of living, and in many cases families assume that such withdrawal is inevitable, and provide support as the person concerned becomes increasingly dependent.

The National Centre for Ageing and Sensory Loss was established in 1988 to promote the interests of those Australians who are experiencing or are at risk of incurring a sensory change as an outcome of the ageing process.

As has been stated previously, many more people are living to an advanced age in the developed countries of the world, and as people age the likelihood of change in vision and hearing increases significantly. Such changes vary in degree and do not necessarily create problems, because many people consciously or unconsciously develop ways to adapt and adjust to changes of this nature. Those who suffer impairment of both vision and hearing, however, are at risk of becoming isolated and dependent as such losses may have a negative impact on relationships and interpersonal communication.

Families and others concerned need to understand and to recognise signs that indicate change in vision and hearing so that they can assist an older person to effect adjustments aimed at compensating for such changes. It is important that the individual, as well as the family, is aware of the need to seek informed advice to prevent further loss, to determine the degree of the problem and to ensure the initiation of appropriate action.

There appears to be a lack of information in Australia as to how many people suffer significant

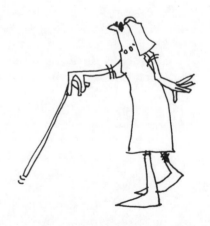

degrees of loss of both vision and hearing in the process of ageing. In a survey conducted in America (Kirchner 1985) it was reported that 87% of those who had a severe visual impairment and were 65 years of age and over also had hearing impairment.

Elderly people are at a disadvantage in that they lack experience with the modern technology which is available and of help to those who are younger, such as computers, teletype equipment, low vision aids, hearing aids and other devices. Old people are often unable to adjust to the use of modern technical aids and generally are not interested in learning sign language or braille. This presents a problem for families and others in their efforts to help individuals thus impaired to adjust and maintain their independence and every day activities.

The principal aim of this chapter is to address changes in vision and hearing. Many old people experience change in the other senses also — taste, touch and smell — which may affect their enjoyment of living.

VISUAL IMPAIRMENT

The common causes of visual impairment are:

- Age-related macular degeneration
- Cataract
- Diabetic vascular disease
- Glaucoma
- Retinal detachment.

Macular degeneration in various forms is the most common cause of the deterioration of vision in elderly people. A presenting feature is the distortion of vision, such as alterations in the depth of perception, the judgement of distance and the size of objects. Commonly, there is loss of reading ability, perception of colour and of vision in bright surroundings.

Degeneration usually progresses slowly and affects one eye some years before the other. Even when visual acuity is reduced to legally blind status, it is usual to retain limited mobility, as, for practical purposes, a degree of light perception remains.

Cataract can be defined as an opacity in the lens, which may or may not affect vision. There is a high prevalence of cataract in elderly diabetics, but surgery and the provision of a replacement lens may be effective.

Diabetic vascular disease may manifest itself as a transient, painless, third nerve palsy with complete recovery within 3 months, or diabetic retinopathy which is more common and more serious.

Glaucoma is characterised by increased intra-ocular pressure which may be heralded by haloes, disturbance of vision, eye ache, headache and vomiting. Urgent action is required to obtain expert ophthalmic advice.

Retinal detachment may occur in elderly people as in younger age groups, and may present with segmental or total visual loss in one eye, which is usually painless and rapid in onset. Immediate action is again required in seeking expert advice.

Signs of visual impairment

Changes can lead to:

- A decline in the management of business affairs
- Frequent dialling of wrong telephone numbers
- Loss of confidence in the use of household equipment
- Problems in locating items that have been moved

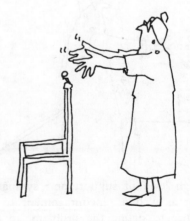

- Problems in walking, with hesitancy, stumbling, shuffling and bumping into furniture

- Deterioration of personal presentation, food stains on clothing and poor grooming
- A change in reading patterns — papers and books taken into bright light or held in unusual ways
- Requests for someone to read mail or address letters
- Change to radio rather than television or placement of a chair very close to the television screen
- Difficulty in focusing on small close objects, which may result in squinting to see things more clearly, while depth perception may have changed leading to accidents with broken glass and china, and serious falls related to steps, street curbs and uneven ground
- Reluctance to leave the house
- Declining to join in social outings
- Changes to shopping by ordering by telephone
- Requests for doctor to visit at home.

The social and emotional impact of visual impairment has been the subject of extensive research. Someone confronted suddenly with a high degree of vision loss may well feel shocked, angry, immobile, lonely and depressed. They will

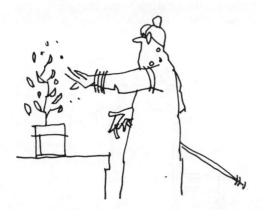

need a high level of support and sympathetic counselling as well as encouragement to seek expert advice to define the problem, to bring about all possible improvement and to assist in the restoration of an independent pattern of living.

Assessment

In seeking expert advice the first point of contact is usually the individual's general practitioner, who should carry out a medical examination that includes the eyes and ears. In the case of visual impairment, the patient should be referred to an ophthalmologist with a note describing the problem, relevant medical history and current medications.

Following assessment, the ophthalmologist should explain the findings to the person concerned, and, as appropriate, a family member, and should advise on the need for medical or surgical intervention, on the possible outcome, and on the assistance that is available to enable the maintenance of an independent pattern of living. Referral to a low vision clinic may well be the appropriate option.

Low vision clinic

A low vision clinic is an assessment and resource centre of considerable value to the visually impaired because access is ensured to expert knowledge and counselling, aimed at achieving the best possible use of residual vision.

The majority of those seeking the help of a low vision clinic are referred by an ophthalmologist. Others may be sent directly by optometrists and general practitioners for assessment by the clinic's ophthalmologist. Following such assessment they should be referred in turn to the clinic's coordinator of services, provided that their residual vision, however minimal, is sufficient for them to benefit.

Steps should be taken at this point to ensure that health problems other than vision are addressed and, where possible, remedied. For instance, those with impaired hearing should be seen by the audiologist, the aim being to maximise the use of residual hearing. Also, aspects of general health may require attention before addressing the problem of impaired vision.

The coordinator of services should invite newly referred people and supportive relatives to attend an information session at the clinic before joining, to enable them to gain insight into the programme and to gauge the value of the services offered.

The clinic should be staffed by a multidisciplinary team of health professionals, supported ably and effectively by groups of volunteers trained to assist in a number of areas. The professional team should include an ophthalmologist, to fully assess the eye condition and the degree of visual impairment, and an optometrist, who is responsible for the evaluation of the degree of sight remaining and, as appropriate, the prescription of low vision aids. These include:

- Spectacles to correct the deficits of eye focus and to reduce glare
- Telescopes to improve distance, intermediate and near vision
- Hand-held and stand magnifiers for near vision, some with built-in illumination
- Special purpose optical appliances designed for particular tasks
- Advice regarding 'non-optical' magnification such as closed circuit television
- Computer equipment modified to assist people in employment situations.

An optometrist needs additional post-basic training to work effectively in a low vision clinic. The problems of people with low vision are complex and varied, and require careful assessment and the precise prescription of appropriate aids to meet individual needs. Even magnifying glasses need to be prescribed if they are to be of optimal value to the person concerned. This applies equally to all the aids listed above.

Also required is an orthoptist, who is responsible for the training of people in the use of the low vision aids, both in the clinic and in the home situation; a welfare officer, who offers information and support for people coping with visual impairment (this service may extend to family and friends); a social worker who is in a position to counsel visually impaired people and their families and to advise them of benefits to which they could be entitled, of community resources and services and about programmes designed specially to assist the visually impaired; an audiologist, who assists those people with a hearing impairment; an occupational therapist, who is concerned with assessing the ability of people to function independently in the normal activities of daily living, and in devising the means or providing the aids to enable them to do so; and an orientation and mobility instructor, who assesses the needs of individuals and assists them to achieve an optimal level of safe independent mobility.

Coping strategies

Relatives and other close contacts need to be fully informed so that they are able to understand the most effective means of assisting someone with impaired vision to manage safely and independently.

Visitors to such a person's home should introduce themselves clearly, and ensure that the purpose of their visit is known. They should also seek the views of the individual as to his or her wishes and perception of need for assistance.

If help is offered and accepted within the house the sighted person should:

- Respect the order and location of personal possessions, furniture and household goods. If items need to be moved this should be done in conjunction with the person concerned, making sure he or she is in agreement with the need for change, and quite familiar with the relocation.
- Ensure that neither loose rugs or other objects are left free standing on the floor as these could cause tripping.

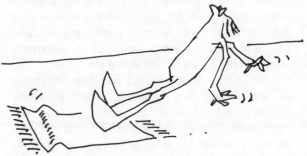

- Ensure that electrical flexes do not trail and that the plugs of kettles and other appliances are safe.
- Ensure that the room doors are left either wide open or closed and that doors of cupboards are closed.

These are general points with which relatives and friends can help, and it would be wise for them to suggest the installation of smoke detectors, as people with low vision and a possibly diminished sense of smell would be very vulnerable in the event of fire.

A visit to the home by an occupational therapist may be of help, also, as such therapists are trained to assist people to overcome disabilities; they are able to teach them to manage the normal activities of daily living by adapting the environment and providing them with appropriate aids.

Together with the person concerned the therapist may suggest the rearrangement of furniture to facilitate safety and ease of movement within living areas, bearing in mind the need for orientation and familiarisation. Advice may be given on the need for the installation of hand rails by steps or stairs, by bath and toilet, and the devising of means of making both the bathroom and kitchen safer. Non-slip mats are advisable in showers as well as in baths, and in homes where toilets are remote or inaccessible it may be possible to suggest the installation of a commode or chemical toilet in an appropriate location.

The edges of garden steps should be painted in a non-slip contrasting colour, and a simple hand rail installed.

Within the house the therapist may ensure that lighting is appropriate to the individual's needs, and well directed in working areas. The telephone is of major importance and the therapist should ensure visibility of the dial by fixing a white collar with large numbers around it, or placing tactile digits on press button phones, and marking the emergency digit ('0' in Australia) distinctively. The householder may be helped to prepare a personal telephone directory on whiteboard or a large pad, with important numbers printed in a size legible to the one concerned. This should be retained near the telephone. The need for an amplified phone may also be considered.

If the person living alone is frail, the installation of a personal emergency alarm system may be suggested as this enhances the feeling of safety. A number of good systems are available.

The kitchen is a high-risk area for people with loss of vision, but even more so if they have impairment of hearing and sense of smell. The therapist may introduce devices to enhance safety and give instruction in the use of aids.

Kitchen

- Tactile markers may be applied to the 'off' position of knobs on stoves
- Storage jars in pantries should be marked in a manner that makes them identifiable
- A range of devices can be provided to assist in the safe preparation and measurement of food
- Safe methods of boiling and pouring water can be taught
- Electronic devices can be made available to assist visually impaired people to pour the required amount of water into cups
- Use of new equipment, e.g. microwave ovens
- Talking scales

Toxic substances

Detergents and other toxic substances should be labelled in a manner suitable for clear identification by the visually impaired person and kept secure in a designated place.

Medications

It is important to:

- Ensure that labels with large print can be read by the individual, otherwise a tactile system recognisable to the one concerned should be applied to identify the content and instructions about use.
- Advise on the availability of special containers divided into compartments for times of day over 7 days. (Such containers may be filled by a local pharmacist, a community nurse, or by a competent family member.)
- Make known the availability of such aids as a 5 mL medicine measure, which can be obtained to replace the lid of a medicine bottle. The bottle is simply upturned and the tap turned to dispense exactly 5 mL of medicine into a receptacle.

Aids to writing

- Templates for completing or signing cheques
- Line frames to assist in letter writing
- Whiteboards and special markers

Aids to reading

Means of magnification have been mentioned previously. Advice could be given on the availability of closed circuit television systems that enable books or documents to be viewed at up to × 30 magnification of the print size.

In general terms the use of contrasting colours within a home can be of value. A simple example is the use of china which is of a colour that contrasts with the table cloth, thus helping to locate the position of the plates and cups.

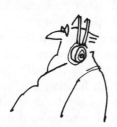

Interests and activities

Many people with impaired vision enjoy listening to the radio and have access to a wide range of programmes from music and drama to sport and world news.

One very important service provided by the Association for the Blind is the manning of special radio networks by volunteers who provide a service for the 'print handicapped' by broadcasting the content of newspapers, magazines and journals, and items of interest in a number of different languages.

Municipal libraries as well as resource centres provide access to a wide range of books in large print, to tapes and talking books, and even videos prepared specially for those with visual impairment. Some videos are of value to relatives and care givers as they assist in the understanding of problems of not only those who are blind or have impaired vision, but also of those with hearing loss and other disabilities.

Other information is available from organisations and resource centres concerning opportunities for recreation, sport and holidays for those who are visually impaired.

HEARING IMPAIRMENT

People, in general, are able to comprehend the effect of the loss of vision, and sympathise readily with those so impaired. Deafness, however, often gives rise to impatience and visible irritation with the one affected, and in some situations, such as in plays or so called comedy programmes it may be used as a subject for ridicule or to typify old age.

As with loss of vision, the onset of hearing impairment can be very gradual and older people often accommodate the loss by changing their behaviour. When a hearing loss becomes apparent the person concerned needs to be encouraged to seek advice. It is important to identify the cause, and where possible to prevent further loss. In some cases the ability to hear may be improved by medical treatment. For most hearing impaired people the use of hearing aids and devices provides great benefit.

Causes

The most common cause of increasing deafness in ageing people is presbyacusis (a sensorineural hearing loss), which does not respond to medical or surgical intervention.

According to Marshall (Warne & Prinsley 1988), it is estimated currently that approximately 40% of all individuals over the age of 65 years experience some degree of hearing impairment. At 65 years of age one person in three has a significant hearing impairment, while at 80 years of age the incidence increases to one person in two. Hull (1982) reported that as many as 80% of those who reside in nursing homes may experience hearing impairment of sufficient degree to interfere with communication.

Sensorineural hearing loss may reduce the older person's ability to hear high pitched sounds and to discriminate between consonants. Speech may well be heard as garbled and muffled.

Asymmetrical hearing impairment may cause difficulty in localising sounds. There may also exist a delay in the processing of speech, which means that the older person needs to be given time to respond to communication.

The negative impact of hearing loss may lead to feelings of loneliness, inadequacy and dependence. Relationships with others may be limited particularly in the areas of business, personal friendships and social contacts. Stone (1987) commented that 'Hearing impairment strikes at the very essence of being human because it hinders communication with others. It restricts the ability to be productive; it reduces constructive use of leisure time; it limits social intercourse; it affects physical and mental health; it often leads to poor self-image and to isolation and despair'.

Signs of hearing impairment

Changes in behaviour that may indicate a loss of hearing include:

- Loud speech resulting from an inability to hear one's own voice when speaking normally.
- The head being held in a position different from normal when the hearing loss is in one ear in an attempt to enhance the capacity to hear.

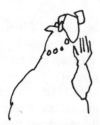

- A chair being moved in order to face the speaker to help lip reading, or the head being tilted towards people as they speak.

- The person concerned asking continually for comments to be repeated.
- Conversations or directions being met with a look of blankness or an inappropriate response indicating that the words were unheard or misunderstood.

The person concerned often notices the changes in ability to hear conversations in noisy environments such as restaurants and shopping centres. The individual may find it difficult to identify the source of a voice or to hear high pitched sounds, such as the ringing of the telephone. Such people may withdraw from social interaction due to embarrassment caused by their difficulty in hearing. They may organise their lives in a manner aimed at reducing the need to respond to others verbally. Relationships often become strained when communication is no longer warm and spontaneous.

Loss of hearing together with an impaired ability to concentrate may even lead relatives to mistake such changes as an early sign of dementia. With changes in hearing it is important that expert advice be sought to define the problem and to enable the discussion of possible options.

Assessment and rehabilitation

In Australia, following referral by a medical practitioner, veterans whose hearing problems may be attributed to service in the armed forces, and pensioners who have medical entitlement, may obtain hearing aids free of charge from the National Acoustic Laboratories. Such people may also obtain batteries and maintenance of their aids free of charge. People without such entitlement have to be referred to audiologists practising privately.

In either case, an audiologist would examine the individual and carry out tests to determine the degree and nature of the impairment, and would advise on the measures which may be taken. Where appropriate and if the individual is agreeable, arrangements may be made for attendance at a rehabilitation clinic. Such attendance enables assistance to be given with the aim of achieving the optimal use of residual hearing. The most suitable type of hearing aid and the need for other devices should be considered and pre-scribed after due consideration of the wishes of the person concerned. Advice should also be given verbally and in writing about the care, use and maintenance of hearing aids to ensure achievement of the best results possible.

Hearing aids

The design of hearing aids has improved mark-edly in recent years, but in deciding on the type to recommend it is necessary to consider the motivation, visual acuity and manual dexterity of the individual.

There are four basic types of aid all of which are composed of similar components: a micro-phone to convert sound into electrical energy; an amplifier to increase the electrical energy; a receiver to convert the energy into sound for delivery into the ear; and a battery to provide the power.

One type of aid, which has long been familiar, is the body aid. This consists of a small case worn on the chest to house the microphone, amplifier and battery. A cord attached to the case takes the amplified signal to the receiver. Such aids can be handled more easily by people with poor manual dexterity such as those with arthritis, or who suffer poor vision, because the controls are relatively large and more accessible. The microphone, however, can pick up unwanted noise from clothing and many find this type of aid unattractive.

A behind-the-ear aid is commonly used as is an in-the-ear aid. Both require finger dexterity as the on/off and volume control switches are very small.

One other type is incorporated in the frame of spectacles with the volume control in the arm of the frame. In this case it is necessary to keep a reserve pair of reading glasses on hand, as these are required when changing batteries or cleaning the ear mould of the aid.

It is important to encourage people to persist in the use of such aids, and to have realistic expectations of them. Following their initial introduction there is a need for regular review and adjustment by an audiologist, particularly during the first 6 months. It is also important

that a relative should attend these sessions to gain an understanding of the instructions given for the use and care of such aids, and to gain an appre-ciation of his or her own role in communication.

Hearing devices

There are many devices available which can assist people with hearing impairment whether they use hearing aids or not:

- Alerting devices to draw attention to a telephone or door bell ringing

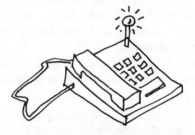

- Hearing devices to amplify sound for the listener linked with the telephone, radio or television set
- Audio loops for amplification at meetings or concerts.

The relatives or contacts of the person con-cerned need to learn how best to communicate and to help by encouraging the person to con-centrate and to listen.

Communication

People with hearing loss should be encouraged to be assertive and not to hesitate in advising con-tacts of their difficulty in hearing, and of the most effective means of establishing communication. Extraneous noise makes it very difficult for such a person to understand what is said, so it is best to talk on a one-to-one basis, to choose a quiet location, to sit face to face, and to allow time for the discussion of matters of concern or interest. The relative or carer needs to moderate the voice and enunciate words clearly and unhurriedly. The use of the individual's name prior to making an important statement stimulates interest and enhances attention. Relatives should be prepared to listen, to assist in resolving problems, and to ensure that points of importance are understood. In situations where there is doubt a notebook and pen should be used for clarification.

Coping strategies

Reference has been made to programmes of rehabilitation. The benefit of these is enhanced if a relative or close supporter of the one concerned is involved also in the programme.

The hearing impaired person can be taught to develop good listening habits, to understand the difference between hearing and listening, and to realise that although it may not be possible to improve one's hearing it is possible to improve the ability to listen.

Hearing can be enhanced by 'speech reading', which is defined by Marshall (Warne & Prinsley 1988) as:

the ability to gain visual information from the lips (lipreading) and also from facial expressions, gestures and a knowledge of the environment in which the conversation is taking place. As most hearing impaired people are able, with suitable amplification, to obtain some auditory input, the definition of speech reading can be expanded to include an ability to integrate auditory and visual information . . .

Such a person can also learn about strategies aimed at the manipulation of the listening environment to his or her best advantage. Consideration is given to where best to sit in a meeting, cinema or restaurant; how best to reply when unable to hear, and how to advise friends or contacts of the need for visual and auditory cues during conversation.

Those providing care for elderly people with loss of hearing need to understand the effect of such impairment and how best to reassure and communicate. In some situations a warm smile and clasp of the hand will do much to dispel unease.

DUAL IMPAIRMENT

Losses of vision and hearing have been addressed separately, however, a great many elderly people suffer losses in both of these vital senses, but loss in one area usually precedes the other. There appears to be a dearth of written material on this subject, and service programmes are not well developed to assist with the considerable difficulties faced by old people with dual sensory loss.

As the number of people suffering dual sensory impairment increases so does the need to develop services and expertise to assist in ameliorating the problems that ensue. The impact of loss of both vision and hearing is difficult to imagine as is the complexity of the experience for an older person.

It is very important that as specialist teams such as those working in low vision clinics and aural rehabilitation develop expertise, that their knowledge be shared, not only with families and volunteers, but with care givers in the community also, such as home helpers, district nurses and staff in day centres and residential care.

Community support services

Losses of hearing and vision limit access to information, and people suffering such loss need help to obtain the services they require. These include help with cooking, cleaning, home maintenance and gardening, as well as with personal care and grooming. A visiting nurse can advise on safety and maintenance of health and nutrition, as well as assisting with medications and personal hygiene. Volunteers can provide a valuable service by reading mail, writing letters and accompanying people to appointments or for the purpose of shopping.

Innovative services need to be developed to enable the increasing numbers of older people, many with loss of hearing and vision, to be supported safely and satisfactorily in the community.

Where there is general access to telephones the network can be used very effectively, not only for those with sensory loss, but for anyone living alone who is housebound and disabled.

Audio conferencing, a service provided by Telecom, was developed to facilitate group discussion between people in varied locations, often at great distance. It has been used extensively for business purposes and by the media. Eight years ago arrangements were made by the Association for the Blind to use the telephone link-up component to establish contact with and between groups of impaired people to enable them to interact with professional staff and each other on a regular basis.

Telelink increases the opportunity for such isolated people to have contact with others, to air matters of mutual concern and to establish emotionally supportive relationships. Many people cannot leave their homes without assistance, the cost of transport is high and many find such journeys physically and emotionally tiring. By engaging them in group work within their home environment, they can answer their telephones fresh, rested and free from visible disabilities. Many people with impaired hearing are able to participate in a Telelink group as there is no extraneous noise and the style of feedback provides additional support, through directed discussion, with clarification as necessary.

Such contact by professional staff, even on a once a week basis, can facilitate intervention when people seek support, and this can assist in preventing deterioration or the occurrence of a crisis situation. This manner of contact is reassuring to those concerned and helps individuals to resolve problems at their own pace, within their own home environment.

Telecare is a monitoring service which also provides social support. Many frail elderly people fear that they may become incapacitated alone and with no help at hand. This fear leads many to seek residential care. The certainty of knowing the telephone will ring once or twice a day is reassuring for the person concerned as well as for family members who live at a distance.

This service can range from a daily, 3 minute safety check call to a longer social call when news items can be discussed, medication reminders given and community activities suggested.

The arrangement basically is that volunteers at a central location make one call a day at a predetermined time to a number of people. If people know they will not be home to receive the call they are asked to inform the organiser. If the telephone rings more than 10 times without answer the call is repeated three times with intervals between. If there is no response, a routine checking procedure is followed: Telecom is asked to check the line; an agreed contact neighbour is asked to visit, and if unable to gain access contact is made with the local doctor to enquire about admission to hospital; if that fails the police are notified.

Personal emergency call systems are of great value for people alone and at risk and information about them is readily available.

Day centres

Special day centres with programmes to meet the needs of older people with loss of vision and/or hearing are of great value. They provide a break from care for relatives, and a change of environment and opportunities for social interaction and the learning of skills for the one attending.

Activities may include handcraft such as pottery, leatherwork, sewing, basketry, woodwork and fibrecraft; discussion groups and music; and cooking and gardening. Services may include assistance with personal care, podiatry and hairdressing and physiotherapy, occupational therapy and counselling.

Residential care

When people with significantly impaired vision and hearing require and seek supervised residential accommodation, relatives or those assisting with the transfer need to be aware of the impact such a move will have on the individual concerned. In assessing possible options consideration should be given to:

• Location and proximity to known community, relatives and friends.

• Design of building — whatever the total size it is desirable that such a home be divided into areas of domestic scale and design; is without steps and stairs; has special hand rails and floor surfaces that indicate location; makes use of contrasting colours of walls and doors; has appropriate lighting and acoustic ceilings; has provision for the use of Telecoil on hearing aids for meetings, television and radio, as well as space to install some personal possessions to enable the individual to identify personal space.

• Policy of the establishment. Residents should have freedom of choice concerning decisions that affect them, access to privacy and maximal independence. Visitors should have freedom to visit and to accompany residents on planned outings away from the home. Staff attitudes and an adequacy of provisions should enable appropriate support and care. Activity programmes should exist to provide an opportunity for social interaction, diversional activities and special interests. Spiritual well-being should be provided for by access to a priest or minister if desired.

It is important that people seeking accommodation be informed fully of the options or option and, if feasible, given an opportunity to visit to gauge their own feelings in the matter before a decision is made. In a new environment the individual is likely to feel detached and anxious, to lose motivation to communicate and to become disorientated. He or she may experience a deep sense of loss of privacy and control over life and become depressed. Following transfer there is a need for special support by relatives and care givers to assist in familiarisation with strange surroundings and an altered pattern of living.

REFERENCES

Davis H, Silverman S R 1970 Hearing and deafness. Holt, Rinehart & Winston, New York

Hull R H 1982 Rehabilitative audiology. Grune & Stratton, New York

Kirchner C 1985 Data on blindness and visual impairment in the U S: a resource manual on characteristics, education employment and service delivery. American Foundation for the Blind, New York

Luey H S, Belsner D, Glass L 1988 Beyond refuge: coping with losses of hearing and vision in late life. Helen Keller Centre for Deaf/Blind, Boston

Myklebust H R 1966 The psychology of deafness. Grune & Stratton, London

Stone H E 1987 Adjustment to post lingual learning loss. In: Kyle J G (ed) Adjustment to acquired learning loss: analysis, change and learning. Centre for Deaf Studies, Bristol, pp 102–104, 116

Warne R W, Prinsley D M (eds) 1988 A manual of geriatric care. Williams & Wilkins, Sydney

10. Psychiatric disorders in later life

Edmond Chiu

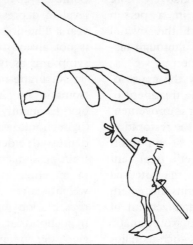

Psychiatric disorders are especially disturbing not only for the individual concerned, but also for close relatives and friends. In ageing people conditions such as depression can be treated effectively, as can the underlying causes of many states of acute confusion, but changes in personality and behaviour which develop insidiously over a long period of time, culminating in dementia, are quite devastating, particularly for a spouse who is also ageing.

Most elderly persons are basically psychiatrically well. Community surveys have identified about 25% of the elderly population as having a psychiatric disorder that warrants intervention. Dementia and depression are by far the most common disorders detected in such surveys but other organic and functional disorders are not uncommon. The behavioural manifestations frequently overshadow the less obvious features of psychiatric disorders, thus leading the observer to fail to investigate the presence of conditions that can be treated effectively. An understanding of such psychiatric disorders in later life will therefore assist management and achieve an improved quality of life for the elderly.

ORGANIC PSYCHIATRIC DISORDERS

Dementia

Dementia by itself is not essentially a psychiatric disorder unless the behavioural component of wandering, agitation and aggression becomes an obstacle to management. The majority of patients with dementia are cared for without the necessity of involving psychiatrists, non-medical psychiatric staff and psychiatric facilities. The management of such behavioural difficulties will be discussed later in this chapter.

Delirium (acute brain syndrome)

This is often misdiagnosed in hospitals and residential facilities. It can occur in between 9% and 25% of elderly patients in hospital. There are many causes of delirium but it develops commonly in those with underlying brain disease, various forms of infections, cardiac failure, drug and alcohol intoxication, endocrinological disorders and nutritional deficiencies. It is frequently mistaken for dementia as the symptoms of altered state of consciousness, decline in attention and concentration, impairment of recent memory, restlessness, confusion and behavioural disturbance are very similar to those indicating the onset of dementia. However, the relatively more abrupt onset of the condition in a person previously cognitively intact and the overall appearance of ill health warrants a thorough history taking and physical examination as well as laboratory investigation to identify the cause of such an acute brain syndrome. The treatment of the cause should lead to recovery or improvement in most patients with delirium and the restoration of normal living. However, the most important reason for investigation and energetic treatment of the physical cause of delirium is the potential for death to occur if the cause remains untreated.

During the state of delirium, management of the behavioural aspects requires symptomatic treatment with major tranquillisers such as haloperidol and thioridazine. However, these need to be used judiciously.

Organic psychosis

An organic delusional state can occur as a result of any assault on an ageing brain. Such a delusional state is frequently accompanied by hallucinations, more often visual than auditory, fearfulness, and aggressive behaviour consistent with reactions against delusional attacks. Organic psychosis is frequently associated with a mildly altered state of consciousness manifest through lowered concentration, attention and orientation. Such illnesses as head injuries, cerebral vascular lesions, endocrinological disturbances, electrolyte imbalance (particularly hyponatraemia), infections, and sometimes unspecified severe chronic pain, need to be investigated as possible aetiological factors. The psychosis usually settles when the basic organic aetiology is successfully treated. Symptomatic treatment of the delusional state is effected by the use of standard antipsychotic medication. Prognosis for organic psychosis is usually favourable. However, prevention of further episodes needs to be vigorously pursued by energetic management of the physical aetiological factors.

FUNCTIONAL PSYCHIATRIC DISORDERS

Depression

Some 15–20% of elderly people will suffer some level of depressive illness during their declining years. The presentation of such depressive illness is not always in line with the classical textbook symptoms as typified by the younger adult. The 'importuning behaviour', the preoccupation with 'somatic' or physical symptoms without pathology, frequently leads to a mistaken diagnosis of 'hypochondriasis' and 'hysterical behaviour'. The depressed elderly person, apart from suffering from pessimism, lower mood, lower activity, loss of appetite, insomnia, loss of interest, loss of weight, and constipation, has the additional presentation of increased somatic concern, hypochondriacal preoccupation and an exaggerated dependence on others. Such behaviour, which is out of context with the personality of the person, should alert the carer to a possible diagnosis of depression and the need for informed advice and treatment.

Treatment of the elderly person with depression varies from the usual strategy for the younger adult. Elderly persons do not tolerate the standard tricyclic antidepressants as well as the younger person. The anticholinergic side-effects of dry mouth, postural hypotension, tremors, sedation and confusion limit the use of most of the available tricyclic antidepressants. The problems of glaucoma and prostatomegaly are contraindications to their use. The coexistence of cardiac impairment in the elderly person is a further problem. Monoamine oxidase inhibitors (tranylcypromine), a newer tricyclic antidepressant, dothiepin, and doxepin have been shown to be useful. However, severely depressed elderly persons frequently require treatment with electroconvulsive therapy (ECT) which can produce dramatic and life saving results.

Attempted suicide by a depressed elderly person must be taken very seriously. The suicide rate among depressed elderly people is much higher than that of the general population. Any elderly person who has depressive mood, inappropriate feelings of guilt for past minor misdemeanours, ideas that he/she deserves to die and be punished by hell fire, and a general nihilistic attitude towards life, family and property should be assessed thoroughly for suicidal ideation, and the depression must be treated energetically. Suicide among the elderly is preventable if depression is diagnosed early and treated effectively.

Anxiety states

Apart from the environmentally induced anxiety in an elderly person whose mobility and participation in community life have been reduced, some elderly persons develop a chronic anxiety state with panic attacks and phobic symptoms. Although this is relatively uncommon, those who suffer such anxiety disorders must be diagnosed and treated. The proper differentiation between a normal person with environmental anxiety and a psychiatrically ill person with anxiety and phobic states depends very much on the vigilance of the observer who needs to recognise when such symptoms go beyond a normal reaction to the immediate environment.

Although unrestrained use of benzodiazepine drugs is to be avoided in the elderly, in those with anxiety state and phobic disorders the careful use of anti-anxiety agents of the benzodiazepine group can frequently restore the person to mental health and tranquillity. Psychotherapeutic treatment with behavioural and cognitive strategies is also extremely helpful and should be used in conjunction with pharmacological treatment.

Paranoid disorders in later life

Late onset paranoid disorders (paraphrenia) present with firmly fixed paranoid delusions of harm, burglary, assault by imaginary maleficent persons, or by relatives and neighbours. This behavioural change causes considerable problems for carers. No amount of persuasion or reassurance will alter the elderly person's complaint against those persons who are 'doing harm' to him/her. These people usually are in full possession of their faculties, with no evidence of any cognitive or personality change and apart from this isolated area of abnormality, they present as totally rational, reasonable and sensible individuals. The constant complaints to police, trusted relatives and neighbours, as well as regular letters to politicians and bureaucracies can lead to considerable social disruption and ill feeling.

Frequently, such persons refuse offers of help which they interpret as further evidence of interference in their lives and this reinforces their paranoid ideation. Enforced psychiatric treatment is often needed. They are usually non-compliant with antipsychotic medication and the use of depot injections of antipsychotic agents are often the only choice left in delivering effective treatment. They can cause considerable disruption to themselves, to their families, the neighbourhood and to community service agencies. For those who accept treatment, albeit reluctantly, the prognosis for return to some quality of life is quite good. Those who continue to be non-compliant with treatment remain a problem to the community.

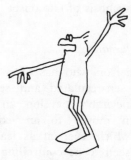

Behavioural disorders in elderly people

One of the most challenging issues in the extended care of elderly people is the understanding and management of what is frequently referred to as a 'behavioural problem'. This label, more often than not, places the elderly person in a situation of gross disadvantage by virtue of the negative connotation inherent in such a description. In the context of the provision of care a person with a behavioural problem is seen as too much trouble and upsetting to others. Adverse reactions that may be aroused in the community can lead to these people being branded as 'aggressive, disruptive, attention seeking, uncooperative and difficult'. In general they do not fit in well with the desirable, well ordered environment of peace and tranquillity, or the trouble-free nature of an ideal home or extended care facility.

Therefore, in order to provide the best quality of life to such people, and the carers and others who live with them, a basic understanding of behaviour manifestations in this context, the effect such behaviour has on others and the management strategies that can be adopted are crucial.

Major causes of 'behavioural' disorders

1. Adjustment disturbances
2. Exaggeration of previous personality traits
3. Acute brain syndromes (delirium)
4. Dementing processes — especially frontal lobe impairment
5. Depression
6. Organic psychosis
7. Paranoid psychosis of late onset

Adjustment disturbances

The elderly person who has been living in an independent, self-regulated and self-controlled home, will inevitably develop an adjustment reaction when moved to an extended care environment which, even at its least restrictive best, will be seen to be controlling and dependency producing.

The previously passive dependent personalities will adjust well to such a change and will be seen as 'nice', 'good', 'well settled' persons. Those who have been fiercely independent will behave in such a way as to present as 'difficult' or 'demanding'. Their need for privacy and control over their own daily lives will frequently be in conflict with the 'good order' and regulated peace expected of a 'good facility'. Personality conflicts between the elderly person and staff lead to constant power struggles which further escalate disturbances and increase intransigence in both parties.

Experienced and sensitive staff have, over time, learned how to negotiate and compromise without seeming to be either 'pandering' or 'inflexible'. The narrow road of 'give and take' is an extremely delicate and difficult one to travel.

Exaggeration of previous personality traits

Commonly observed in elderly people is the exaggeration of previous 'not so nice' personality traits till they may become a source of behaviour problems. In some elderly persons the 'nice' traits are retained, but are frequently overshadowed by 'the nasty bits'. This is aggravated by any brain impairment, whether it be a dementing process, cerebral vascular lesion or toxic brain syndrome.

An understanding of the premorbid personality traits by taking a history with care from available relatives is essential. This is to enable previous 'nice' traits to be enhanced while at the same time developing strategies to deal with the problems expressed. Frequently, relatives will be able to pass on strategies that have proved successful and suggest new methods and solutions.

Acute brain syndrome (delirium)

The most common cause of sudden behavioural change in the elderly is the development of an acute brain syndrome. The combination of sudden behavioural change with delirium, confusion and general deterioration of function should alert the carer to the possibility of an acute brain syndrome, with common causes of infection, transient ischaemia attacks, polypharmacy, inappropriate compliance, physiological changes due to the intercurrent illnesses and interaction with over-the-counter preparations.

Dementing processes

The death of neurones in a dementing process produces increasing levels of confusion and functional deterioration. These by themselves do not always lead to problematic patterns of behaviour. However, when the frontal lobes are significantly affected, the consequential behaviour may create very real problems.

Behaviour consequent upon frontal lobe impairment. The actual impairments listed below are commonly viewed in a negative manner, and the behaviour resulting from such impairment can readily be misinterpreted and thus produce hostile reactions in staff and family carers.

- Disinhibition of social/sexual behaviour
- Lack of social judgement and appropriateness
- Apathy and volitional loss
- Emotional incontinence or labile affect
- Irritability with aggressiveness
- Urinary incontinence
- Inability to plan, sequence and change sets
- Perseverative incoherent talk

In elderly persons whose premorbid personality was that of a 'nice' person, the change to this level of function carries further difficulty with carers who remember the person as he/she was and the comparison is thereby much more painful and hard to accept.

Depression

Frequently the presenting symptoms of depression, particularly that of hypochondriacal concern and importuning behaviour, are mistaken as behavioural problems. The proper identification of depressive illness and its subsequent treatment will remove this problem and potential misinterpretation.

Organic psychosis

The delusional state with the accompanying behavioural response to hallucinations and the fear of harm, can produce very aggressive actions against others. Therefore, it is important to identify such delusional states of organic origin, and to treat actively the cause of the behavioural change.

Paranoid disorders of late onset

Such persons are difficult to manage if general persuasion and cajoling fails to succeed in obtaining cooperation with treatment. Frequently, it becomes necessary to undertake involuntary treatment. In some patients, where behaviour is not disruptive to health, safety and community good order, it may be appropriate to leave well

alone and to provide whatever community support services are acceptable to that individual.

Because an elderly incontinent person may be a high-risk candidate for nursing home admission it is essential to monitor progress carefully and on a continuing basis to prevent relapse and avoidable dependency.

MANAGEMENT ISSUES

- What is the problem?
- Who has the problem?
- Who needs treatment?

To select appropriate management strategies to deal with behavioural disorders in the elderly it is necessary to address the above questions. It must not be assumed that the 'patient' is the answer to all three questions. More often than not the patient is only part of the problem. The answers to these three questions include the patient, the carer, the extended care community and the environment of extended care. Above all, the basic attitudes of everyone in the extended care community play a crucial role in developing appropriate, successful strategies which enhance the quality of life for all without detracting from the autonomy and dignity of everyone involved.

Attitude management

Any existing negative stereotypes towards the elderly will be reinforced when confronted with behavioural problems. This will inevitably exacerbate any difficulties in an extended care environment with perpetuation of such negative interaction between the carers and the elderly. Such an unhelpful environment will create a vicious circle of negative reinforcement on both sides. Therefore, the establishment of a *positive non-judgemental and accepting atmosphere* will be central to any specific management strategies to deal with such behavioural disorders. This must be underpinned by intelligent cognitive understanding of the psychological, social and physical bases of behaviour disorder which can only be achieved through understanding and sympathy on the part of the carers.

Management of physical environment

With most behavioural disorders attention to the adaptation of the environment through a simple commonsense approach can bring many benefits to the elderly person concerned. Colour schemes, using simple uncomplicated visual cues assisted by contrasting colour coding of functional areas, and bright well lit rooms, can reduce the level of confusion and disorientation. Spaciousness, allowing people 'room to move' and more than adequate 'personal space' between each other will assist in the reduction of aggressive behaviour. Sound-proofing and dampening of noise by soft furnishings as well as designing rooms with minimum echo effect can contribute to less irritating noise. Provision of well appointed 'quiet areas' where aggressive and noisy persons may be temporarily separated from others will reduce the 'mass effects' of one person's behaviour causing others to react negatively in a chain reaction. Such a quiet area can also be useful in managing those persons with 'twilight syndrome' (the diurnal, evening disturbances of behaviour often found in persons with brain impairment) and 'sleep-reversal'. Era-appropriate furnishings and designs for the elderly enhance familiarity and stability as against feelings of strangeness and unease in an environment of modern design. The range of environmental adaptation for older people with behaviour disorders is limited only by the common sense of the carers and the sense of innovation and resourcefulness. The advice of intelligent and practical-minded, well elderly people should be sought. The management of wandering by well designed functional and visually appealing landscaping such as the use of fast growing shrubs as environmentally appropriate safety barriers can enhance the quality of life as well as managing unsafe behaviour.

Pharmacological management

When the cause of the behavioural problems has been identified as of a 'medical' aetiology, the appropriate use of medication should be vigorously pursued in those conditions in which pharmacological treatment has demonstrated a good response. The treatment of depressive illness with antidepressants (e.g. dothiepin, tranylcypromine) and psychosis with antipsychotics (e.g. haloperidol, thioridazine) has restored many elderly persons to a better quality of life. In severe depressive illness, ECT has been life-saving in some persons and in others restored the joy of living. In acute brain syndromes, apart from using tranquillisers to manage the acute behavioural disturbance (e.g. haloperidol, lorazepam, chlormethiazole), medication should be used very carefully and judiciously. Noctural agitation often responds to chlormethiazole, the twilight syndrome can be effectively managed by using thioridazine at about 4.00 p.m. in anticipation of the behaviour. The use of lorazepam, a short-acting benzodiazepine for daytime agitation, has been found to be helpful. For behavioural disorders with more social and psychological components, medication should only be used as a last resort, if at all.

Social management

Attitudes to the social environment of any elderly person suffering behavioural disorder, in combination with management of the physical environment, can enhance improved relationships despite the behavioural disorder. Social interaction based on mutual respect, trust, understanding and acceptance will provide a firm basis for positive response from the behaviourally disturbed elderly person even in the presence of gross impairment of cognitive and intellectual function. Even the most severely affected dementia sufferers will respond to human warmth, expressions of care and the explicit demonstration of 'tender loving care'. On the opposite side, non-acceptance and negative attitudes will be perceived, recognised and a negative response generated, which will result in a vicious circle of mutual dislike and discord. The maintenance and enhancement of a positive social environment surrounding the elderly behaviourally disturbed person must hold a high priority in developing strategies of care.

Psychological/behavioural therapy

In many extended care facilities, the use of behavioural therapy techniques has been introduced. Such techniques have good results when practised with a positive attitude in a caring social environment of unconditional positive regard. Punitive strategies have no place in behavioural therapy, which should deploy repeated positive reinforcement as its central operational style. Behaviours that are socially unacceptable because of the effect on other elderly persons and because of their intrinsic maladaptive or unsafe characteristics should be handled with an attitude of caring, albeit without any positive emotional feedback (but *not* negative emotions). On the contrary, socially contributory behaviours are reinforced by very positive emotional responses so that they are encouraged to continue towards positive behaviour. At no time should the elderly person be treated as a child, in anyway infantilised nor patronised because of his/her behaviour. The carer must look behind the behaviour to see a person to be dignified by being treated with the maximum measure of human warmth and positive regard.

Caring for the carers

When the problem belongs to the care providers and they are in need of treatment, then this should also be pursued, vigorously. It is of little benefit to the elderly if the care providers are not given appropriate care. In order to do this the care providers need to be supported, encouraged and helped by:

- Attitudinal change and review
- Knowledge and understanding
- Adaptable working environment
- Support networks
- Affirmation and challenge
- Participation and contribution.

The care providers, under the strain of caring for behaviourially disturbed elderly persons, are constantly challenged by such behaviour to review their attitudes towards the individual as well as the elderly as a group. Such review should be encouraged and facilitated by me. practical administrative and educati available in each extended care envirc unsupported review by a carer of his attitudes often leads to guilt, depres and demoralisation with resultant burn-out. The regular update of knowledge based on advances in medical and social sciences and psychology as applied to the elderly will provide a wider and wiser base for innovative caring strategies and help each carer to reach a deeper understanding of the elderly person's behaviour. An adaptable, flexible and sensitive working environment which takes due note of each carer's personal and psychological needs will produce a sense of being valued. A wide support network outside the framework of the extended care environment, i.e. in the carer's personal and social life, will provide the opportunity for 'recharging batteries', learning about life, growing as an individual and bringing to the caring task knowledge, experience and wisdom so gained. Affirmation of the caring task well done with gentle supportive challenge to do better will enhance self-esteem. The warm inner glow can be a very motivating drive for the carer. The opportunity to participate and contribute in the development of strategies for caring which are derived from the above experience, when added together, will generate a large mass of information to enable better care for elderly people. Therefore, caring for the carers will bring not only better morale, but improved quality of life for the elderly person concerned.

Conclusions

Behaviourally disturbed elderly people are currently seen in a very negative light. A change of attitude is needed to provide them with better quality of care and improved quality of life. The carers need to be able to identify the causes of such behavioural expressions and provide specific and general management strategies. This requires knowledge, understanding and experience in the delivery of care. Further, carers should be stimulated by themselves being cared for and challenged to bring to their caring task wisdom, sensitivity and innovation.

11. Assessment

Bernard Worsam

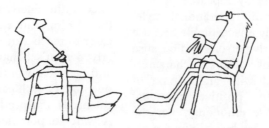

Perceptive and informed medical and psycho-social assessment is the *vital* factor in planning appropriate action when any person, particularly one who is elderly, presents with a health problem, or seeks assistance.

Assessment (and periodic review) is, therefore, the keystone in enabling provision of an effective ongoing health service for the elderly and other disabled people.

THE NEED FOR ASSESSMENT OF AGED AND DISABLED PEOPLE

Those elderly people who retain independence only with difficulty, or who lose independence in some areas of functioning, can generally be shown to have more than one active disease process. Common serious disease processes are: heart disease, cerebrovascular disease, malignancy, arthritis, diabetes, depression, delirium and dementia. These and other disease processes are likely to produce multiple disabilities, and such combined disabilities may then exceed the individual's ability to compensate, leading to dependency on others for help.

While most elderly people remain independent, those with serious disabilities place a major strain on relatives and friends, and tax the resources of health and welfare providers. Adverse social factors contribute to reduce independence, but disproportionately in those with physical and mental disabilities. Conversely, the minor changes of normal ageing seldom produce a significant contribution to dependency.

Disabled and dependent elderly people are 'recycled' by general hospitals, geriatric centres, nursing homes, local doctors and other community agencies and welfare services. Despite extensive involvement with care agencies, it is common that no comprehensive plan of management is made. Instead, each agency may make a diagnosis and initiate a treatment plan in isolation and with little subsequent sharing of information. While this problem of fragmentation of care is obvious in the general hospital–geriatric centre–nursing home sequence, it is still more a difficulty in the area of community care. Here, the effects of fragmentation of care are often hidden, but are of bewildering complexity and likely to defeat all attempts at consistent and rational care. The many components of domiciliary care are often provided by autonomous agencies who may have no functional links with local doctors, general hospitals, geriatric centres or welfare agencies. Where 'non-integrated' patterns of care prevail, each component of domiciliary care makes a diagnosis centred on the service requested, rather than on the patient's total needs, disease processes, prognosis and likely outcome. The slender information of a medical nature provided to the domiciliary service in a referral letter is unlikely to provide any functional information or general care plan.

Dependent or potentially dependent disabled elderly people often need the opportunity to have disabilities reduced and independence maximised through a programme of restorative care. This may be provided at home, through day care or through a restorative care (rehabilitation) ward. Full diagnostic information must be obtained to direct such activity, and both an immediate and continuing care plan formulated. This central pool of information can then be drawn upon by other involved agencies. The extent of incoordination of care may be reduced by such a system without threatening the independence of the agencies involved. A variety of approaches have been described as effective (Atkinson & Curran 1988, Hendriksen et al 1984, Mold et al 1987).

PRINCIPLES OF ASSESSMENT

Even though diagnosis is fundamental to offering care, the scope of diagnostic interest is often narrow; diagnostic effort may be solely directed to identification of the current new pathological problem. Even when continuing or past disease problems are acknowledged, there may be no attention given to describing the functional effects of those diseases present. Further, the critically important social accompaniments of disease and functional loss may be overlooked. The term 'assessment' is now widely used as a description of a particular type of diagnosis, where disease identification (with its underlying pathology and aetiology) is added to by a measurement of functional loss, and evaluation of social factors. Whichever term is preferred — diagnosis or assessment — the key issue is not the name but the underlying principles and methods.

When the clinical methods of diagnosis are applied to short-term illness, Occam's razor — looking for the best single reason for the abnormalities recognised — is usually effective. The process is disease–organ–system-oriented, the time scale is short and relates to immediate needs, and the process generally involves one observer acting in a 'medical' way.

The elderly and others with continuing disabilities fit this diagnostic approach poorly because social problems, multiple diseases and the effects of normal ageing are commonly present. Even 'inactive' diseases may continue to produce the limitation of function we call disability. As has been pointed out (Dornhorst 1981), the important question is not 'What shall we call it?' but, instead, 'What is going on?'. A functional assessment to determine what is going on must cover physical, mental, social and environmental aspects. The tunnel vision imposed by using a 'presenting complaint' as the focus of review must be discarded in favour of a more comprehensive approach.

A holistic orientation will ensure that the evaluation is made against the background of the patient's lifestyle, understanding, life view and expectations. The data that are sought should take into account ongoing needs as much as immediate ones. Clearly, such a broad process of diagnosis demands some type of multidisciplinary approach. Indeed, social aspects are likely to be quite as important as medical ones, and the diagnosis may need to be expressed in terms of 'disturbed social functioning' as well as disturbed anatomy and physiology.

Such an assessment is general rather than specific: it relates to no one problem in isolation, takes a broad view of the patient's functioning, and is not confined to any one health care discipline.

Purpose

The purpose of assessment is to establish a knowledge base that will allow effective and fully appropriate care — care which answers the patient's real needs. Active and specific treatment may be required for some problems, but for others, more general supportive care. Treatment, both active and supportive, may be delivered by doctors, nurses, therapists, social workers, relatives or community workers. Whatever the treatment or care programme, it will be directed toward an improvement in function, i.e. improved independence and quality of life. Specific goals of treatment can be set since the database should allow a treatment programme that is precisely tailored to the person's needs. The client's own goals and expectations are best incorporated in the plan when assessment information and a knowledge of available care resources are appropriately presented; only then can real choice be exercised. It is important that the client has opportunity to make full use of the remaining capabilities; only as an active participant is the person able to gain full advantage from the assessment.

Process

By enquiry, observation (including physical examination) and measurement, assessment data are collected (often over a period of time and in a number of contacts) and then brought together into some type of construction. Adequate data, correctly interpreted, will give a picture of the patient's disabilities and capabilities, dependency, the reasons for functional change, and some idea of likely progress — a prognosis. Because functional information is so important, some tests of performance will generally be part of the assessment: examples are a mental function test and examination of gait. Many measurement tools have been described (Dickinson & Young 1990, Applegate et al 1990, Wade & Collin 1988). The use of 'disability language' (Lefroy 1980) has been promoted as a tool to improve analysis, planning and care by focusing on both disabilities and capabilities.

Problem definition is the very basis for correct intervention and must precede action; the initial action will be to set realistic goals for care and formulate a beginning plan of care. In all this activity, it is essential that reversible factors — medical and non-medical — are identified and treated; a positive approach should also be made to irreversible change which can often be controlled and accommodated with a well-judged approach.

Diagnosis is made difficult by the complex nature of abnormality present; for the doctor, insidious onset, atypical disease patterns, and the presence of deafness and confusion all reduce diagnostic accuracy (Berman et al 1987, McCallion et al 1987, Wroblewski et al 1986, Day et al 1987, Puxty & Andrews 1986).

Method

Although an assessment team may be established with a separate identity, it is more appropriate for the team to be the mobile arm of a comprehensive geriatric service. In either case, assessment staff carrying regional responsibility for care of the disabled aged provide a consultant service to the primary referring agent, usually the client's own doctor. Although the team is in some way limited by using a medical entry point, it is common for the client, relatives or staff of community agencies to participate in initiating the referral.

The primary team may include a consultant physician in geriatric medicine, social worker, nurse, occupational therapist and physiotherapist. Sometimes a psychiatrist and community psychiatric nurse will be members of the team; alternatively, a parallel psychiatric assessment team may exist.

Other team members, who are involved by referral from members of the primary team, include the speech pathologist, podiatrist, dietitian and psychologist. The team should be based at a hospital with investigation, day hospital and inpatient facilities, and the team should have access to (and preferably responsibility for) day hospital places and hospital beds for continuing assessment of the client with complex problems, general medical care and rehabilitation. The team should also have links or appointments to suitable community bases such as community health centres, and, where facilities are separate, an established relationship with the area psychiatric service.

Wherever possible, assessment should be made in the patient's own environment, and in a way that allows the patient to exert some control over the process. (Assessment of the actual home environment is dealt with in detail in Chapter 15). While the maxim 'better diagnosis equals better care' is a useful guide, an extensive 'routine' assessment that is imposed on the person may be so disruptive as to produce disability and damage. Part of the philosophy of assessment is that minimum well judged intervention be used. For this to be possible, senior staff are very much to be preferred to junior 'assessment officers'. The judgement and experience of senior staff will often allow an adequate database for goal-setting and initiation of care, without the client being serially assessed by many staff or shifted from the home. Care should be taken to enlist the client as a full participant in the assessment and care process (Hayman & Howe 1988).

The assessment team cannot be effective if it is so closely tied to one agency as to only have on offer those resources managed by that agency. It is essential that the assessment staff present advice regarding care which is related to the full range of community resources. If a team is limited to giving 'one agency' answers, the options put forward may only relate, for example, to residential care.

Consistent with the consultative process, the assessment staff must report to the local doctor. Involvement of the local doctor in the care plan should be mandatory; it is desirable that some members of the assessment team also act as part of the inpatient and day hospital treatment team. Flexibility of approach can be maintained by using an 'overlapping' team model, good communication, and an adequate resource base for the team. Communication should extend to the patient, relatives and the staff of other agencies involved.

Occasions for assessment

When should people be assessed? Comprehensive diagnosis is likely to be of special benefit when applied to certain 'at risk' people who are still living in their own home: those who are 'failing to thrive' or whose relatives are coping with difficulty; those, who have an abrupt change in social circumstances; and those who have a variety of 'risk events'. Such risk events are: repeated falls, episodes of despondency, reduced mobility, episodes of confusion, episodes of giddiness on standing and episodes of incontinence. Those who have major events such as stroke or hip fracture should also be assessed, as formal restorative care is almost certainly indicated and underlying provoking conditions may be exposed. Partly-dependent people discharged home from general

hospitals after episodes of general disease are at particular risk.

Whenever a change of accommodation is suggested, particularly toward institutional living, assessment should be mandatory (Brocklehurst et al 1978, Rafferty et al 1987, Kalra & Foster 1989). When long-stay care in a nursing home appears necessary, assessment brings a variety of benefits (Golding et al 1987, Lazarus & Gray 1988). Diagnostic intervention should not be delayed until there is a crisis; a preventive approach should be taken.

Providers of community support such as home help will often recognise clients with general needs, or who are showing evidence of failing mental state or failure to thrive. Such service providers will be aware if multiple drug therapy is being used, or if sedative or other psychotropic drugs are being used in quantity. Dependent 'at risk' clients so exposed should be referred with their knowledge and agreement to the assessment staff of a geriatric service for comprehensive diagnosis.

Staff of community care agencies, in undertaking assessment of their own clients, apply similar skills, philosophy and methods. However, 'service-specific assessment' is a limited and special type of assessment rather different from general assessment, when the outcome is more open. Such service-specific assessment is best applied when it is related to the general assessment process, and not used as an alternative.

Outcome of assessment

The outcome of a general assessment programme will be a rationalisation of health and welfare activities for the aged and disabled; in particular, duplication of diagnosis and care should be reduced. More effective use should be made of general practitioner services, general hospitals, rehabilitation wards, day hospitals, domiciliary and other supportive care, welfare services and voluntary care. Studies have shown that careful assessment will uncover much unreported and undiagnosed disease — and will also identify many non-medical problems because of its nursing, social work and paramedical components (Jonsson & Halldorsson 1981). Openings for preventive care are exposed and unnecessary disability avoided. General practitioner and non-medical community resources should be made more effective, both because of better understanding of the needs of the client and because of the entry to wider resources which are advised or provided by the assessment staff and their backing geriatric service and hospital.

COMPONENTS OF AN EXTENDED CARE SERVICE

Patient assessment is of limited value unless there is access to appropriate solutions. Short-term admission to an acute general or psychiatric hospital, rehabilitation or treatment on an in-patient or day hospital basis, care at home with the support of domiciliary nursing or community welfare services, and short- or long-term care in hostel or nursing home are often required.

It is essential that the use of such services and facilities be on the basis that they meet individual need and are accessible, available, and appropriate and that their use is coordinated.

As previously suggested, it is important that there be a central pool of information. It is also essential to have effective liaison between the assessment team and the general practitioner, family and other carers; this liaison activity may be undertaken by assessment team members, the

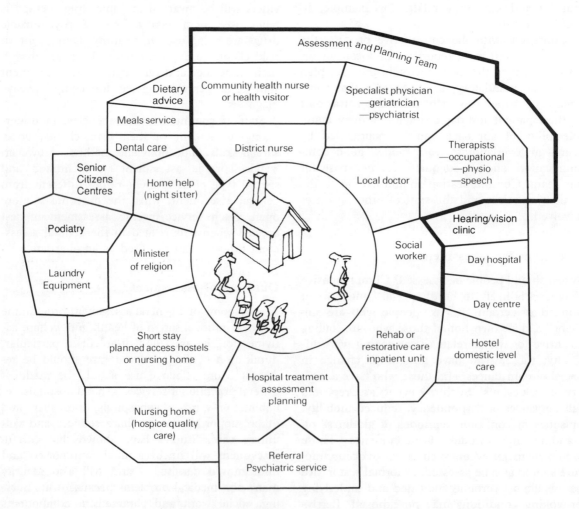

Fig. 11.1 Components of an extended care service.

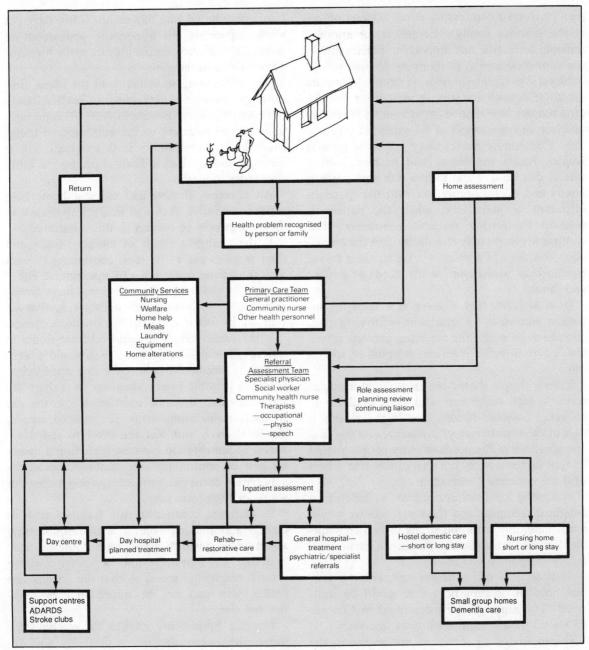

Fig. 11.2 Range of options required following patient assessment.

general practitioner, community nurse, social worker or health visitor. It is also vital that the needs of the client are reassessed on a continuing basis so that changing needs are recognised and met.

Figure 11.1 shows the components of the service and Figure 11.2 the range of options required in a system of extended care. The interrelationship of these components, and the importance of their availability in ensuring adequate and appropriate action, needs elaboration.

The first point of referral when a health problem occurs is usually the general practitioner, who may have been alerted to the need for help by a concerned community nurse, welfare officer or the person's family. The general practitioner remains an active and important participant in the care programme, in its many phases.

Nurses, in their various roles from community health or domiciliary nursing to acute or psychiatric nursing intervention, treatment and care, are involved in every aspect of the extended care system. Community nurses carry out an important liaison, health promotion and problem-solving role in this context and form a link with patient, family and doctor, as well as with the specialist physician or geriatrician when the patient is referred for further medical assessment. The community nurse may also draw upon the knowledge and skills of a social worker to assist in the psychosocial assessment of the needs of patient and family.

It is desirable that if there is a need for inpatient admission for treatment or investigation, admission be under the assessing geriatric physician's care in either a general hospital or special unit.

Elderly people should not be isolated from the services, high technology and skills available in an acute hospital. Health care of the elderly is part of the mainstream of medicine, and the special approach to the needs of older people should be well understood by doctors, nurses and others who are concerned with their care.

Following inpatient assessment, in which paramedical therapists and the social worker would participate, problems and strengths can be identified, and plans made for treatment, restoration and/or supportive continuing care.

Transfer to a rehabilitation unit within a general hospital or geriatric centre could be indicated. The range of skills described in Chapter 13 would then be drawn upon as necessary.

Depending on the extent of improvement, the support available and wishes of the old person, a decision is made whether discharge home, with access to the services shown in Figure 11.1, is appropriate. It may be necessary for the patient to continue with a treatment programme in a day hospital which is staffed with similar therapists to those of the rehabilitation unit. Attendance from

home may be on one day or up to five days per week depending on a periodic assessment of need. Alternatively, a plan may be made for some form of residential care.

The continuing surveillance of the home situation by the community nurse in his/her liaison and, as necessary, treatment role, is important, as is the involvement of the occupational therapist whose responsibility it is to create a safe environment in which a disabled person can function independently.

An effective, flexible and efficient home help service is another factor of major importance in assisting people to remain in the community.

If the changing needs of elderly people and their families are to be met, continuing contact with the liaison nurse must be maintained, either directly or indirectly, through home help, family member or meals-on-wheels deliverer, so that action can be initiated should the situation change.

If the anxiety is to be removed from frailty in old age, it must be possible to give old people and their families an assurance that appropriate action is possible in any situation. It is therefore important that there be coordination in the use of the various components of extended care at the local level, and that the involved staff have access to appropriate services, including a hospital bed or continuing care facilities, hostel for supervised domestic care, or nursing home for short- or long-term care.

In planning continuing care facilities such as hostels and nursing homes, it is desirable that attention be given to achieving a domestic scale in design, and that these units be scattered within normal residential areas, so that old friends can readily visit and not be intimidated by institutional size.

Nursing home care should be reserved for those with irreversible major disability and dependency, and with careful assessment and planned use of such facilities, excessive provision can be avoided. There is a need for flexibility of use, such as shared care with families through short-term planned admissions, to enable the same quality of support and care in the terminal period as is described in Chapter 18.

Conclusion

Better diagnosis is the only way to bridge the gulf that exists between average practice and high quality care for those who are elderly and disabled.

The provision of available, high standard assessment presents many challenges. Some of the issues are: funding, staff training, confidentiality, team relationships, relationships with community agencies, general practitioners and hospitals, and even such practical matters as the written form of assessment.

It is important that assessment is not seen as an alternative to a medical approach, and that any assessment includes a serious medical diagnostic component. Reversible disease must be identified, or any care offered will be deficient. The whole process of assessment must be a disciplined one, in which methods appropriate to local circumstances and resources are used.

REFERENCES

Applegate W B, Blass J P, Williams T F 1990 Instruments for the functional assessment of older patients. New England Journal of Medicine 322: 1207–1213

Atkinson R, Curran J T 1988 The geriatric assessment project in Tasmania. Australian Journal on Ageing 7: 21–24

Berman P, Hogan D B, Fox R A 1987 The atypical presentation of infection in old age. Age and Ageing 16: 201–207

Brocklehurst J C, Carty M H, Leeming J T, Robinson J M 1978 Medical screening of old people accepted for residential care. Lancet ii: 141–143

Caird F I, Judge T G 1979 Assessment of the elderly patient, 2nd edn. Pitman Medical, London

Day J J, Bayer A J, Pathy M S J, Chadha J S 1987 Acute myocardial infarction: diagnostic differences and outcome in advanced old age. Age and Ageing 16: 239–243

Dickinson E J, Young A 1990 Framework for medical assessment of functional performance. Lancet 335: 778–779

Dornhorst A C 1981 Information overload: why medical education needs a shake-up. Lancet ii: 513–514

Gallo J J, Reichel W, Andersen L 1988 Handbook of geriatric assessment. Aspen, Rockville

Golding R, Lugon M, Hodkinson H M 1987 Confirming long-stay status. Age and Ageing 16: 13–18

Hayman A, Howe A 1988 Client participation and advocacy in geriatric assessment. Australian Journal on Ageing 7: 15–23

Hendriksen C, Lund E, Stromgard E 1984 Consequences of assessment and intervention among elderly people: a three year randomised controlled trial. British Medical Journal 289: 1522–1524

Jonsson A, Halldorsson T 1981 Domiciliary assessment of geriatric patients in Reykjavik. Gerontology 27: 89–93

Kalra L, Foster C J 1989 Multidisciplinary assessment of applicants for sheltered housing. Age and Ageing 18: 271–274

Kane R A, Kane R L 1981 Assessing the elderly. Lexington Books, Lexington

Lazarus R, Gray L 1988 Clinical characteristics and outcomes in a cohort of patients who were assessed as in need of nursing-home care. Medical Journal of Australia 149: 410–415

Lefroy R B 1980 Assessment of disabilities. Medical Journal of Australia 1: 635–636

McCallion J, Canning G P, Knight P V, McCallion J S 1987 Acute appendicitis in the elderly: a 5-year retrospective study. Age and Ageing 16: 256–260

Mold J W, Steinbauer J R, Wunder S C, Small B 1987 outpatient multidisciplinary geriatric assessment I. Journal of Oklahoma State Medical Association 80: 367–371

Puxty J A H, Andrews K 1986 The role of chest radiography in the evaluation of the 'geriatric giants'. Age and Ageing 15: 174–176

Rafferty J, Smith R G, Williamson J 1987 Medical assessment of elderly persons prior to a move to residential care: a review of seven years' experience in Edinburgh. Age and Ageing 16: 10–12

Wade D T, Collin C 1988 The Barthel ADL index: a standard measure of physical disability? International Disability Studies 10: 64–67

Wroblewski M, Mikulowski P, Steen B 1986 Symptoms of myocardial infarction in old age: clinical case, retrospective and prospective studies. Age and Ageing 15: 99–104

12. Drugs and elderly people

John Hurley

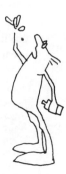

Medications, whether prescribed or acquired, can create many problems for elderly people, whether they live alone, and are forgetful, or are patients in hospitals or nursing homes. This important subject has, therefore, been covered in some detail.

A significant proportion of elderly people suffer from a multitude of illnesses, diseases or complaints. Consequently, multiple drug remedies are common. These may be prescribed by a doctor or other authorised health care professionals. Often, though, they are off-the-shelf preparations prescribed by the elderly person or a well meaning relative or friend. Monitoring programmes have indicated that elderly people are disproportionately greater consumers of drugs. One study indicated that some 80% of elderly people admitted to a hospital were already receiving regular drug therapy. Another study reported that about one-third of elderly people received four to six different drugs at one time.

Unfortunately, the incidence of adverse drug reactions increases with age. Studies have shown that some 6% of people under the age of 60 years sustain an adverse reaction to a prescribed drug, while in the over 65 years population, this incidence is in the order of 15%. Adverse drug reactions in the elderly age group are becoming a problem of significant dimensions as the num-

ber of elderly people increases, especially those over 80. It is in this latter group that toxic drug levels are more likely to occur. The number of elderly people admitted to hospital because of drug-induced causes is extensive, reportedly in the vicinity of 12% of all persons over 65 years.

A glance through many medical and pharmacological journals in the past decade indicates that apparent interest in the effects of drugs on elderly people is growing. Although many departments of geriatric medicine, in particular, have stimulated a great deal of work in this area there is, still, considerable ignorance of the potential problems associated with the prescription of drugs for elderly people. Since medical practitioners especially will become exposed more frequently to these problems as the elderly population increases, it is essential that they become more aware of the difficulties and hazards concomitant with drug prescribing.

The effects of therapeutic agents should be of concern to other health care staff as well because they are associated, often more directly, with the daily care of elderly people. Nursing staff, for example, should be aware of drugs that may produce confusional states; paramedical staff ought to understand the problems of postural hypotension and know the drugs that may produce it. Domiciliary nurses and other health care staff who visit a person at home need to be familiar with problems related to compliance with prescription instructions as well as the side-effects of the more common drugs. In these ways problems may be detected earlier and action taken to prevent unnecessary deterioration. Close liaison between the general medical practitioner and other health care staff is essential to facilitate such monitoring.

PHARMACOKINETICS

With advancing age there is a definite change in pharmacokinetics — the ability of the body to manage drugs. In general, this change leads to individual variations resulting in decreased tolerance for many drugs and in a prolonged duration of action. There are five main factors that may influence the effect of drugs: absorption, metabolism, distribution, receptor sensitivity and excretion.

Absorption of drugs, that is, how a drug is assimilated from the gut after ingestion, is probably little affected by age. There are, however, some situations where the simultaneous use of different drugs, especially in elderly people, may influence efficient absorption. For example, there is reduced tetracycline absorption when this drug is taken in association with antacids containing salts of aluminium or magnesium.

The *metabolism* of therapeutic agents is carried out primarily in the liver. There may be an age-related reduction in the microsomal enzymatic action of this organ. Consequently, a lesser amount of some drugs may be metabolised resulting in a hazardous amount remaining free in the bloodstream. Propranolol is one of a number of drugs metabolised less effectively by the liver in old age. Inefficient metabolism may be shown as an increase in the half-life of various drugs. The half-life is the length of time taken for half the drug dose to be metabolised and eliminated from the body. Diazepam, for example, has a half-life of some 30 hours in a young person but in a 90-year-old person the half-life approaches 90 hours. Therefore, if diazepam is ingested by an elderly person in a regular daily dose as for younger people a build-up results. Undesirable effects such as depression or falling may ensue.

The hepatic changes in regard to drug clearance in the elderly population are constantly being researched and reviewed. The current situation seems to suggest that there is a reduced clearance of many drugs. It would seem that this is more marked in females and particularly involves those drugs that are metabolised through oxidation, such as diazepam, propranolol, theophylline and nortriptyline. Drugs that do not use the oxidative route and undergo metabolism by other means, such as oxazepam and temazepam, may be less affected by the ageing process.

The *distribution* of drugs within the body also reflects age-related changes. Elderly people tend to become fatter as they age, in that body fat increases as a proportion of total body weight. This is significant because it means that fat-soluble substances may be contained in a larger reservoir. Diazepam is lipid soluble, for example, and will have a longer, effective duration in an elderly person. Elderly people are also drier, with total body fluid, especially plasma volume and extracellular fluids, depleting with age. Thus, there is a smaller volume of fluid to dilute drugs. In addition, there is a tendency for the serum albumin level to fall in a chronically ill person, and this may be associated with a reduced ability of the albumin present to bind drugs. An example of the latter is the decreased binding of warfarin in elderly people. The consequences of this reduced binding ability is an increase in the active free drug and this may result in dangerous effects.

Receptor sensitivity may vary with age. This may explain the increased likelihood of delirium in elderly people. Likewise, the markedly increased incidence of postural hypotension, for example with tricyclic antidepressants, may fall into the same category.

The kidneys are the primary organs concerned with the *excretion* of drugs. Age-related deterioration in kidney function is common. Renal blood flow and glomerular filtration decrease significantly, often in the vicinity of 50%. There is also a concurrent reduction in tubular excretion. Thus, the elderly kidney has little functional reserve capacity. Consequently, any insult will reduce performance further. This is particularly common in cases of dehydration, hypotension and cardiac failure, all conditions that are found frequently in elderly people. The reduced capability of the kidneys to excrete drugs is a major factor in the development of toxic drug levels and adverse reactions. This needs to be considered very carefully when prescribing drugs for elderly people.

Managing drug regimens

Many elderly people have difficulties when trying to manage drug regimens without assistance. Poor compliance is common. In part, this may be due to lack of understanding, the prescriber having failed to explain adequately enough to ensure comprehension. However, there are a number of other problems that may lead to erratic drug ingestion.

The elderly person may have an impaired memory which results in failure to comply with instructions. Frequently, this problem is compounded by the complexity of the regimen instituted. It is not unusual for an elderly person to have several different drugs prescribed, each having a different schedule. With forethought, it is possible to regulate the majority of drugs to a once or twice a day regimen. It has been demonstrated that some 25% of elderly people are unable to manage reliably a schedule of more than three drugs and every effort should be made to limit the total number of drugs in use. By simplifying the regimen, compliance can be increased readily.

Impaired vision is another common problem associated with poor compliance. Drug contain-

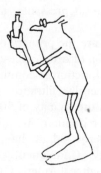

ers ought to be clearly marked with instructions typed, not handwritten. The regimen instructions need to be clear and in adequate detail. The use of 'as directed' alone on the label is not appropriate for elderly people.

More attention may be given to the size, colour and shape of the tablets being prescribed. By varying these parameters so that each drug is quite different from the others, the chances of taking the wrong ones can be reduced. There may still, however, be confusion with colours if the pharmacist uses brown bottles or opaque containers.

The packaging of drugs is of great importance when considering compliance with the regimen. The prescriber needs to consider the ability of the elderly person to manage the container. Many child-proof bottles may be elderly-proof as well. This is a particular problem for people with arthritic hand conditions, poor coordination or one functional hand. Bubble packaging and tear-off containers are also difficult. The most satisfactory container for most elderly people is palm-sized, screw-topped and transparent.

Specially designed dispensers are commercially available, many are divided for each day of the week and further subdivided for time sectors of the day. One dispenser may be prepared with a week's supply of drugs. If an elderly person can cope with this dispenser a great deal of danger may be removed from the situation. Such devices should be considered for use when compliance is a known problem.

THE PRESCRIPTION

The path that the prescribing medical practitioner follows in geriatric medicine is often complicated and hazardous. Because of multiple symptoms and problems it is a simple matter to fall into the trap of adding to the list of prescriptions. In conjunction with considered prescribing, the medical practitioner should review medications regularly with the aim of discontinuing drugs that are no longer necessary. This pruning exercise frequently results in a much improved patient.

Many elderly people require medications. A few simple rules may assist in the intelligent use of modern drugs, many of which do bring great benefits to people who need them.

- Make a careful diagnosis
- Prescribe only when necessary
- Prescribe as few drugs as possible — a maximum of three is a good rule
- Prescribe once or twice daily doses, if possible
- Prescribe different shaped and coloured tablets if possible
- Begin with a low dose and increase slowly — a good rule of thumb is one-third the dose suitable for a person half the age
- Use palm-sized, screw topped, transparent containers
- Have clearly typed instructions on the container, never use the phrase 'as directed' without accompanying detailed information
- Regularly review with the objective of withdrawing therapy
- Be aware of the side-effects of drugs and their duration of action

Common problems in prescribing

Drugs for the cardiovascular system

Many of the drugs used in the management of disorders of the cardiovascular system may produce toxic symptoms mainly because of the reduced renal clearance of such medications. Digoxin is a frequently used drug for cardiovascular problems. When it is used in conjunction with a diuretic the frequency of toxic side-effects increases because hypokalaemia may be produced by the diuretic. Hypokalaemia, in turn, enhances the toxic effects of digoxin. The plasma half-life of digoxin also increases in old age, another reason for care in its use.

Criteria for the use of digoxin vary between countries and indeed between prescribing medical practitioners. It is most commonly used in controlling atrial fibrillation. Recent studies indicate that in many cases the dose used is sub-therapeutic. It would seem that digoxin should only be used for specific reasons in old people and the correct dosage ascertained through monitoring of the serum levels.

It should be remembered that digoxin toxicity in elderly people may present as a confusional state as well as the more usual signs such as cardiac dysrhythmias including coupled beats, bradycardia and tachycardia. Nausea, vomiting and weight loss also may be symptoms of digoxin toxicity.

Diuretics are used with marked frequency in the drug regimens of elderly people. It is not uncommon to find an elderly person on long-term treatment for ankle oedema, the cause of which has never been ascertained and which could have been managed in other ways. Diuretics are a potent cause of hypokalaemia which, in itself, can give rise to confusion, weakness and postural hypotension. Further problems associated with the more powerful diuretics may be incontinence and, on occasions, falls in association with rushing to the toilet.

The problem of acute or chronic retention is frequently found in elderly men because of an enlarged prostate: a diuretic does not help the situation. It has been shown that high doses of diuretics may worsen lower limb peripheral vascular ischaemia. Increased blood viscosity secondary to reduced fluid volume has been suggested as the cause of further deterioration in blood flow. The lesson to be learned is to prescribe a diuretic only if necessary and to review the person's progress regularly with withdrawal of the drug frequently considered. One study found that of 54 long-term elderly patients who ceased diuretic therapy, only eight needed to recommence therapy later.

Hypotensive agents are a potent cause of adverse drug reactions in old people. The main danger is the precipitation of postural hypotension with its associated problems of weakness and falls. The fact remains, however, that recent papers, in particular the European Working Party relating to blood pressure in older people, have clearly shown the benefit of treating elevated blood pressure. The level of blood pressure at which treatment is recommended to commence is 160/90 mmHg or above. Several studies have shown that total mortality increases with higher, systolic blood pressure whereas the situation is less clear for raised diastolic pressure. However, controversy regarding the benefits of treatment of hypertension in the 80-year-old age group, particularly men, remains.

The first line of treatment for hypertension is usually a thiazide diuretic which is effective on its own in many instances. The second level of treatment is now debatable in that new and generally expensive drugs are less troublesome and are safer to use than drugs previously available. So favourable are their haemodynamic and biochemical characteristics that there are advocates for choosing such medication as first line treatment. Such newer drugs are angiotensin-converting enzyme inhibitors, for example, captopril, and calcium-channel blockers such as nifedipine.

The taking of blood pressure on a regular basis is mandatory before and after commencing therapy. This must be done with the elderly person both lying and standing. Failure to do so may result in missing the fact that there is a significant drop in blood pressure when moving from lying to sitting or standing, even to dangerously low levels.

Drugs for night sedation

Changes in sleep patterns are common as old age progresses. There is usually a reduction in phase four sleep, which is that part of sleep associated with slow, deep wave patterns on an electro-encephalograph. There is also a reduction in rapid eye movement sleep, in which the electro-encephalograph shows a faster and shallower pattern, an increase in pulse rate, respiration rate and cerebral blood flow. The number of awakenings at night usually increases and their duration progressively extends. In addition, there is a tendency for elderly people to take longer to go to sleep. Unfortunately, these phenomena are exaggerated in elderly people with dementia.

The use of sedatives is common, often because the doctor is pressured to prescribe by apparently insomniac patients. The alternative to a drug prescription is an explanation of the effects of normal ageing on sleep and advice about coping appropriately. The elderly person should keep active during the day and avoid naps near the time for normal sleep. A person awakening at night and unable to return to sleep ought to be advised to

rise and undertake an activity before attempting sleep again. Further, the avoidance of stimulants before retiring may improve the chances of sleep. Caffeine and alcohol are two common stimulants that may have a disturbing effect on the sleep pattern of many people.

If such advice and reassurance fails, prescribing a night sedative may prove necessary, on a short-term basis only, and with care being taken in selecting the drug. It is preferable to use a preparation with a short half-life to prevent accumulation and consequent 'hangovers'. Accumulation most likely will occur with regular nightly doses of a drug with a half-life in excess of 16 hours. Consequently, it is necessary to be aware of the half-life of the prescribed medication and the expected half-life for the age of the person using it. Those with appropriate short half-lives include chloral hydrate, chlormethiazole and temazepam. Most of the benzodiazepines and barbiturates have half-lives in excess of 16 hours. Nitrazepam should not be used because its half-life is in excess of 20 hours. Also, there may be problems with a variable rate of metabolism in different individuals. Elderly people appear to be especially sensitive to the benzodiazepine group of drugs and this may lead to increased drowsiness and impaired reaction times, particularly when arising from the bed. Falls and other such accidents may be a direct consequence of the use of benzodiazepine.

In summary, night sedation should be avoided if possible. When necessary, it ought to be prescribed on a short-term basis and be a drug with a short half-life.

Drugs used for tranquillisation

The most commonly prescribed tranquillisers for elderly people are drawn from the phenothiazines and benzodiazepines, and great care should be taken in the selection of the specific drug to be prescribed.

In the phenothiazine group, thioridazine is the first choice because it produces fewer side-effects in elderly people. This is because of its short half-life and limited tendency to create problems with postural hypotension. The dosage should be tailored to meet the needs of the elderly person.

Often, it is preferable to commence with a 10 mg dose scheduled at the time of day or night when the behavioural disturbance begins to be demonstrated. A slavish three times a day regimen is not required in many instances.

Of the benzodiazipine group, oxazepam has a shorter duration and is preferable. It may be used in a similar fashion to thioridazine, tailoring the dose to suit the individual elderly person. Diazepam has a prolonged action in most elderly people and should be prescribed in smaller doses than normally used for younger adults or be avoided if possible. The benzodiazipines are generally used in controlling anxiety states and preferably should only be used short-term for this purpose. The use of this group of drugs in people with Alzheimer's disease is best avoided as it may cause dysinhibition with resulting deterioration in behaviour.

In both groups the more powerful preparations should be reserved for situations in which the elderly person presents grossly disturbed behaviour. The use of more potent agents such as chlorpromazine or haloperidol too early in the confusional state may worsen it or result in over sedation. The old adage of start low and build slow fits well in this situation.

Drugs used for depression

Clinical depression is a common problem encountered in geriatric medicine. It may present in many ways other than the classic form. Often, the elderly person complains of physical ailments but depression is found to be the basis. On occasions depression masquerades as dementia. As the rate of successful suicides increases with age it is essential that depression is recognised, diagnosed and treated.

Tricyclic antidepressants are the most frequently used therapeutic agents but these drugs have side-effects that pose special problems. For example, postural hypotension is a common complication of this therapy, resulting in apathy and falls. If tricyclic antidepressants are used, even in low doses, it is important to monitor blood pressure carefully, both lying and standing. Other complications include confusional states, constipation, and retention of urine.

When the decision is taken to use a tricyclic antidepressant, it should be started in low dosage. The dose may then be increased gradually until a level is attained which suits the needs of the individual. Once or twice daily therapy with the major dose at night is recommended.

There are a multitude of tricyclic antidepressants available. Prescribing medical practitioners need to be very familiar with information about the potential complications each has for elderly people to ensure selecting the safest. Tetracyclic antidepressants that are less likely to produce postural hypotension and anticholinergic side-effects are now available; included among these is mianserin, but its rare effect of bone marrow depression should be kept in mind.

Monoamine oxidase inhibitors may also be used in the treatment of depression. However, the complexity of their interaction with other drugs and foods containing tyramine, as well as the frequency of multiple medications for elderly people, makes their use in this age group quite hazardous. The problems are complicated by the dangers of unreliable drug and dietary compliance due to memory impairments. If these drugs must be used they need to be carefully started and closely monitored.

Drugs for diabetes mellitus

Maturity onset diabetes is the most commonly encountered variety of diabetes mellitus in elderly people. Blood glucose levels tend to increase with age. There has, however, been controversy about the normal levels for elderly people. Various parameters have been suggested including a blood sugar level of 11 mmol/L 2 hours after the midday meal or a fasting blood sugar level of 8 mmol/L. Results at and above these levels should be considered as possibly indicating diabetes. Further investigations such as a glucose tolerance test may then be carried out to confirm the diagnosis.

Diet is the mainstay of therapy in diabetes mellitus. In elderly people it is frequently all that is necessary to produce satisfactory control. Drug therapy may be required to complement the diet when that alone is insufficient to return the blood glucose levels to normal. Sulphonylureas are the most widely used group of drugs. The majority of these are metabolised by the hepatic system. Chlorpropamide is an exception in that it is removed unchanged via the renal system and this drug is best avoided since renal impairment may be undiagnosed and lead to unexpected and severe hypoglycaemia. The choice of drug, as in many other situations in geriatric medicine, rests with the duration of action of the preparation. It is preferable to prescribe a shorter acting sulphonylurea in the first instance, such as tolbutamide or glipizide.

Biguanides have been criticised because of the danger of lactic acidosis; metformin appears to be free of this side-effect, and is a useful addition when sulphonylurea drugs give inadequate control. Very few elderly people require insulin except in situations where the diabetes has been a very long-term condition. Insulin-dependent diabetics who have survived into old age are usually very aware of their disease and appreciate the problems. However, their insulin requirements often decline with age, and the therapeutic regimen should be kept under active review.

All hypoglycaemic agents may lead to hypoglycaemia which can masquerade as confusion, especially at night. Care must be taken to diagnose this problem correctly and not make the error of apportioning blame to old age or a dementing process. Chlorpropamide is particularly prone to producing hypoglycaemia due to its prolonged action.

Drugs used for parkinsonism

Anticholinergic drugs have been used in the treatment of parkinsonism for many years, but are capable of causing confusion, glaucoma, or retention of urine. Amantadine is also capable of causing confusion, hallucinations and nightmares. Levodopa combined with decarboxylase inhibitor is less likely to cause difficulties but hypotension and confusion may still occur. Starting with a low dose and gradually increasing is the appropriate approach to therapy, watching for dyskinesia during the process.

Drugs used for anticoagulant therapy

Warfarin is a drug which must be used with considerable care in the management of thrombotic disorders in elderly people. Protein-bound warfarin is inactive. However, because of lowered albumin levels in some elderly people there is a decrease in protein binding of warfarin, and a consequent increase in the amount of free active drug in the system. This danger is increased by the use of drugs that compete for protein-binding sites. Small doses and careful monitoring are essential to avoid the development of dangerous prothrombin times with the associated hazard of bleeding.

Drugs used for infections

The reduced glomerular filtration rate usually accompanying old age leads to reduced excretion of antibiotics. Sometimes this is helpful but in other situations it may be harmful. For example, the reduced excretion of penicillin may be an advantage in the event of a severe infection because less drug may be needed. Drugs that may result in harm are the aminoglycosides including streptomycin and gentamicin, which are known to produce renal damage and ototoxic effects. It should be noted that ototoxic effects of aminoglycosides may be enhanced by the concomitant use of frusemide. Tetracyclines which are widely used are dangerous where there is renal impairment because they aggravate the problem of uraemia, especially when dehydration is present. Nitrofurantoin should also be used with care in the presence of renal impairment. Further, it ought not be used long term because of the danger of peripheral neuropathy.

Table 12.1 indicates the expected half-life in hours for some of the more commonly prescribed drugs. It is essential that the half-life be considered before prescribing the drug to an elderly person.

Guidelines for prescribing

The changes associated with age result in the body handling drugs in a different way and the

Table 12.1 Some drug plasma half-lives

Drug	Half-life (hours)
Chlormethiazole	3–8
Chloral hydrate	8–11
Barbiturates	
Amylobarbitone	20–27
Pentobarbitone	22–24
Phenobarbitone	48–144
Phenothiazines	
Chlorpromazine	16–32
Thioridazine	9–24
Benzodiazepines	
Oxazepam	6–18
Diazepam	20–95
Nitrazepam	20–30
Flunitrazepam	25–30
Temazepam	4–8
Antidepressants	
Amitriptyline	15–40
Imipramine	4–12
Nortriptyline	18–35
Desipramine	12–54
Mianserin	6–11
Oral hypoglycaemics	
Sulphonylureas	
Acetohexamide	2–5
Chlorpropamide	24–42
Glibenclamide	10–16
Glibornuride	5–12
Gliclazide	8–12
Glipizide	3–7
Tolbutamide	4–10
Biguanides	
Metformin	1.5–3

Establishing the person's current drug-taking habits is vital. As with multiple disease, so too multipharmacy is not uncommon. It is not unusual to find elderly people on several drugs of the same type for the same condition, not infrequently prescribed by different doctors, each ignorant of the other's involvement. The most common in this category would be diuretics, tranquillisers and antidepressants. Another problem may be the prescribing of a number of drugs each with the same side-effect. Most common, and most devastating, in this regard are drugs with anticholinergic actions. Box 12.1 describes those effects while Box 12.2 lists the common drugs in the anticholinergic group.

Box 12.1 Some consequences of anticholinergic drug action

Confusion	Hypotension
Constipation	Pupillary dilatation
Dry mouth	Tachycardia
Glaucoma	Urinary retention/Incontinence
Hallucinations	

Box 12.2 Some drugs with anticholinergic actions

Anticholinergics
Benzhexol (Artane)
Orphenadrine (Disipal)

Phenothiazines
Chlorpromazine (Largactil)
Thioridazine (Melleril)
Metoclopramide (Maxalon)
Prochlorperazine (Stemetil)

Miscellaneous
Disopyramide (Rhythmodan)
Propantheline (Probanthine)

Tricyclic antidepressants
Imipramine (Tofranil)
Doxepin (Sinequan)
Amytryptyline (Tryptanol)
Nortriptyline (Allegron)

---

same processes may lead to the elderly persons themselves misusing their prescribed drugs. In the latter case, poor memory and complex regimens may lead to poor compliance in that too much or too little of the drug issued may be taken. It is clear, therefore, that careful thinking before prescribing is important.

In the first instance, a *definitive diagnosis* must be made. Following a diagnosis, a decision is required as to whether drug therapy is indicated. In some cases, drugs may be avoided as non-drug therapeutic regimens are available. Hypertension may be managed initially with a regimen of exercise and weight loss and drug therapy used where this fails. Diabetes mellitus may respond to dietary measures so that there is no need to use oral hypoglycaemic agents or insulin.

The district nurse is often aware of the multitude of drugs present in an old person's home and should have no hesitation in notifying the medical practitioner in relation to this. The district nurse may also be aware of other drugs that are part of self-medication about which the medical practitioners may be unaware. Bringing all drugs to the initial consultation or following admission to hospital is of great benefit in assessing the overall situation.

Having reached a diagnosis and decided that drugs are necessary, then prescribing appropriate medication is the next step. A knowledge of the altered action of drugs in elderly people will be of advantage to the prescriber. It is especially valuable to be aware of those drugs that are prone to produce adverse drug reactions. It is known, for example, that central nervous system depression is more common in older people when larger doses of benzodiazepines are used; thus, using smaller doses is preferable. Certain other drugs are better used in reduced dosage, for example, haloperidol (Serenace) and thioridazine (Melleril), the former because of its propensity to produce extrapyramidal signs and the latter because confusion may occur with higher doses. In 1981 the World Health Organization recommended that certain drugs should be avoided where possible in old age; a selected number are shown in Table 12.2.

Table 12.2 Some drugs best avoided in old age (after WHO 1981)

Drug	Problem
Barbiturates	Confusion
Chlorpropamide	Hypoglycaemia
Chlorthalidone	Incontinence
Nitrofurantoin	Peripheral neuropathy

In general terms the ageing process tends to result in many drugs having a prolonged duration of action and a higher plasma level for a given dose. It would seem logical, therefore, to use the lowest dose that is effective. Often the individual dose itself may be reduced but, just as effective, in some cases, is the use of the recommended dosage less frequently, for instance twice a day rather than three times daily. Where the latter is possible it often aids compliance, another benefit. The appropriate monitoring of blood levels of drugs is now increasingly available and is a valuable aid to therapy in some cases.

Since elderly people frequently have multiple diseases requiring multiple therapies it is imperative for the regimens to be kept as simple as possible. It is often necessary in the acute phase of an illness to use a multitude of drugs in a complex regimen but once the acute problem is stabilised it is possible, and necessary, to simplify the maintenance therapy. Many drugs can be withdrawn once the acute episode is over; drugs such as digoxin or diuretics that were initially necessary may no longer be required once the precipitating acute disease has been dealt with. To ensure the elderly person's comprehension the number of drugs should be kept to a minimum. Time needs to be spent explaining the treatment plan, and the reasons for the prescription. The pharmacist can be of singular value in this educative role. The district nursing staff should also be involved in this process, if appropriate, as the therapeutic plan may need to be explained to a relative or friend as well as the elderly person.

To assist compliance it may be necessary to ensure that the form of medication is appropriate. A liquid or dissolving form of a drug may be more easily swallowed by the older person.

Constant review of the medical therapy is essential, and the opportunity to discontinue medication no longer considered necessary must be taken as soon as is practicable. The tendency to continue medication unnecessarily often occurs when several medical practitioners are involved or when junior medical staff are involved in follow-up in outpatient departments.

Those caring for elderly people need to be aware that drugs are more likely to produce adverse drug reactions in older people, and to be alert to those reactions that occur most commonly (see Box 12.3). The manifestation of adverse drug reactions may involve many systems; neuropsychiatric disorders are particularly common, being caused by a considerable number of drugs. With this in mind, care needs to be taken when prescribing, especially when the disease process is asymptomatic, since powerful drugs may add iatrogenic problems to an already complex situation.

Ignorance regarding drugs is common among elderly people and their relatives. Education of

Box 12.3 Some adverse drug reactions that may be experienced by elderly people

Biochemical	*Gastrointestinal*
Hyponatraemia	Nausea and vomiting
Hyperkalaemia	Ulceration
Hypokalaemia	Diarrhoea
Fluid retention	Constipation
Hyperuricaemia	
	Geniurinary
Cardiovascular	Incontinence
Dysrhythmias	Renal impairment
Hypotension	
Cardiac failure	*Haematological*
	Marrow depression
Central nervous system	Haemolytic anaemia
Confusion	
Seizures	*Skin*
Hallucinations	Rashes
Insomnia	
Depression	
Parkinsonism	
Tradive dyskinesia	
Peripheral neuropathy	

the elderly person and their carers should be given high priority; involving nurses and pharmacists in this matter is most useful.

Managing medication personally requires understanding by the elderly person so some form of self-medication should be attempted in the hospital prior to discharge. While this often occurs in rehabilitation units, it is nearly impossible to arrange in acute hospital wards. However, an effort to explain the action of drugs and the importance of compliance should be made prior to discharge from hospital. The more complex the regimen, the more likely it is that errors will occur. Similarly, signs of impaired memory are associated with poor compliance. In these situations, relatives and the district nurse may need to be involved in supervising the elderly person's medication regimen.

Monitoring the elderly person's compliance with the prescribed regimen can be enhanced through the use of diaries or by having a relative regularly check a commercially available dispensing device that may be loaded by the pharmacist, relative or district nurse.

The increasing number of aged people in the population means larger numbers attending for medical care. Often this takes the form of medication. It is clearly important that all members of the medical team are aware of changes that occur in drug response and the vulnerability to adverse drug reactions that occur with ageing.

REFERENCES

Bursztyn M, Gavras I, Favras H 1989 Hypertension in the ageing patient: implications for selection of drug therapy. Journal of the American Geriatrics Society 37: 814–818

Campion E W, de Labry L O, Glynn R J 1988 The effect of age on serum albumin in healthy males: report from the normative ageing study. Journal of Gerontology 43(1): M18–20

Castleden C M, George C F, Marger D, Hallet C 1977 Increased sensitivity to nitrazepam in old age. British Medical Journal 1: 10–12

Castleden C M, George C F 1979 The effect of ageing on the hepatic clearance of propranolol. British Journal of Clinical Pharmacy 7: 49–54

Hurwitz N, Wade O L 1969 Intensive hospital monitoring of adverse reactions to drugs. British Medical Journal 1: 531–536

Hurwitz N 1969 Predisposing factors in adverse reactions to drugs. British Medical Journal 1: 536–539

Kales A, Scharf M B, Kales J D, Soldaids C R 1979 Rebound insomnia: a potential hazard following withdrawal of certain benzodiazepines. Journal of the American Medical Association 241: 1692–1695

Macklon A F, James O, Rawlins M D 1979 Hepatic metabolism of diazepam in relation to age. Clinical Science 56(3): 14

Nolan L, Kenny R, O'Malley K 1989 Need for reassessment of digoxin prescribing for the elderly. British Journal of Clinical Pharmacy 27: 367–370

O'Malley K, Crooks J, Duke F, Stevenson I H 1971 Effects of age and sex on human drug metabolism. British Medical Journal 21: 607–609

Wagner G 1967 Drug accumulation. Journal of Clinical Pharmacy 7: 84–88

Williamson J, Chopin J M 1980 Adverse reactions to prescribed drugs in the elderly: a multi centre investigation. Age and Ageing 9: 73–80.

13. Restoration and rehabilitation

Doreen Bauer

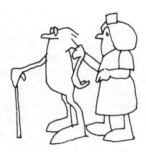

The quality of the initial phase of care of an elderly person following an acute episode such as cerebrovascular accident, major surgery or amputation, is of vital importance in setting the stage for recovery and motivation towards rehabilitation.

Professional staff in acute hospitals who are concerned with direct patient care (doctors, nurses, social workers and therapists) need to share a common knowledge and understanding of the principles and practice that underlie the approach to rehabilitation and restorative care, with their counterparts in the field of extended care. Such knowledge, and the achievement of close liaison between the acute field and those working in geriatric assessment and rehabilitation units might well improve the quality of life and lessen the dependence of many more people.

RESTORATIVE CARE

Restorative care is the term applied to a system of services for people experiencing functional problems in the recovery stage of a physical or mental illness. There are a number of features of such services.

• An organised approach which includes the elements of assessment, general medical care and rehabilitation.

• An opportunity for the person to develop abilities to function adequately or at the maximum level of potential independence.

• A process which requires the planned, progressive withdrawal of support or assistance for success.

• A team approach which depends upon the active participation of the person and the family.

• A detailed, individual process which is problem related and goal orientated.

The cry of one frail, elderly lady in a nursing home has been echoed by countless others: 'Please tell my daughter I want to go home, please'. But she can't go home. Her health, her family and her society failed her several years earlier. Now it is too late. A fractured femur signalled the end of self-reliance, prompting the envelopment of her life with the mantle of defeat and dependency. Postoperative confusion and incontinence were, unfortunately, interpreted as irreversible symptoms of senility. Institutionalisation was considered the only solution. Perhaps this outcome was inevitable. Who knows now?

In a geriatric programme, restorative care is a system of services provided for elderly people who are disabled or unable to function competently in their normal life roles. The extent of disabling problems in elderly populations is usually subject to speculation because objective data are, generally unavailable. It has been estimated that some 20% of people over the age of 65 years may have problems that require the assistance of a comprehensive geriatric service. A disability, or more commonly disabilities, due to physical, mental, economic or social factors usually precipitates the call for help. As age progresses the likelihood of disabling conditions increases.

To complicate this picture, there does not appear to be any concrete evidence that one can, with accuracy, predict a person's potential for overcoming the effects of a disability. Thus, the number of elderly people who may benefit from restorative care is difficult to estimate. Further, many elderly people fail during the first assessment to show much promise for functional improvement because their emotional state is too fragile. Given a period of positive, reassuring care some may, later, become candidates for a restorative care programme.

The success rate of a restorative care programme is also difficult to measure. Frequently, cure or return to normal are not realistic goals. Gains are often quite small but they may make the difference between dependency and a degree of self-reliance. An important aspect of the definition of restorative care is the 'opportunity to develop abilities to function adequately or at the maximum level of potential independence'. When cure is the goal the period of intensive rehabilitative activity may be prolonged inappropriately, the elderly person perhaps wasting precious days being maintained in the hospital setting, the elderly person and the family perhaps becoming institutionalised. Further, when the overall aim is to return to normal many elderly people are rejected as possible candidates for rehabilitation because the potential improvement in function is regarded as too slight to be worth the effort. Any increase in competency, no matter how small, is very worthwhile. This subjective judgement, unfortunately, is not adequate alone to demonstrate the value of restorative care. With so many competing appeals for a share of society's limited resources benefits in economic terms must be forthcoming. Procedures for measuring the results of restorative care, especially in terms of reduced demands for continuing care beds or staff, should be a priority for service planners.

DISABILITY

Disability is an all too common feature of the lives of many elderly people. Stereotypes exist in literature and theatre, the press, jokes and popular myths. Disabilities due to deafness or poor memory are used frequently to portray old age. Many people, unfortunately, see old age itself as a disability. One of the primary aims of a geriatric service is to deal with all the implications of disability, both real and imagined, upon the lives of elderly people as individuals and as a group.

A disability is an incapacity to function competently, to interact adequately with the normal environment. An interference with the smooth, purposeful undertaking of any function may be considered a disability, whether temporary or permanent. The word 'function' contains a host of notions — grasping, walking, manipulating, perceiving, exploring, thinking, communicating, learning, caring, and sharing. The ability to function competently in the vast range of daily living activities may be thwarted by physical, psychological, social, economic or environmental difficulties.

The problems that may create a disability come in various guises. They may be temporary or permanent, single or multiple, simple, complex, static or progressive. A physical disability may be overshadowed by psychological or social problems to such an extent that amelioration of the physical condition is, initially, inconsequential. Further, the same problem may have dissimilar effects on various people. Because of this, many rehabilitation philosophers believe that it is incorrect to consider the defect or the impairment as being the disability. Numerous people with impairments live full, active, productive and contented lives. Others with similar problems succumb to dependency. If the impairment is the same the question is, then, obvious. Why is one able and the other disabled?

Rehabilitation philosophers stress the personal nature of disability in answering the question.

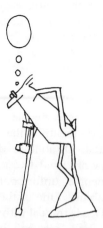

Disability is not the actual impairment but rather the person's reaction to it. The reaction is often coloured by the responses of family, friends and society. Each person's reaction is unique based upon pre-disability personality, developmental skills, social and cultural attitudes, abilities to solve problems and take responsibility.

REHABILITATION

People, whether elderly or not, may be assisted to conquer the effects of these potentially disabling problems fully or partially. The term usually applied to the process of overcoming the effects of disability is rehabilitation. The philosophical and technical basis of rehabilitation has developed significantly in recent decades. Today, it is viewed by many as a specialist service, the process requiring special units, special staff and special procedures. This is, in some ways, unfortunate. Many people, particularly elderly people, are being denied planned rehabilitation because they do not have access to the special units, staff or procedures. If special units or special staff are not available others must use the skills and talents they possess to stimulate or assist the disabled person to strive toward independent activity. Instincts may not always lead to correct procedures. Maybe the wrong reflexes will be stimulated after a stroke but the person walking with a typical, if undesirable and possibly avoidable, hemiplegic walking pattern is a far more humane story than would be that same person senile, contracted and confined to bed while life ebbed.

Each elderly, disabled person is an individual with unique needs, reactions and responses. Regardless of the degree of disability or the complexity of the problems, the same principles of restorative care may be followed by a specialist rehabilitation team, a domiciliary care team under the leadership of the general medical practitioner, the staff of an acute care ward or a nursing home unit.

Basically, restorative care may be considered a philosophy, an attitude rather than a technique. Specialised units may be staffed by people who are committed to the principles of restorative care and are not distracted, usually, by other caring approaches such as acute care, continuing care or hospice care. Specialised staff of special units are skilled facilitators of aspects of the rehabilitation process when the person is unable to undertake adequately some functions alone. Often, particular knowledge or skills are required to assist a person to achieve the most effective rehabilitation possible. Often, certain skills and talents are required to stimulate the level of motivation necessary to initiate the rehabilitation process.

Specialised units, however, are not essential for the application of the principles. In fact, acute care hospitals may contribute more effectively to the care of elderly people if the principles of restorative care are applied early in the convalescent stage of their stay. Many elderly people are discharged directly from acute care to home without any opportunity to discover functional problems that may have resulted from the pathology which caused the admission, from the procedures which may have been undertaken or from the enforced dependency which hospitalisation seems to require. Too frequently, elderly people are discharged home without adequate functional skills and break down before they have had a chance to regain full independence. It is, further, unfortunate that many elderly people sustain a shock when transferred from an acute care hospital to a geriatric rehabilitation unit.

Adjustment problems on transfer often delay progress unnecessarily. It is difficult for many to move suddenly from an atmosphere pervaded by night clothes and efficient 'let me do it for you' attention to an environment that demands day clothes and aims at functional independence even if it is a struggle. This shock could be diminished significantly if staff of the acute care units progressively practised the principles of restorative care from the earliest stages of recovery.

Often, the earlier restorative care is implemented the greater the chances for success. There should not be any programme delays due to organisational planning such as waiting for a bed in a rehabilitation unit. The programme ought to commence wherever the person is waiting: hospital or home. If necessary, staff from the rehabilitation unit could be available to undertake the commencement of the process or to assist others to start. When delays occur which are not related to the elderly person's condition, problems may be compounded and the potential for improvement reduced. Of course, it is rarely practical to attempt active participation while the elderly person is medically unstable. Preventive techniques should be practised while waiting for the convalescent stage to begin.

PREVENTION

The prevention of avoidable complications following the onset of pathological conditions is an essential element of the restorative care process. Immobilisation of an elderly person in bed should be avoided if at all possible. The effects of prolonged bed rest may be seen in most systems of

---

Box 13.1 Potential consequences of prolonged bed rest

Loss of joint mobility — contractures

Reduced muscle strength — weakness

Retarded endurance

Predisposition to venous thrombosis

Pressure sores

Urinary tract dysfunction — incontinence

Respiratory complications — pneumonia

Development of osteoporosis

Dehydration and electrolyte imbalance

Boredom and reduced motivation

Emotional deterioration

---

the body. Box 13.1 indicates some of the more common problems for which measures for prevention are necessary.

Contracture of muscle and joint structures are an all too common consequence of lack of adequate active or passive movement. The knee is the joint most often affected when an elderly person is maintained in bed. Inappropriate positioning leads to low back discomfort which the person attempts to relieve by bending the knees. Careful positioning with adequate joint support plus daily full range movements must be seen as vital elements in patient care.

Painful shoulders also occur with unfortunate frequency. A common cause of this problem is staff persistence in attempting to move dependent elderly people by lifting them under the axilla. Staff and families must learn appropriate transfer procedures which have been developed specially to protect the joints of elderly or dependent people while also being safe for the person assisting.

Pressure sores, incontinence, venous thrombosis, pneumonia and confusion are, often, avoidable complications of bed rest. Patient care regimens must specify the measures to be taken to prevent these problems. They should not be left to 'commonsense'.

The responsibility of the restorative care service in the area of prevention is not, however, limited to the avoidance of complications in the preconvalescent period. The prevention of disability producing problems ought to receive greater attention if the service is not to be swamped by the number of people in need of help.

The possibility of reducing pain or loss of normal function resulting from inefficient, inappropriate or decreased physical activity is gaining recognition. Postural deformities, back pain, cardiac deficiencies and osteoarthritis could be less common if people were taught and motivated to care for themselves. Respiratory diseases, rheumatoid arthritis, congenital perceptual problems and ageing need not become major limiting disorders if detection, education, correction and motivation could be established early. It is becoming increasingly evident that incontinence is a significant feature in the development of disability because of its role in falls and depression, which lead to a decrease in social and physical activity. Treatment of the causes or effective management of the consequences are possible in the majority of instances (see Ch. 7). Personnel who work in restorative care have a detailed awareness of the consequences of the failure to prevent disability. They should, therefore, have a great deal to contribute to the development of preventive programmes.

Staff who work with elderly people need a comprehensive understanding of the more common physiological and psychological features of the ageing process. Often, the prevention of problems is dependent on this knowledge. For example, many elderly people experience progressive deterioration in kinaesthetic sensation, especially in their feet. If an elderly person needs to watch the feet while walking, therapists must consider carefully their attempts to break the habit. They must also counsel the elderly person about walking in the dark.

Vision changes provide another example of the need for staff to understand common ageing processes. One aspect of vision, the ability to discriminate colour and shape, has particular implications for safe mobility. A grey concrete verandah with grey concrete steps to a grey concrete path may be a hazard for people with deteriorating shape and colour discrimination. Precautions such as brightly coloured paint stripes on the step edges may prevent an elderly person from falling down, or more commonly, up the step.

The scope of preventive programmes is, seemingly, limitless. They are the responsibility of restorative care as well as of all other areas of the geriatric service.

THE RESTORATIVE CARE PROCESS

Essentially, restorative care is an adaptive process designed to overcome the effects of disability. There are six basic steps in the process: assessment, problem identification, planning, implementation, evaluation and discharge. Restorative care, though, is not always a clear six step recipe. Figure 13.1 illustrates how complicated the process may be. However, if the six steps are kept in focus it may be possible to fol-

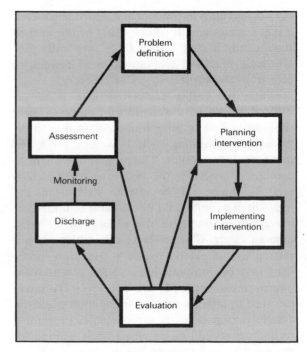

Fig. 13.1   Restorative care process

low each problem through to a satisfactory solution.

Assessment

Data collection through detailed assessment is the first step in the restorative care process. Elderly people frequently present a multiplicity of problems, some readily obvious, others hidden. Each problem should be explored fully to ensure the completeness of the assessment process. It is not enough to focus on the presenting medical diagnosis. In restorative care the 'whole person' philosophy must be practised. For example, an elderly person may be admitted to the programme following a fractured femur. The problems related to this condition may be complicated by deteriorated vision, kinaesthetic defects, hypotension or other such ageing changes. If the assessment focuses on the fracture and fails to examine these other areas the elderly person may learn to walk only to fall again.

Sometimes a problem may not be that which is presented by the elderly person. There may be a complaint of chronic joint pain which is, in fact, the acceptable manifestation of the pain resulting from loneliness. Another elderly person may be unable to use public transport supposedly because of mobility problems but really because of shame at being a disabled person. An elderly man may be assessed as being dependent in dressing skills. This may have nothing to do with his physical disability. Perhaps it results from the fact that his wife insists on doing it for him. It is, therefore, essential that assessment is a detailed process, the assessor carefully working through the data maze.

The principles of assessment have been described in Chapter 11. Appropriate restorative care requires the strict application of these principles. Although the initial assessment may appear to place priority on the presenting disabilities it is important to consider the functional abilities the person retains. Often the restorative care programme is built upon regimens to strengthen these abilities to overcome the negative effects of disabling problems which cannot be corrected.

Assessment data may come from many sources, all members of the team contributing to the total picture. Observed information frequently needs to be verified by testing before it is accepted. For example, one member of the team may report that the elderly person needs significant assistance from two people to get out of bed. On careful functional assessment in a normal environment, as opposed to a hospital environment, it may be found that the elderly person is quite capable of independence in this activity. The person presenting the initial report may have assumed that the elderly person was dependent and failed to provide an opportunity to demonstrate independence. The need to verify data through functional testing cannot be over-emphasised.

It is especially important to undertake a detailed home assessment as early as possible in the restorative care process. Realistic planning requires a very clear picture of the home environment so that training is appropriate. There is little point in teaching an elderly person to use a bath in the hospital or rehabilitation unit if the bath is of a significantly different height to the bath at home. Even more so, there is no point in training the person to be independent in the

bath if there is no bath at home. The same applies to kitchen training. A carefully planned rehabilitation kitchen which bears little, if any, resemblance to the home kitchen is not a satisfactory place to test or train kitchen skills. Of course, it is not possible to have training facilities that simulate every peculiarity which may be found in the homes of elderly people. It is practical, however, to have training facilities that reproduce aspects of normalcy, which may be modified to represent the individual's home situation. The tendency to develop idealised training facilities in rehabilitation units needs to be considered more carefully by programme planners. It should also be noted that it may well prove more cost-effective to undertake part or all of the functional training in tasks such as kitchen duties in the person's own home environment.

Assessment is not a once only task. Rather, it is a dynamic procedure going on throughout the whole restorative care process. New information may be discovered at any time, new information which may colour or change goals.

The assessment format used may vary with the resources of the service. Checklists, scoring forms and computer programs are common. Care must be taken to validate such forms and lists to ensure that the data are comprehensive and reliable; to be sure that adherence to formats does not blind the assessor to the real problems. Box 13.2 indicates the primary areas of functional activity

Box 13.2 Primary assessment areas	
Communication	Initiative
Memory	Decision making
Emotional status	Attitude to disability
Motor skills	Family relationships
Transfers	Social attitudes
Mobility	Home environment
Feeding	Financial status
Dressing	Vocational status:
Grooming	employment
	homemaking
Bathing	leisure
Bladder control	
Bowel control	

which may be considered in a comprehensive assessment. Within each area the depth and scope of examination will be determined by the problems presented by each individual and the skills of the person undertaking the assessment. Experienced professional staff are usually in the best position to undertake a comprehensive assessment because they should be able to react to clues, following leads in appropriate depth, sidestepping areas that may be of little consequence.

Assessment findings may be easier to manipulate if rating scales are developed to add a measurable dimension. Such a rating scale may be simple or complex depending on the skills of the people undertaking the assessment. The five point scale described in Box 13.3 may be a useful

---

Box 13.3 Functional rating scale

1 Complete independence — able to live alone as he or she wishes

2 Dependent in an adapted environment — able to live alone if special needs are met

3 Semidependent — able to care for him or herself with assistance from another person to perform some activities

4 Dependent — requires assistance from another person for most activities

5 Severely dependent — unable to participate in own care at all

---

basic tool which can be modified to suit the service. It needs to be pointed out, however, that services wishing to participate in evaluation and research projects, comparing results with other services, must use assessment scales that have been validated and found to be statistically reliable.

Problem identification

A problem is a functional incompetency or anything which prevents a person from functioning effectively. While medical diagnoses are very important for planning appropriate medical intervention throughout the restorative care processes, it is essential that problems are defined in functional rather than medical terms. A diagnosis

of rheumatoid arthritis, for example, may have major implications for the independent functioning of one person. Then again, the problems resulting from the disease may be minimal for another. Attempting to plan a restorative care programme on the basis of the medical diagnosis alone is, thus, inappropriate.

Problem identification should consider both actual and potential disabilities. This is particularly important in progressive diseases.

Problems should be organised in a list of priorities. Learning theory suggests that it is very difficult to learn too many tasks or activities at the same time. Elderly persons, particularly, need to help establish the priorities since they are likely to work harder on the problem they have recognised as being of most importance.

All problems should be recorded in a format that will promote team planning and evaluation. 'The problem orientated medical record' (Weed 1969) describes a process of particular usefulness, especially as it promotes one comprehensive record to which all participants contribute. To ensure the most effective record it should be remembered that a problem is something about which someone does something. It may be corrected, modified, considered or ignored. Once a problem is noted it should be followed by a statement of action or not, to facilitate later evaluation.

Planning intervention

Once problems have been identified and documented it is possible to begin planning solutions. This is best done as a team activity with the elderly person and the family participating. Many a well constructed plan has failed to materialise because health care personnel applied the 'we know best for the patient' principle. Unfortunately, the blame for failure usually is placed upon the patient or family, not on the staff who are probably more at fault. Each disabled elderly person ought to select a rehabilitation objective that is suitable for the person's situation and needs. Staff are, more appropriately, advisors who contribute knowledge and experience to assist the elderly person to work wisely.

The programme plan should be based on a positive approach to learning. The disabled person has to learn to explore and appreciate a new or changed body environment. At the same time staff and family members have to learn to stand back, to allow the disabled person to try to solve problems independently, to guide rather than to do. This approach takes time, needs patience and insight. It is not, however, a unique approach. Most parents realise the need to allow children to learn from experience even if they, the parents, could ease situations. Parents who attempt to do everything for their children are considered mistaken and foolish. The same applies in restorative care.

Planning requires the establishment of goals. Aimlessness or idealism are impractical in restorative care. Without a definite target the elderly person and the staff do not know for what they are striving. The goals established by the elderly person, the family and the staff need to be rationalised and be based on reality. Conflict in goal setting often has a disastrous effect on the progress and outcome of a restorative care programme. If the elderly person craves self-reliance while the family prepares for dependence difficulties will follow. If the staff consider wheelchair independence to be an attainable goal while the elderly person declares that walking or nothing is the aim, little progress will be made. Where the elderly person has aspirations that appear to exceed the potential assigned by the staff or family it is important to allow the higher goal to predominate. Eventually, either the elderly person will accept the fact that the goal is unattainable or, not uncommonly, the staff or family will be forced to revise their opinions. Little will be gained by staff who attempt, openly or discreetly, to force the elderly person to acquiesce.

Goals of independence, however, ought not to place excessive demands on an elderly person, demands which drain energy and emotional resources that may have been spent more usefully otherwise.

It is, further, important that the expectations of the personnel who may be responsible in the future for the elderly person in a continuing care setting are consistent with the goals of the restorative care programme. It is not uncommon for an elderly person to struggle to gain semi-independent skills such as walking with assistance only to be denied the opportunity to practise later. Some continuing care staff do not have time, skill or motivation to maintain the level of ability no matter how slight. It is essential, for the well-being of the elderly person, that these deficiencies are rectified.

While goals should be based on reality it is often difficult to predict accurately the outcome of intervention. Long-term goals need to be established early to assist everyone involved to aim in the same direction. Such goals, however, should not be considered sacrosanct. There ought to be opportunities for goal revision at any stage of the process.

The major goal outcomes that are considered most commonly are:

- Restoration to full independent living at home or with a family
- Restoration of some independence in self-care functions to lessen dependence on the family, plus educating the family
- Restoration of some independence in self-care functions to maintain self-respect in a continuing care facility, plus teaching the staff new skills if necessary.

Short-term goals are, perhaps, more important because they give more precise and attainable aims. By establishing such goals, and achieving them, many elderly people are encouraged to strive. For example, the long-term goal of independent, functional walking may seem an impossible dream to the elderly person who has sustained a fractured hip. Walking with assistance in the ward within, say, two weeks, followed by walking in the garden, around the block, around the shops over the next several weeks, may be attainable, phase by phase.

An essential element of goal setting is the establishment of a time frame. When will accomplishment of a task be achieved? Experienced personnel should be able to make this judgement. If the goal has not been achieved in the time frame one must then ask why. Is it because the task is not possible; the therapy not effective; the time too short or what? Such review and evaluation is important to ensure appropriate therapy and appropriate striving.

Prevention of disability is an important goal of the restorative care process. It may well prove that an attempt to restore one function may, in fact, mitigate against the overall success of the process. For example, an elderly person may be unable to walk independently because of the effects of a stroke. This condition may be complicated by another pathological problem which suggests a limited life expectancy. The prolonged hospitalisation required for the person to regain safe, independent walking may be outweighed by the potential psychological disabilities which result from the absence from home and family.

Implementation of intervention

The procedures that may be employed to restore function or to gain as much improvement as possible will, of course, depend on the problem. Specialist staff may possess particular knowledge, skills and talents that facilitate more effective restoration. However, other personnel who do not have them must not give up without trying, especially if admission to a special rehabilitation unit is not possible. Further, special knowledge should not be further than a telephone call away. Most geriatric units have staff available and willing to assist others learn appropriate procedures.

Intervention may include:

- Medical management
- Training to restore normal function
- Training to restore function within the limits of the disability
- Training to use other abilities to overcome the effects of the disability
- Training to use devices or aids
- Adaptation of the environment to facilitate function
- Family education
- Staff education
- Dealing with social problems
- Solving economic problems.

It is beyond the scope of this book to detail the intervention techniques that may be used in a restorative care programme. The accompanying bibliography lists books that deal with procedures. It is important to remember, though, that information about rehabilitative techniques often needs modification before it is applied to the care of elderly people. Again, an indepth knowledge of the ageing processes will assist people to use the available information appropriately.

Evaluation

Regular evaluation of progress, a planned activity involving the elderly person, the family and the staff, is an important feature of restorative care. By measuring progress against initial assessment information and goals it is possible to determine programme continuation, revision or termination as well as the effectiveness of particular procedures.

Precise records are necessary to facilitate accurate evaluation. Attempting to rely on memory to measure progress is hazardous. Further, staff changes may destroy programme continuity if there is not an accurate documentary process. Video recording is becoming an increasingly common way to measure progress. It needs to be remembered, though, that some elderly persons may be distressed when confronted by their image on a screen, either because of the disability or dishevelled dress or grooming.

Adequate records, especially problem documentation, help to ensure that all problems have something done about them. If some action about a problem is not intended the record should state the reason. Effective evaluation needs to be able to measure progress or not for each problem if an accurate picture of the elderly person is to be presented.

Discharge

The restorative care process is an approach guided by principles. It is not a recipe that follows a schedule. Although discharge is the last step in the process, planning for it must begin as early as possible. While the restorative care process is active and progressive the elderly person should be encouraged to continue working toward the established goals. Once these have been attained the process is, of course, terminated. However, if the elderly person reaches and maintains a performance plateau short of the long-term goal discharge should be considered on revised terms. The restorative care process ought not be prolonged unduly with dependency upon the procedures replacing the original aim of independence.

Discharge from an inpatient restorative care unit should be a carefully planned procedure. In the majority of instances the elderly person will be discharged to home in the community, perhaps alone or with a spouse, perhaps to live with family or friends. The home situation will, of course, dictate the planning steps.

• Inpatient discharge plans need to provide for all necessary preparations:

  — home alterations
  — installation of aids
  — training in drug management
  — referrals to all required services
  — programme continuation as an outpatient, usually in a day hospital
  — appointment of case manager or advocate to assist with managing ongoing care.

• Inpatient discharge to home alone ought to be preceded by progression through minimal care and self-care. This may take place in special units that reproduce domestic conditions. Where such facilities do not exist, staff should make efforts to simulate such. This may take the form of progressively increasing periods at home with diminishing supervision. Alternatively, staff may withdraw assistance, especially with domestic duties such as bed making, meal preparation and room cleaning. Hospital policies that demand dependence on staff, for instance during bathing, until the moment of discharge should be carefully reviewed to ensure that the safe discharge of the elderly person has not been compromised.

• Elderly persons who are to manage their own drug regimens ought to be given the opportunity to practise while an inpatient. The usual practice of drug management by nursing staff until the moment of discharge needs to be reviewed. Unless the elderly person is given this opportunity staff will have no chance of discovering and correcting compliance problems.

• Inpatient discharge to home with a spouse or relatives should be based on a planned education programme to ensure that they understand what is expected of them.

• Outpatient discharge from a day hospital should occur when the goals have been reached or a plateau is established. Discharge may be to an alternative form of day care such as day centre or socialisation group. Therapy-centred day hospital care ought to be guided by restorative care principles and not be prolonged indefinitely.

• Discharge from restorative care may involve referral to a maintenance programme supervised by continuing care staff — domiciliary, day centre or nursing home — to ensure that positive gains are continued.

• An elderly person's discharge from restorative care should be accompanied by reassurances of continued monitoring and later re-admission if the situation warrants. Sometimes, gains cannot be maintained and another burst of intensive therapy may be necessary.

• In some instances discharge from restorative care will be to a continuing care programme. Similar planning steps should be undertaken. The continuing care staff will need to know the elderly person's abilities and the skills gained. They may need some instruction in the use and maintenance of aids which the elderly person will continue to use. The restorative care staff will enhance the elderly person's transfer if a member of the team visits the new facility to discuss the transfer.

REFERENCE

Weed L 1969 Medical records, medical education and patient care. Case University Press, Cleveland, Ohio

14. Team concepts

Doreen Bauer

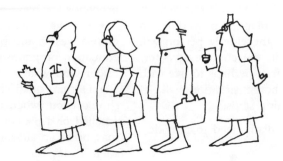

The complex nature of the approach to rehabilitation and restorative care has been covered; for these aims to be achieved, close working relationships and understanding must exist between all those involved in the achievement of optimal independence for an individual. This includes the one most concerned, as well as the family, the local doctor, and the many others whose interrelated roles are described in this chapter.

Geriatric care is a fertile field for the curious and imaginative professional mind that is stimulated by the challenges inherent in a 'whole person' philosophy. Because geriatric care is concerned with the often interrelated influences of health, economic and social dynamics upon an elderly person it cannot be effective if it focuses on one apparent problem. People who work in geriatrics must have an awareness of the multifaceted nature of this person-orientated service. Without an appreciation of the consequences of disturbances in one or more areas of total functioning it is difficult for the care giver to unveil the complete problem-asset portrait of an individual person. Without a willingness to search beyond the presenting complaint for the background causes the obvious solution may fail to alter the situation positively. Further geriatric or extended care is a process which encompasses the broad spectrum of health and welfare services including education and prevention; diagnostic, hospital and ambulatory care; home care, rehabilitation and institutional care. Such a programme requires coordination and integration of services. It is, however, dependent upon the active participation of the elderly person, the family and the service personnel in assessment, planning, implementing and evaluating (Fig. 14.1). Whether the service staff consists of one person or many people the need for a team approach is inescapable.

A significant proportion of elderly people will not need the help of an organised geriatric programme because their personal resources are adequate, permitting a full and independent life until it ends. The great variety of problems that may cause other elderly people, or families, to seek help have led to a proliferation of health and welfare disciplines in a geriatric service. Of those who do need assistance, not all will require the intervention of the many and various skills which these disciplines may provide. Such skills, however, ought to be available when required.

Current concepts of geriatric care, as well as other similar programmes such as rehabilitation, stress the necessity of organising the contributory disciplines in a coordinated, cooperative manner. This 'team' approach is widely recognised as a basic element in effective care.

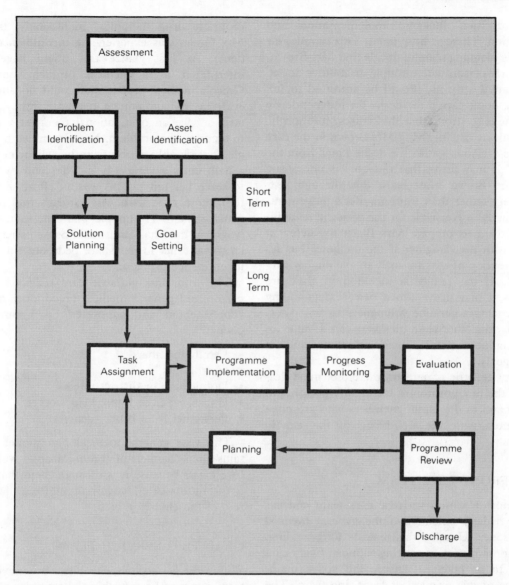

Fig. 14.1 Team action

There are a number of team structures in geriatric care, each constructed according to need as well as to availability of personnel. The centre or focus of the team is always the elderly person or the elderly person and the family. Unfortunately, the health care system has tended to develop according to the philosophy that health care workers 'do for' people rather than 'do with'. It is not uncommon to find people being treated who do not understand the problem, the treatment or the potential outcome. Often medical practitioners appear to believe that they are too busy to spend time in detailed explanations. Many tend to leave this function to nurses who, often, are constrained by rules that demand that only the medical practitioner may disseminate information.

An effective geriatric programme recognises the importance of the full participation of an informed elderly person and family in the care process. This participation is possible only if they are included, deliberately, in all aspects — planning, decision making, implementation and evaluation. There is little point, for example, for the care planning team to decide that Mrs Brown, an elderly person with multiple disabilities due to rheumatoid arthritis, should be admitted to full nursing home care if the desire for independence at home is so strong that she refuses, stubbornly, to acquiesce. By involving Mrs Brown in the care process everyone knows the desired goal from the outset. It may prove that this goal is unrealistic but Mrs Brown must learn this through self-discovery rather than from another's judgement.

Similarly, it is useless for the geriatric rehabilitation team to prepare Mrs Black for living at home with her daughter if the daughter has no real intention of making such an eventuality successful. If the family is included in the care process it may grow into a new understanding and develop a genuine willingness to try. Alternatively, the other team members can develop an appreciation of the daughter's reluctance and set other goals.

Every geriatric care team, therefore, must designate the first position to the elderly person and the second to the family members who are most concerned with the well-being of the elderly person.

THE FRONT LINE TEAM

The most common geriatric care team consists of the elderly person and the general medical practitioner. Usually, this team is longstanding, based on a history of trusting support. Every care ought to be taken to ensure the active maintenance of this primary or front line team. The general medical practitioner carries a great deal of responsibility and needs to honour it by keeping up-to-date with knowledge pertaining to the care of elderly people. An understanding of the breadth of geriatric care and a willingness to call in consultants if the situation appears to require further assistance are also essential.

Mrs Green, for example, had been maintained satisfactorily for many years by her general medical practitioner. Apart from various acute conditions which responded to treatment Mrs Green had chronic osteoarthritis of both hips. The resultant pain was controlled by various, ap-

propriate drug therapies. Increasingly, though, Mrs Green was experiencing incontinence accidents. At first glance this might have been interpreted as a medical problem but Mrs Green's medical practitioner could find no such evidence. By summoning assistance from the geriatric service an occupational therapist was able to focus on the problem. Mrs Green had to struggle considerably to rise from her chair, negotiate a hall, cross a verandah and descend two steps to reach her toilet. This was an effort and often took more time than Mrs Green's frail bladder could sustain. A suitable platform to raise the height of her chair and make rising easier and a chemical toilet in her spare bedroom solved her incontinence problem.

The front line geriatric care team of elderly person and general medical practitioner may be supplemented and supported by a variety of people:

- Family members
- Neighbours
- Domiciliary or district nurse
- Housekeeper or home help worker
- Personnel from other agencies.

The wise general medical practitioner maintains open channels of communication with such care givers because it is through them that there is the means of effectively monitoring the progress of the elderly person.

GERIATRIC SERVICE TEAM

Within the geriatric care facility a more extensive team ought to be available to help elderly people in need of more comprehensive assistance. Again, such a team must have as its focus the elderly person and the family. It cannot be overstressed that the active participation of these people in the assessment, planning, programme implementation and evaluation phases of geriatric care is fundamental. A variety of health care disciplines may provide additional team members, the range depending upon the employment practices of the facility. Each discipline brings particular knowledge, skills and talents to the service. Planners need to be aware of these and ensure their availability according to the programme objectives.

The general lack of understanding of the potential contribution of many of the newer disciplines needs special attention.

The most commonly required health care workers in the geriatric service team are:

- Audiologist
- Dentist
- Dietitian
- General medical practitioner
- Geriatrician
- Nurse
- Occupational therapist
- Orthotist
- Physiotherapist
- Podiatrist
- Prosthetist
- Recreation therapist
- Social worker
- Speech pathologist

The word team, by most definitions, refers to a joint action. Today, the term is used most commonly in reference to sport. A geriatric care team will be enhanced if it models its organisation and activity upon a successful sporting team. A premier football team, for example, consists of a certain number of skilled people who combine under the leadership of a captain and the direction of a coach to play the game according to the rules. The team trains and practises; studies and plans; shares and supports. A selfish prima donna who attempts to star alone usually leads the team to failure.

A geriatric care team is a similar alliance of disciplines. To be effective it must have a common philosophy to which all are committed. This philosophy ought to be documented so that every member of the team has the opportunity to understand it. A team that promotes the last resort concept of institutional admission will have a different philosophical base from the team that believes that it is easier to look after disabled elderly people in clusters. A geriatric rehabilitation team that is committed to returning elderly people to home as soon as they are safely functional has a different philosophy from the team that strives for normal function before considering discharge. If team members work according to various personal philosophies disjointed action will result with frustration preventing cohesion.

A team must be an alliance of peers who participate in democratic decision making. Freedom to discuss, suggest and argue must be fundamental. Team members may need to practise or train in this activity. It should not be taken for granted that the act of forming a team will automatically result in easy communication. Democratic decision making has to be supported by the willingness of all team members to accept the decision. Too many people believe that they function in a team structure because they meet in a conference once a week. They do not, however, necessarily recognise the importance of commitment to the team decision. For example, a team meeting may decide that Mr Jones is to be discharged to his home and the care of his wife on Friday. If one member of the team continues to dispute this decision and proceeds to counsel Mrs Jones that admission to nursing home care is more appropriate, chaos will ensue.

Usually, a team has a manager to coordinate talents and responsibilities and to arbitrate in deadlocked issues. Traditionally, the team manager has been the senior medical practitioner. There is no reason, however, why this management function should not be conferred on someone else, on the most suitable person who has leadership skills and abilities. Designation of leadership to someone other than a medical practitioner does not, in any way, diminish the medical practitioner's responsibility for controlling the medical management of the elderly person, or diminish the medical practitioner's authority in matters of medical decision making.

The team may choose to function under the case manager model, where a particular person is designated the team leader for a particular patient. This case manager would have responsibility for coordinating the entire programme for the patient and the authority for ensuring that others fulfil the goals established by the team.

The most common approach to team care, though, is that of conjoint goal setting and progress evaluation with the members working out their disciplinary plans independently, if interrelatedly. Mrs Smith's story illustrates this approach.

Mrs Smith was admitted to the geriatric re-habilitation unit following surgery for a fractured neck of femur. The team medical practitioner, nurse, occupational therapist, physiotherapist, dietitian and social worker undertook their various assessments. At a team meeting the findings were pooled, problems identified and goals set. Each worker then planned a specific care programme according to the orientation of the particular discipline.

- Medical practitioner: intervention for medical problems, parameters for weight-bearing progression.
- Physiotherapist: exercise, transfer training, walking re-education.
- Nurse: personal care, monitoring physical and emotional status, liaising with relatives.
- Occupational therapist: functional activities, home modifications, recreation.
- Dietitian: weight-reduction programme.
- Social worker: referrals to domiciliary care agencies.

A timetable scheduled Mrs Smith's day with appointments for physiotherapy and occupational therapy governing the time of rising, bathing, having visitors, participating in recreational activities. Regular team meetings noted Mrs Smith's progress.

Such an approach to care, although common, has some major deficiencies. Mrs Smith was slotted into the therapy schedule where there were vacancies. No attempt was made to obtain advice from nursing staff about the time of day when Mrs Smith was most active in response to her body clock. Because Mrs Smith was portered to the physiotherapy department for her exercises and walking training the nursing staff were transporting her around the ward in a wheelchair long after she could walk with supervision. The medical practitioner saw Mrs Smith in bed and did not realise that difficulties the therapists were having with her stability were due to postural hypotension. The occupational therapist was frustrated by Mrs Smith's apparent lack of enthusiasm for her session each afternoon. The intensive physiotherapy sessions each morning were consuming a disproportionate amount of her energy reserves. These, and many other problems, resulted from a lack of cooperative total care planning.

Some teams have found that the most satisfactory results eventuate from cooperative planning. The assessment findings are pooled in a comprehensive problem list. Solutions to these problems are determined through team discussion. Then a 'patient/client care plan' is prepared — not a nursing care plan, or a physiotherapy care plan. Then, and only then, do the team members decide who is the most appropriate person to carry out each aspect of the plan.

For example, perhaps an identified problem for Mr White was an inability to bathe safely. The solution was to teach Mr White to use a hand-held shower while sitting on a bath seat. This was the method of choice in the rehabilitation unit because his home bathroom would require such a method. Usually, it is the occupational therapist's role to teach this functional activity. Ideally, the occupational therapist will undertake this therapeutic programme at the time Mr White chooses, perhaps after breakfast, perhaps just before going to bed. The occupational therapist will not, satisfactorily, practice in the middle of the afternoon with Mr White fully dressed and pretending to function. If this is the only time the occupational therapist can offer it would be better to leave this training function to the team nurse. The nurse may need specific guidance from the therapist about methods and equipment. In a team this guidance will be sought readily and given freely.

Lest it be imagined that role transposition is usually in the direction of the therapist to nurse, another example may demonstrate the possible two-way nature of teamwork. Mr White needed to produce a midstream urine specimen at 11 a.m. each morning for four days. According to the timetable he was away from the nursing unit at this time, scheduled to be working in the physiotherapy department. The team nurse had three choices for resolving this problem.

1. Mr White could return to the ward, thus curtailing his physiotherapy.
2. The nurse could leave the ward and the other patients and go to the physiotherapy department to collect the specimen.

3. The nurse could teach the physiotherapist the procedure and provide the necessary equipment.

In an effective team the third choice will be the most appropriate.

PRIMARY THERAPIST TEAMS

Another team arrangement that has considerable merit, especially in domiciliary care, is based on the 'primary therapist' concept. The functions of this team are clearly divided into two parts:

1. decision making, including assessment, planning, goal setting and evaluation
2. programme implementation.

The decision-making component involves all appropriate team members while the programme is implemented by one person. The team will decide which member has the most to contribute at a particular time and will assign the primary therapist role to that worker.

For example, Miss Grey was referred to the domiciliary team by the rehabilitation team because of continuing disabilities due to rheumatoid arthritis. Her assessed needs were:

- Bathing assistance
- Monitoring wearing splints on each wrist and a brace on her left knee
- Monitoring drug compliance
- Provision of bed sheets and towels on a weekly exchange basis
- Supervising an exercise routine.

The member of the domiciliary team most appropriate for these functions was the district nurse. As the 'primary therapist', the district nurse undertook the roles of the medical practitioner, physiotherapist, occupational therapist and orthotist, reporting as required to them during team meetings.

Sometime later Miss Grey sustained a flare-up of her rheumatoid arthritis. The decision-making team determined that carefully controlled exercises plus rest and an increase in medications were the programme priorities until the condition stabilised. The physiotherapist was the key person at this time. Therefore, the physiotherapist assumed the 'primary therapist' function, assisting Miss Grey with her shower, monitoring the drug compliance, delivering the laundry as well as supervising the exercise and rest regimen.

Such a concept is still quite novel but it will become common as increasingly scarce and costly resources demand the wisest utilisation of personnel. It is too expensive, in terms of finance and time, to have a number of people from different disciplines visiting the one client when one could undertake all the tasks. It will be necessary for participants of such a team approach to be willing to transpose roles, to accept advice, to consult and to teach. Unfortunately, many professional people tend to guard their roles and functions jealously, disputing any suggestions that another can be effective. These people need to be reminded that the primary therapist concept has been practised for generations. Many a relative has been, and is, a most effective primary therapist.

TEAM MEMBERSHIP QUALITIES

People who wish to be effective in team care need to recognise the implications and decide if this method of functioning is really for them. Some people work best independently, in isolation. This is a fact of life. These people may learn to work in the team situation if they make a deliberate attempt and if the other members appreciate the potential difficulties. Others, however, find it impossible to function in a cooperative. They should seek employment in an area that facilitates independent functioning.

Team members need to demonstrate a variety of qualities:

- To be willing to involve the elderly person and the family as equals in all aspects of care
- To be flexible and able to cope with the unexpected
- To be able to accept the elderly person's rejection of the team's advice
- To have an understanding of the concepts that apply to their own disciplines as well as an appreciation of the roles of other disciplines

- To be willing to recognise that each is dependent upon others for successful programmes
- To be aware that staff conflict and tension affect the progress of the elderly person
- To be innovative and unencumbered by jurisdictional disputes.

TEAM COMMUNICATION

Communication is the key to successful cooperative action. An effective team needs to meet formally on a regular basis. Such a meeting ought to be considered sacrosanct by the members and only missed in an emergency. In such an event the missing member must still contribute, either in a written report or through a colleague. Corridor conversations, while important in cooperative action, are not adequate substitutes for a formal meeting.

Team meetings need ground rules that all members understand. It is usually helpful to have these documented so that new members can prepare for full participation on joining the group. These rules are also important to ensure that no one member dominates the team.

Communication needs a common language to assist all participants. Disciplinary jargon should be avoided. Medical information with its special language is apt to become distorted by non-medical people. Since it is often difficult to avoid using such language it is important that a deliberate attempt be made to validate accurate understanding, especially on the part of the elderly person and the family. It may be necessary to prepare elderly people and the families for team participation to lessen their anxiety when confronted by a group.

To facilitate communication the 'problem orientated medical record' is a most appropriate method for documenting the work of the team.

TEAM ACTION AND ROLES

The members of a geriatric care team bring skills and talents to the programme for an individual elderly person according to their interests and experiences as well as the philosophy of the particular discipline to which each belongs. Members often have a great deal in common. Usually, role overlapping is unavoidable because there are no clear lines of demarcation, no definite boxes to surround each discipline. Because there are so many variations in team composition, often depending on the objectives of the service, it is not possible to describe a standard team. Further, individuals often bring a particular approach to the practice of a discipline, making precise descriptions difficult.

15. Care in the community

Doreen Bauer

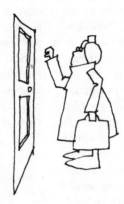

Community care is one of the main pillars of the system of extended care. Without a balance of effective and supportive community services many more people would become institutionalised.

Appropriate services need to be developed further and distributed equitably in all communities if the imbalance between institutional accommodation and the opportunity to receive appropriate care at home is to be redressed.

COMMUNITY CARE PROGRAMMES

Home care is not, contrary to popular belief, a new concept in health care. Since the beginning of time people have been cared for at home by others who have assumed responsibility, whether willingly or not. Today, by far the major share of home care is undertaken by innumerable husbands, wives, relatives, friends and neighbours. Recognition of the enormous contribution of this vast army of home carers is, unfortunately, rare.

Community care programmes have been developed in response to the needs of people who wish to remain at home and who do not have access to appropriate home carers either in terms of people or skills. Currently, concepts of home care and programmes to facilitate it are receiving a great deal of attention, especially as they relate to the care of frail, disabled or ill elderly people.

It has been clearly established by research and by experience that most elderly people prefer to remain in their own homes. When circumstances force an elderly person to consider alternatives the last resort choice of institutional living is made with great reluctance. Ownership of territory, even if actually rented, is a guarantee of security with strong implications of autonomy and control. Most elderly people strive, often fiercely, to maintain an independent relationship with the usual known environment. Frailty or disability may jeopardise this relationship by preventing the person from behaving competently in one or more areas of functioning.

It is important that when changes in health or level of independence occur, it should be possible to refer the elderly person for perceptive medical and psychosocial assessment, to ensure that appropriate action ensues, whether it be simple problem-solving advice, admission to hospital for restorative treatment, provision of support services at home, or, as a last resort, institutional care. Increasingly, society is accepting the premise that many people wish to and can be maintained in their own homes despite frailty or disability.

However, as this humanitarian premise gains acceptance, governments are being confronted with serious financial problems. The seemingly insatiable demands of health and welfare programmes have consumed a greater share of the total resources than is deemed to be appropriate. The cost of institutional care has escalated beyond the available financial resources. The growing number of potential institution users, whether of acute hospitals or continuing care facilities, has forced governments to re-evaluate their approach to meeting the needs of people, especially of frail, disabled or ill elderly people.

Care at home is no longer considered an alternative to institutional care; it is, rightly, the first approach to be considered. Increasingly, services and facilities are becoming more flexible, available to be used to match assessed needs as and when they are required.

A domiciliary care programme needs to be comprehensive, coordinated and continuous, with clearly defined relationships with other facets of the overall geriatric care network. It must provide services that are appropriate, available, accessible and acceptable. The proliferation of agencies providing services has created a major challenge for health and welfare workers who must ensure that each individual client's needs are met with an appropriate type and level of service. A number of management systems may be considered to assist with coordination.

The development of geriatric assessment teams is considered a valuable step in the coordination process, the independent team of specialist health and welfare personnel being seen as an entry point into the system. In the past, services might have been prescribed to solve an apparent functional difficulty without the benefit of comprehensive assessment and problem identification. For instance, inadequate nutrition might have been managed by referral to the delivered meals service. More adequate assessment, however, may have identified more basic problems such as inability to use an old cooking stove, difficulties with shopping, or depression, problems which could have more appropriate solutions than delivered meals (Table 15.1).

Finding the most satisfactory solution should be facilitated by a comprehensive approach to assessment, problem identification and solution planning, the elderly person being provided with a range of options from which to select a desirable service. The role of the geriatric assessment team in the planning and coordination of individual client programmes is still subject to debate but there is increasing evidence that the team has a valuable and cost-effective contribution to make, especially when it acts as an independent agent concerned only with the best interests of the elderly person.

Table 15.1 Problem: nutritional deficiency and how to overcome it

Cause	Possible solution
Chemistry dysfunction	Diet, supplements
Lack of knowledge	Education
Lack of cooking experience	Training — acquirement of basic skills
Lack of equipment	Advice, assistance
Lack of budget skills	Advice, assistance
Shopping problems	Transport, shopping
Loneliness, lack of motivation	Companionship
Poor teeth	Dental care — regular check-ups
Disability	'Meals-on-wheels'

Case management is another well established process, one person being assigned the responsibility for overseeing the total programme. The actual structure of the case management concept, however, is still subject to debate as various systems are evaluated. The case manager may be just responsible for coordination but, increasingly, the case manager is being delegated brokerage responsibilities. In this role, the case manager has the authority to purchase services from various agencies according to the agreed needs of the individual. This financial authority gives the case manager the power to supervise the programme, ensuring appropriate standards.

Considerable work still needs to be done to determine the most effective, including cost-effective, manner of implementing case management. Clearly, though, it is desirable to have one person acting as the client's primary contact when a variety of agencies are involved in service provision. Without such a formal approach it is difficult, if not impossible, to ensure coordination when agencies have independent objectives, their own staff and administration, and their own identity to defend.

Most essentially, the services must undertake energetic community education programmes to overcome widespread consumer ignorance. Many people have little information about the available options. Even when programmes are known, many people have access problems because they do not know how to reach the service.

A primary area for coordination lies in the transition from hospital to home. It is imperative that liaison between the acute hospital and the domiciliary programme be formally established, someone from the domiciliary programme being fully involved in the hospital discharge planning process for any elderly person who is at risk. It would be helpful to develop a risk scale which is a mandatory measure applied to every hospitalised person aged 70 plus. (Such a scale should be similar in concept to the Apgar scale applied to every newborn baby.) Such a scale would alert hospital staff to the potential for problems and ensure more adequate assessment and intervention planning before the discharge was effected. Too frequently, elderly people are discharge from hospital unable to cope adequately. Hospital staff need to be aware that failure to plan appropriately for discharge makes life very difficult for the elderly person, the family and the domiciliary services. The need for better planning will become increasingly evident as hospitals strive to reduce length of stay. It is, therefore, in the best interests of the hospital to cooperate fully in the development of improved approaches to discharge planning.

Service objectives

The following general objectives will be common to most coordinated domiciliary care programmes.

- To discover people with unmet or underserviced needs.
- To identify specific problems by competent, comprehensive assessment.

- To determine strategies that will assist to solve or cope with the problems.
- To facilitate the delivery of services, either directly or through other agencies, ensuring that the services are effective and maintained as long, but no longer, than necessary.
- To function as the focus of a range of service agencies which have mutual goals and which may be effective only in a coordinated endeavour.
- To monitor and evaluate the programme constantly and adapt to rapidly changing circumstances. Establishing new programmes, altering the direction of established ones, and realigning priorities within the scope of limited resources must be an ongoing process.
- To undertake a planned, continuing staff education programme to assist in the maintenance or improvement of competency.
- To provide staff with ongoing support and supervision, recognition and appreciation.
- To accelerate public education to develop a greater appreciation of the spectrum of age-related matters in elderly people, in families, and in the about-to-become elderly, and to improve society's competence in decision making.
- To influence community decisions on matters related to the care of elderly people.

A suitable programme to serve a community must be planned. Planning demands answers to fundamental questions. A quantitative and epidemiological approach is essential. It is not enough to know that frail, disabled or ill elderly people can be cared for at home. Planners must have some idea of the number of people in need of assistance and the types of assistance required. Studies must be undertaken to identify people already using institutional resources and determine if they would, in fact, have benefited from a restorative care or treatment programme and been more appropriately managed at home. Research is also necessary to demonstrate that hospital programmes and beds in use could be reduced to such an extent that savings will exceed the cost increases associated with a home care programme. Research is required to determine at what point it should be decided that the cost of maintaining an individual at home exceeds an acceptable level and alternative institutional care be therefore appropriate. Research is required to identify gaps or overlaps in the current service. The number and type of people required to provide care must be based on fact not belief. Questions related to standards of education, disciplinary mixes and case-load levels must be answered factually and realistically rather than emotionally.

Considerable attention is being devoted to research in these areas and a good deal of evidence is being considered in Australia as well as in many other countries. It is essential that all the players in the system look at this research dispassionately, agreeing to changes as the evidence dictates.

NEEDS

A number of issues should be considered in any general discussion of the needs of elderly people. It must be remembered that people do not fit a standard pattern. Each person is a unique human being, who should be approached and appreciated as an individual. Research may develop a list of needs that are commonly demonstrated by elderly people. Planners must not forget that not all old people will demonstrate these needs and not all old people will have the same depth of need. Care must be taken to ensure that there is no suggestion, either deliberate or accidental, that old people form a homogeneous group.

Another issue relates to differentiating between 'needs' and 'wants'. Commonly the words are

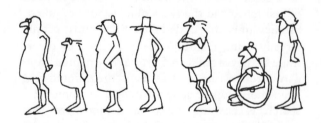

used synonymously but discrimination is essential. A need is a requirement, recognised by an observer: e.g. he needs a balanced diet. A want is something perceived by the subject: e.g. I want meat every day. Everyone knows about the elderly person who needs supervised accommodation but wants to remain in his or her usual, acceptable squalor. When defining the specific needs of an individual it is essential to involve him or her in the assessment process and the ensuing interpretation. Unless there is rationalisation of the planner's concepts of 'his/her needs' with the recipient's judgements of 'my wants', the programme may end with services that will only be used by the weak under duress.

Accuracy in the interpretation of expressed needs is equally important. A person may claim that he/she needs one form of assistance when he/she really wants something else. He/she may be quite unaware of this alternative or may, through implied shame, be unable to express it. Physiotherapy departments, for example, frequently receive elderly people with pain problems for which they demand treatment. Frequently, the pain in the physical sense is the acceptable expression of a deeper, more fundamental pain. Emotional pain resulting from loneliness and depression may not even be recognised. Treatment of the physical pain without solving the underlying problems will only create a person who must depend on the physiotherapy department to meet his/her emotional needs. Other forms of care, perhaps day centre socialisation, could meet these needs more appropriately.

A further complication in determining needs is the fact that conscious consumer wants are limited by experience and knowledge. An individual can only want what he/she knows is available. Manufacturers understand this and spend fortunes on advertising to ensure that people know what is offered and to encourage them to 'want'. People should be fully informed of the range of possibilities available to meet actual needs, if they are to be in a position to make an informed choice.

In many countries, including Australia, the delineation of need and the planning of programmes have to be placed against very complex cultural backgrounds. A culture provides its members with a set of rules expressed in terms of expected behaviours, statuses and roles. Ethnic considerations must, quite clearly, colour the perception of need. Ethnicity, however, is but one of many cultural factors which complicate the task of defining need. Most people belong to one or more subcultures: sex, age, religious, political, occupational, sport, economic, regional and social. Each group or subculture has its set of statuses, roles and expected behaviour, all of which temper the response of an individual. Further, each culture or subculture is evolutionary even if appearing conservative. Keeping abreast of the changes adds a further challenge.

With these provisions in mind, community care needs may be classified into five broad groups: economic, housing, health, welfare and social.

Economic

Economic problems are a common feature of life for many elderly people. Unfortunately, society appears to assume that it costs significantly less to live when one is old. Financial difficulties may not be a new thing in the life of the elderly person. Substandard housing and impoverishment may have been a long-term state either through circumstances or choice. There are, however, an increasing number of elderly people whose income, despite prudent planning, is insufficient to maintain an adequate life at home. Many elderly widows especially are disadvantaged significantly when they are plunged suddenly into the management role previously occupied solely by the husband.

The repercussions of financial problems may be far reaching into most other aspects of the elderly person's life. For example, low income and high housing costs may mean that there is little left for food, clothing or transport with consequential problems with health and social relationships.

Housing

Housing difficulties are a major source of concern for many elderly people. Many wish to remain in the house which has been the scene of their mature life. Sometimes this is substandard without the basic comforts of adequate plumbing and heating. Often this is large and beyond the resources of the elderly person to maintain effectively. Frequently, it is not suitable environmentally for the mobility or functional disabilities that have developed with age.

The current problems might have resulted from attempts to correct previous difficulties. An elderly person might have surrendered the home to move into the home of relatives. This might have proved to be an unfortunate decision but there is insufficient money now to purchase another home. Increasingly, elderly people who have retired to new communities find the decision inappropriate, especially as resort or leisure centres, the most common attractions, are not geared to cope with the problems of old people, should they develop.

Health

Health problems are those most commonly presented by elderly people who require support to live at home. While these cover the full spectrum it is important to note that health problems are frequently an acceptable expression of other difficulties that the elderly person is unable to admit. For example, complaints of pain in the knees due to osteoarthritis may be, much more, a plea for solace from loneliness.

Welfare

Welfare problems are usually associated with interpersonal relationships. Many elderly people are effectively and adequately sustained by family, neighbours and friends. A significant minority, however, do not have such a supportive network upon which to rely. They, then, have problems with shopping, attending to personal business, such as banking, paying accounts, or keeping office appointments with doctors and solicitors. Lone people often have no one to maintain surveillance, to respond to an emergency.

Social

Sociocultural problems are important but still frequently overlooked. The need for meaningful social relationships is primary for the majority of elderly people. It must, however, not be concluded that elderly people want to be associated exclusively with other elderly people. A broad spectrum of relationships from babies through all age groups are needed by most people. Further, many elderly people continue to want to be of service to others, to be involved in community life, to participate in creative activities, to maintain religious affiliations, to enjoy new and novel experiences. Frequently, old age is a time for strengthening the ties to a culture that was left behind on migration to Australia. Failure to meet these needs may have serious consequences for an elderly person.

ASSESSMENT OF THE HOME

A careful examination of the home environment is an essential supplement to the general assessment described in Chapter 11. Before any person attempts a home assessment it is essential to consider a number of vital issues.

1. An assessor may enter a person's home by invitation, not by right. The 'guest in the home of the host' relationship ought to permeate the task. Permission must be obtained to undertake each aspect of the assessment. Considerable care should be exercised to avoid any suggestion of criticism or condemnation which may embarrass the host or the family.

2. A home assessment cannot be undertaken adequately when the elderly or disabled person is absent. The primary purpose of a home assessment is to determine the person's ability to function effectively and safely. Thus, the assessor needs to see the person functioning. Too often a perception of difficulty may not be a reality. Many people, able and disabled, function well despite an apparently poor environment.

3. Undertaking a home assessment by interview is a very hazardous task. Many people find it difficult to recall the details of the home environment which are essential for evaluation. Many people, especially poor elderly people, are reluctant to admit that there are problems, particularly if these are related to poverty. For example, a person may deny any problems with managing the toilet, neglecting to admit that it is located in the garden.

4. It is important to understand the expectations of function held by the person and the family. A person who plans to live alone may have quite different functional expectations from the person who is to live with a family in a quite acceptable dependent relationship. There will be little point in adapting the family home for complete independence if it is not to be practised.

5. Problem solving requires a very informed understanding of the financial resources available to meet potential costs. Bathrooms, for example, are the most frequently discovered problem areas. The cost of modifications, especially if plumbing is involved, may be outside the personal resources of the person or the family. The assessor will need to determine if alternative sources of money are available and if the person is willing to accept such assistance. If the answer is no to either of these questions the assessor will need to plan alternatives. For example, the bathroom may not have an effective source of hot water. A new water heater will be the obvious solution. If, for whatever reason, this proves impossible, then day centre attendances with bathing being one of the activities undertaken may be a satisfactory solution.

6. Solutions for problems may not be developed until the difficulties have been discussed and appreciated as problems by the elderly person. An effective planner will introduce solutions skillfully, in such a way that the elderly person sees them as his or her own answers. An effective planner will not force solutions.

Many detailed home assessment forms have been developed for staff undertaking this task. Such a form is not being recommended here because they have a tendency to blinker the inexperienced assessor who may miss significant factors while seeking form answers. Rather, the following is offered as a reminder list. The ability of the person to function effectively and safely in each appropriate area should be carefully considered.

- Access to the home
  — from the road
  — gates
  — paths
  — steps
  — doors
  — location of letter-box

- Mobility within the living areas
  — safety
  — manoeuverability

- Lighting
  — accessibility of switches
  — strength of illumination
  — location of illumination

- Furniture
  — suitability
  — accessibility
  — stability

- Power points
  — safety
  — accessibility

- Water supply

- Heating
  — safety
  — suitability
  — effectiveness

- Kitchen appliances
  — suitability
  — accessibility
  — effectiveness
  — safety
  — manoeuverability

- Toilet
  — location
  — effectiveness
  — safety

- Bedroom
  — furniture
  — mobility
  — bedside light

- Emergency
  — means of contacting others for help
  — means of escape in case of emergency

- Transport
  — accessibility
  — safety

- Shopping

- Socialisation

An occupational therapist is, usually, the most suitable person to undertake the home assessment. The orientation of this discipline is in functional competence. In the absence of an occupational therapist others may be quite effective if the assessment takes the form of functional observation. Such observation also falls within the ambit of the community health or district nurse. Many problems may have clear and simple solutions. When this is not so, it may be practical to seek the advice of an occupational therapist who may be able to provide some ideas for consideration.

SERVICES

Counselling

Frequently, elderly people and their families are unable to cope with day to day living at home because of lack of knowledge. Problems may appear to be insurmountable because people are unaware of possible solutions. Further, many elderly people continue to view social services as charity. They may need significant assistance from a very understanding person to come to terms with the emotional concepts of welfare. A counselling service may permit people to gain essential knowledge of community resources. Counselling involves problem exploration, need identification and examination of solution options. Counselling implies advising and assisting a person to make informed choices.

Counselling is not the particular prerogative of any one discipline although social workers or welfare staff should have greater expertise. Every person who works with elderly people must have a general understanding of the spectrum of services available as well as the functions of other workers to facilitate referrals.

Education

An elementary feature of a domiciliary care service should be a broadly based public education programme. People must be informed if they are to plan intelligently, to identify problems early and to seek satisfactory solutions. Because there is not a standard approach to domiciliary care throughout Australia each community will have to prepare an individual education programme. Media campaigns, pamphlets and information displays should supplement an active public speaking programme by staff from the extended care service to reach as many people as possible.

Environmental adaptation

An elderly person may not be able to manage at home because aspects of the physical environment do not promote safe or effective functional independence. It may be desirable and practical to modify the environment to correct such problems. Often, solutions are simple. For example, a bath seat and hand-held shower attachment may permit bathing when the physical status of a person prevents him or her climbing into the bath. A chemical toilet in the bathroom may solve the problems associated with the toilet at the end of the back verandah, two steps down.

Environmental adaptations may require:

- someone, most effectively an occupational therapist, to analyse the situation and plan suitable modifications
- . a source of equipment supply
- someone to install aids or undertake structural alterations
- a source of funding.

Theoretically, elderly Australians requiring assistance in one or more of these areas may have these needs met through a variety of government programmes. Unfortunately, the resources available to meet the needs are, as yet, inadequate.

Errands

Lack of mobility may reduce an elderly person's effectiveness in managing his or her affairs. When families or friends are unavailable, such a person

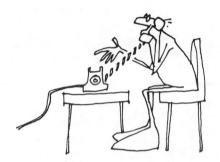

may need a reliable service to undertake a range of tasks upon instruction. Shopping and banking are common requirements but the potential list may be endless.

An organised errand service may be seen as a community solution to this problem. Many people, however, have evolved a variety of measures such as the use of a telephone and a taxi driver to meet their needs.

Family relief

Many families are willing to assume direct responsibility for relatives either in a caring or supervising capacity. When the degree of dependency is high the burden of the task often becomes intolerable. This is particularly so if the family members are unable to pursue their own lives because of the constancy of the caring role. Abdication of responsibility with admission to an institution is often seen as the only solution. The increasing incidence of 'granny bashing', whether physically or mentally, is another expression of the frustration experienced by many relatives in their struggle to maintain an elderly person at home.

These families could be more effective home carers in the long-term if they had opportunities for relief. There are a number of ways in which relief may be provided:

1. District nursing service. This service plays a most important part in enabling a frail incapacited old person to remain at home. District nurses monitor the health and well-being of patients, supervise medications, carry out treatment programmes, assist with physiological functioning, observe changes or risk factors, advise and teach patients and families, and provide terminal care for those who wish to die at home. They also liaise with general practitioners and other health professionals as necessary, and act as coordinators and facilitators within the system of extended care.

2. Home respite care. Reliable people take over the carer's role and tasks for a short period, either regularly or on special occasions. This may range from a few hours to a weekend.

3. Day centre. The elderly person is admitted to a day centre for social stimulation, activity therapy, and supervision. Again, attendance should be tailored to meet the relatives' particular needs. For some, attendance from mid-morning to mid-afternoon one day a week may prove adequate. Others may require longer days, five days a week, to cover the carer's normal working hours.

4. Holiday admission to continuing care. Many families are able to care effectively if they have opportunities for holidays. When alternative home carers are unavailable a temporary admission to a continuing care facility may be a practical solution.

Home maintenance

Many elderly people have been admitted to an institution simply because they have been unable to undertake a satisfactory standard of home maintenance. The anxiety created by unkempt gardens, spouting blocked by leaves, and minor repairs such as dripping taps may be a direct cause of physical and mental breakdowns. The increasingly high cost of commercial services to solve these problems often places them outside the financial resources of elderly people. An organised approach to a handyman service may assist many elderly people to remain at home. Such a service may be:

- freely available through a domiciliary service on appropriate referral
- arranged on a contract basis, the domiciliary service recommending a reliable tradesman who charges an approved fee
- organised by a service club, the domiciliary service recommending people in need.

Housekeeping

A functionally disabled elderly person may be able to remain at home if someone is available to undertake housekeeping tasks. Most, if not all,

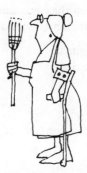

local governments have housekeeping or home help services with trained staff available to undertake a range of personal and domestic duties. The tasks that may be undertaken vary from service to service but, increasingly, the home help is being seen as the primary, personal care provider.

An effective home help service is the heart of the domiciliary programme if the helpers are encouraged to be the status monitors. By reporting the progress of the client to the coordinator of the domiciliary programme the home help may facilitate early intervention in potential problems.

Hospital discharge planning

Planning for discharge to home after a period of hospitalisation is a critical matter. Ideally, discharge planning should commence upon admission. If domiciliary services are anticipated, arrangements need to be made in advance to ensure implementation at the right time. A domiciliary care coordinator or liaison community health nurse, should be a member of the hospital team to identify potential problems and recommend solutions. Being part of both the hospital and the domiciliary service, such a coordinator may ease the transition from hospital to home especially if the patient or the family is anxious.

Nutrition

An effective domiciliary service will have a range of options available for people with nutritional problems. While home-delivered meals are the best known of the nutrition services it is essential to remember that they are not the only service necessary. A nutrition service may involve:

- delivered hot meals
- delivered frozen meals
- dietary supplements
- dietary education
- cooking training
- kitchen modifications or aids
- shopping
- dental care
- companionship.

Communities that do not have access to a 'meals-on-wheels' service have developed a variety of solutions. Subsidised counter lunches at a hotel may be practical. The hotel may prepare and deliver a meal. A neighbour may be willing to cook and deliver a meal for the approved fee. A sharing talents scheme may be possible, where an able elderly lady cooks the meals for an inexperienced man who returns the favour by undertaking simple house maintenance.

Periodic review of status

Many lone elderly people seek institutional care because of anxiety that assistance will not be available when it is needed. An extended care programme should be able to offer such people the security of status monitoring by a liaison community nurse so that help can be made available if and when it is needed. Monitoring visits provide opportunities for:

- education, especially for families
- counselling
- ongoing assessment, particularly of hygiene standards, diet, maintenance of drug therapy, psychosocial status, functional abilities and family or community relationships.

Personal care

Domiciliary care planners are coming to realise that many disabled people are able to be maintained at home if a personal care service is available.

Bathing is a well known service which may be undertaken by a home help or district nurse. The nurse may also have wide ranging responsibility for treatment and health maintenance programmes. Many disabled people, however, need assistance to get out of bed and dressed in the morning. They can then function reasonably independently until bedtime. The availability of skilled people to undertake a valet service appears to be an important requirement of a domiciliary care programme. In Australia, there used to be a tendency to view the skills required for a valet service to be those of a nurse. This was, of course, an expensive solution to a problem which is now being solved by people with less training. Skilled staff such as nurses or therapists may be essential to assess needs and to plan strategies but home help or home health aids are well able to implement the daily programme.

A laundry service may be an essential feature of a personal care programme. Many elderly people cannot cope with the laundering of heavy items such as sheets and towels. Special problems arise when there is incontinence. Families may be able to undertake the general care of an old person, but break down under the constant laundry created by incontinence.

A laundry service in which sheets and towels are delivered on a weekly exchange basis, has proved of inestimable value in keeping many elderly people at home. When incontinence is a problem, special sheets that protect the person from wetness are of value also.

Laundry services should be part of every extended care programme. Informal arrangements, however, between a family and the local hospital may be possible in the absence of alternatives.

Recreation

Recipients of home care services who are unable, or unwilling, to participate in day centre or other socialisation programmes may need assistance to maintain recreative experience. Mobile library, art and craft programmes could well be appropriate. Day trips, visits to church and social functions may be organised directly by the domiciliary service or through arrangements with volunteers. Assistance with planning a suitable holiday would also represent a significant service.

Security

Increasingly, frail elderly people are requiring assistance with security at home. A variety of systems is available. Previously satisfactory methods such as signs in windows or flashing lights are coming into disfavour because they advertise the weakness of the elderly person to criminal elements in society.

More sophisticated electronic devices operated via telephones are proving more suitable for summoning emergency assistance as well as providing daily status monitoring. Although these systems are quite expensive an increasing number of subsidised programmes are becoming available.

Transport

Many disabled people have special transport needs which cannot be met by public transport systems. In many areas there is no public transport available. Frequently, dependency is enforced because of lack of mobility. A domiciliary programme needs to be able to assist people to retain necessary mobility. Services must, however, be planned adequately and have skilled personnel available. Management of people who need transferring assistance is a skill that must be learnt. Similarly, training in the manipulation of a wheelchair will facilitate safe transportation. Physiotherapists and occupational therapists have particular skills in the management of mobility problems.

Treatment

The elderly person at home may require treatment services for one or more problems on a short- or long-term basis. The full spectrum of extended care disciplines may be involved in a broadly based treatment service. The primary therapist model, described in Chapter 14, should be the basis for an effective treatment service.

Welfare

Assistance with problems associated with housing, finances, family relationships and other such social welfare matters is a service commonly required by elderly people striving to live at home. Frequently, difficulties arise because people do not know where to turn for help.

Domiciliary or community care programmes have been developed to varying degrees, in response to the needs of people who wish to remain at home but do not have adequate resources to do so. Theoretically, or idealistically, it is possible to provide services to keep a person in his or her own home regardless of the type or level of disability. Realistically, however, it is necessary for society to develop criteria for reasonableness in terms of resources, both personnel and financial. There is a further need for extensive research into the epidemiology of problems, the primary services required to meet the identified needs and the personnel required to implement programmes in terms of members, education and disciplinary mixes. The consequences of lack of formal coordination in a multiple agency system also demands scrutiny.

16. Care of elderly people with dementia

Penny Phillips

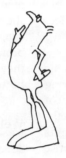

By the year 2000 the increase in the population over the age of 80 years will result in a steady increase in the number of people suffering from organic brain diseases. Although there has been considerable progress in research into the cause of Alzheimer's disease over the last decade, the possibility of prevention or cure is still a long way off. Unless there is marked progress in such research within a few years, leading to prevention or amelioration of this condition, the implications for those responsible for the provision of support and care will be immense.

Confusional states can occur as a symptom of many illnesses in the elderly. In cases where the onset is acute, and mental function previously was normal, it is essential that the underlying problem be determined and treated. In all probability the causative factor would lie outside the brain, and one cause in the elderly with which many nurses are familiar is an acute infection such as pneumonia, the successful treatment of which should lead to the restoration of normality.

Where the onset of confused behaviour, with deterioration of mental function, is progressive over a period of time the problem is usually associated with organic brain disease. Careful medical diagnostic assessment is essential to ensure that identifiable causes within the brain, such as a tumour or subdural haematoma, are addressed. Where no remediable cause can be demonstrated emphasis must be placed on appropriate care for the one concerned, and support for the spouse or family.

Both acute and chronic confusional states are dealt with fully in the section on 'confusion' in Chapter 5 and in Chapter 10. This chapter will deal with the special needs of those suffering from Alzheimer's disease and related disorders and the general term 'dementia' will be used in this context.

SOCIAL IMPLICATIONS

A very high proportion of the elderly people suffering from dementia is living in the community, supported by families. In most instances the immediate provision of care rests with women — either wives or daughters. As the numbers of 'old old' suffering from dementia increase, the burden on their children, also ageing, will increase intolerably giving rise to a high degree of stress.

Dementia may progress slowly over many years, and result in memory loss, disorientation, agitation, wandering, sleeplessness, withdrawal and in some instances communication disorders and aggression. Such problems must inevitably cause distress to the individual concerned as well as to those providing care.

Following retirement many couples adopt a pattern of living that is based on the sharing of interests and activities. As the years go by the daily routine is apt to settle into a regular pattern. Most people can adapt their style of living to accommodate physical illness or disability, but if the mind of one becomes increasingly impaired every aspect of the lives of both are affected. The one who remains competent is conscious of losing that vital companionship which is based on sharing problems, as well as participating in the pleasures and the normal activities of everyday living. Many in this situation feel lonely and have great difficulty in adapting to the changes that are occurring in the personality and behaviour of their spouse.

To quote Enid Levin (1989) '. . . dementing illnesses are tragic, daunting and destructive. By impairing, and at their most extreme, destroying the ability to think, remember, reason, they strike at the very core of a person's being'.

COMMUNITY SERVICES

As stated previously most people suffering from dementia receive support and care in the community from their own immediate families, or sometimes friends. These carers or 'significant others' need informed advice and psychological counselling, as well as access to services appropriate to their needs. Breaks from the care of the demented person through regular attendance at a special day centre, or through planned intermittent admission to residential (respite) care may be of benefit to both people.

Those providing care must, of course, be involved in the planning of systems of support, as must the recipient as far as is possible. However, it is not possible to plan without first defining the needs of the individual concerned and the requirements of the carer(s), while at the same time identifying the resources available to meet those needs.

Community nursing

District nursing is often the first and sometimes the only service involved. While being in a position to provide 'hands on care' through 24 hours

when nursing needs are present, district nurses are also important in their role of encouraging and coordinating the use of other services.

Ideally, district nursing services should have - access (preferably on staff) to consultants such as social workers, physiotherapists occupational therapists and speech pathologists, as well as to nurse consultants in psychiatry, gerontology and continence. These consultants work with staff, patients and other care givers to provide specialist expertise within the home setting. This enables carers to have access to resources at a time in their lives when they have less opportunity to leave home. In some situations, respite in the home can be provided by trained health aids, who act as substitute relatives under the indirect supervision of a district nurse (Royal District Nursing Service 1989).

Municipal services

Home help and meals-on-wheels are two of the many services offered by local councils, and in some areas, in addition to household duties, home helps provide a considerable degree of support and general care. Other services of special value where dementia sufferers are cared for at home include social work counselling, occupational therapy advice and the installation of aids to enhance safety.

A high level of cooperation and communication between district nurses and council service providers is essential if the provision of appropriate services to those who need them is to be assured.

Day centres

Special day centres provide information, care, therapeutic activities and socialisation within local community settings, as well as respite for the care giver.

In multicultural societies it is important to plan day centre activities for cultural subgroups, so that participants can enjoy their familiar language, food and social customs within a supportive environment.

Multilingual social workers linked with such services should have the training and skills to act as counsellors and coordinators.

Assessment

The principles of assessment and the assessment processes described in Chapter 11 are very relevant in this situation, and clearly the family doctor should be closely involved in all phases of the person's programme of care. The process of assessment needs to be documented carefully to ensure the accurate identification of problems. This facilitates the treatment of remediable conditions, the resolution of immediate difficulties, and allows the planning of care to be based on relevant objective data.

Regular review is important to ensure that changes in the client's needs are recognised and met. The family doctor should be able to call on help as necessary from members of the assessment or health care team, such as a social worker, psychiatric nurse, occupational therapist or speech pathologist. This team could assist all those concerned with the provision of care with advice regarding the management of behavioural and interpersonal difficulties, agitation or aggression.

Where there is also a degree of physical disability an occupational therapist can assist in making living space safe and more convenient, with particular attention focused on the kitchen and bathroom. In addition, advice may be given on simple systems of communication with neighbours, but more importantly the special skills of the occupational therapist should be used in exploring activities that may be enjoyed by both the carer and caree, such as painting, handwork, music and the modification of interests previously shared, particularly those involving exercise.

Respite care through day centres and residential accommodation has been mentioned, but periods of relief for lone carers in the home, to allow them to go out and follow personal interests, would be beneficial. If no relative or friend is available, carefully selected volunteers or paid staff could spend time in the home on a planned basis. Such a service should provide overnight care during a weekend or over a longer period to give the carer time to relax. This would be of particular value for supporters of dementia sufferers who are manageable at home, but who become aggressive and upset if moved into residential care. Such services need to be tailored to meet the needs of a particular situation, and thus have to be flexible to ensure that the response is appropriate and of optimal value.

Levin et al (1989) suggest that dementia poses a serious challenge to the advocates of community care, who want to keep old people, including those with dementia, at home, and they raise the question of 'at what cost to families upon whom the policy largely depends?'. They suggest that the success of community care does not have to be achieved at the high personal costs now borne by so many supporting relatives. Their research has shown that standard community services are relevant to the supporters' problems, appreciated where received, and that they can have beneficial effects on the psychological health of some supporters. It was found, however, that of those interviewed many were not aware of the availability of services, or had not been offered services that could have reduced their levels of stress. Information about services in the community needs to be well publicised as does the availability of informed advice.

The coordination of the delivery of effective services and care is difficult to achieve but is important if the best use is to be made of limited resources. In many countries responsibility for the various components of extended care — health services, treatment facilities, community services or residential accommodation — is scattered between public, private and voluntary care sectors, controlled in turn by government legislation and funding, or by local government regulations.

RESOURCE AND SUPPORT CENTRES

There are increasing numbers of government-funded special day centres in Australia for dementia sufferers, which have imaginative and innovative activity programmes. These centres form part of an organised system of care. In addition, the Alzheimer's Disease and Related Disorders Society (ADARDS) provides a network of support for both families and sufferers of dementia. The Society provides a forum in which families and those concerned can meet and talk together, sharing experiences and problems as well as giving mutual support and encouragement. ADARDS provides a counselling service, assists with the management of stress and advises on access to services. ADARDS (Australia) has acted as advocate in drawing to the attention of the Federal Government the special needs of dementia sufferers for funding for special care facilities and services. The Society has also stressed the need for further research in this field. More information on community services applicable to those with dementia is contained in Chapter 15.

RESIDENTIAL CARE

Many sufferers of dementia receiving care at home with planned intermittent admission to hostels or nursing homes progress towards permanent admission when care at home is no longer appropriate or tenable. Those not previously involved in a planned programme of care, based on informed assessment by the regional geriatric assessment team, could benefit from such assessment before permanent admission, as some improvement in physical functioning and management may still be possible.

Within many residential facilities for dementia sufferers, whether hostel or nursing home, the principles of 'reality orientation' are applied. Other approaches may include 'validation therapy' or 'resolution therapy'. Whichever approach is favoured it is important that staff act with patience and tolerance as well as with kindness.

Reality orientation

'Reality orientation', as described by Folsom (1973), is a continuing programme for the dementing elderly person aimed at stimulating awareness of time, place and person. The organisation of the environment is an important feature of reality orientation. Group sessions in a classroom setting are aimed at stimulating thought processes and these supplement activities of daily living. Signs, clocks, calendars, bulletin boards, colour coding and personal possessions all reinforce verbal information.

In a day hospital or institutional situation several important factors contribute to a healthy environment for such people. These include a consistent 'team' approach to care through 24 hours, seven days a week. The provision of appropriate educational programmes enables understanding and influences attitudes of staff and other care givers. Classroom reality orientation also encompasses sensory stimulation and remotivation programmes. Reminiscing is also of value in this context. Whatever the approach, all carers should keep in mind that each individual needs to be assessed and a personal care programme developed for them. As in most areas of life, the quality of the relationship is more important than the purity of the technique (Folsom J et al 1978).

Techniques such as reality orientation and validation therapy are not mutually exclusive; rather it is a matter of degree as to what input is likely to be most helpful and appropriate at any given time.

As well as having a profound effect on the elderly person concerned, confusional states complicate the lives of people involved in care, including relatives and friends, who in turn need to participate fully in whatever approach is most likely to be beneficial to the clients. Reality orientation gives direction to carers (especially hospital and nursing home staff) to assist them in providing a consistent, understanding approach that ensures some continuity of care in a setting where there is often an overwhelming parade of strange faces before the confused person. The presentation of reality at all times can assist such an individual to act appropriately — so the time of day is associated with meal times or an activity group. For some people, or at certain times, information about time, place and person may not achieve any desired response. The important point about reality orientation is that it must be applied consistently by all staff with sensitivity as to what the client can comprehend; time must be allowed to interpret the response. It should be borne in mind that such persons must not be coerced or intimidated and that allowances must be made if they become distressed.

A dementing person needs constant repetition of useful information, such as: 'Yes, Mr Smith, the toilet door is at the end of the green passage' or 'Yes, Mrs Jones, you shall have your lunch at twelve o'clock as promised'. This may seem unnecessary to the care giver, but repetition of basic information represents a lifeline back to reality for the disorientated person. Environmental clues such as night lights and colour coding will assist some clients to negotiate their environment.

Maintenance of orientation

Bold face clocks, and large print calendars are essential for the maintenance of orientation. An 'orientation board' which is set up each day to denote the day, date, weather and special events has been found to be a helpful device. Before such a board is organised it is important to assess the potential users for print size and colour contrast abilities. Residents must be able to read the words on the board. Literacy and ability to read the English are also important considerations in planning an 'orientation board' and where residents are non-English speaking in origin, efforts must be made to enable communication in their own language. Importantly, an orientating device must be strategically placed so that residents will be reminded to read it. The board can be placed in any room used for socialisation and can be also used in the classroom situation. However, where a client is suffering from dysphasia he or she may have difficulty in understanding verbal or written words and may be unable to communicate with others.

An effective organisational environment is dependent upon a commitment to a total team approach by all who come into contact with the person. All staff, including support personnel such as cleaners, as well as the family, clergy, visitors and volunteers must be included in the team processes. The ill advised remark of one person can undo weeks of careful and caring work. Regular, consistent and appropriate information regarding reality and a predictable environment can help people to feel understood and accepted. Reality orientation need not be an expensive exercise. The attitude of care givers is of greater importance to the success of the programme, than is the length of their training.

Reality orientation group sessions provide an opportunity for confused persons with similar levels of cognitive deficits to share appropriate activities with an emphasis on orientation. 'Classroom' sessions can supplement the 24 hour a day reality orientation approach. Severely disorientated people benefit from short sessions each week day morning with a break from routine on the weekends. A maximum of five or six people in a group allows each to receive some individual attention. Ideally, a group leader should have a

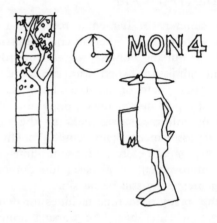

caring consistent approach and be well known to those participating. People who wander may benefit from such sessions but can be disruptive. A second helper is therefore important. Several films are available that demonstrate the value of reality orientation in different settings (e.g. Geri Hall. Managing the unmanageable: a rational new approach to caring for the confused and Alzheimer's patients. Age Concern, Gardenvale).

Personal identity

An elderly person needs to be reminded that he or she is an individual who has worth and value; and carers must remember also that individuality and the contributions made by their elders. Anonymity must be resisted with vigour in any caring programme. Each elderly person has the right to be called by the name and title of choice. It is incumbent upon all staff to ascertain that choice and to avoid using impersonal generalities. Large print name badges may facilitate the correct use of names by everyone.

Time and place

Dementia is commonly manifested by disorientation in time and place. Elderly people in institutions often have significant problems, especially in identifying time. It is important that care givers recall occasionally just how easy it is for anyone to become momentarily disorientated, to fail to remember the date or the day, or to be unaware of the passage of time. A person, any person, who has no calendar, cannot read the newspaper and is not reminded will have difficulty in accurately reporting the date. When days pass by with unrelenting sameness it is difficult to differentiate between Wednesday and Sunday.

Orientation to time and place help the confused person to link where they are to what is occurring, or is about to happen. It helps to prepare them for what is required and what others are doing, e.g. keeping a diary for a confused person provides a reference for recent or planned events.

The passage of weeks may be marked by special days for particular activities, especially if they can be related to habits of the past. Entertainment, food and drink are essential features of a party and need to be provided in a special manner. Unless particular reasons prevail, alcohol can add a festive touch. It is important that a special event be viewed by staff as being special so that they assist the participants to prepare themselves appropriately in terms of clothes and grooming. Knowledge of the participants will assist staff to decide how long in advance the notion of a party should be raised. Because many people in this situation are unable to cope with anticipation, the timing of the announcement is often critical in preventing impatience and frustration. Barbecues, bus trips to familiar places, concerts, shopping expeditions and holidays are other special events that are suitable for many elderly people. It is important, however, when taking such people out into the community that they be protected at all times, especially from behavioural lapses that may reinforce low self esteem. It is also important to ensure that a positive public image of elderly people, in general, is fostered. This does not mean that people with potential behavioural lapses, such as incontinence, should be prevented from participating in activities. It does mean, though, that such people should wear protective clothing and, also, be taken to the toilet as necessary.

Special events are, often, ideal opportunities for involving families in activities as they promote pleasant sharing in more normal functioning and assist in allaying guilt feelings experienced by many caring families. Frequent opportunities to experience the world outdoors are helpful to maintain seasonal orientation. It is difficult to realise that the winter season has arrived if no frost, wind or rain are ever felt. However, a changed environment may create increased anxiety in a person and this may be too stressful and, thus, counterproductive.

Reminiscing is a useful therapeutic tool since some dementing elderly people have a deeper level of disorientation related to time. The past may have greater meaning than the present. Their world may have reverted to an earlier era. Reminiscing about the past ought to be encouraged as it enhances feeling of worth and self-esteem, but care must be taken to bring such discussion back to the present. Staff need to avoid any tendency to participate in the disorientation by supporting the confusion. They can gently help the dementing person to delineate past from present. Some people, however, may not be able to respond positively to such reminders of the present. If gentle correction results in agitation or aggression, then time may need to be spent 'working through' feelings associated with the past.

Incontinence

It is impossible to estimate the annual number of working hours spent by staff in institutions in dealing with the consequences of incontinence. The implementation of measures based on knowledge gained from research into incontinence (Fonda & Wellings 1987) would diminish the problem considerably. Careful assessment, followed by treatment or planned management is essential to lessen discomfort and distress, for both the person and the carer(s).

Incontinence in a demented person may well be the symptom of a remediable underlying cause, which could also be responsible for a heightened state of confusion. It is, thus, very important to investigate the possible cause, as treatment could well restore continence and diminish the level of confusion. If no underlying reason for incontinence can be found it may simply stem from the individual's inability to cope with the environment.

A person with directional problems may become lost when trying to negotiate featureless corridors, or difficulties with sequential thinking may prevent them from associating discomfort in the pelvis with walking to the toilet. Organisational planning may be ineffective and contribute to the person's incontinence. The use of physical restraints or the imposition of barriers to independent movement may prevent a person from getting to the toilet when necessary. Nocturnal incontinence may be associated with the use of sedation, lack of sensory cues, an inability to get out of bed or move in the dark. A new environment may fail to sustain old habits. The person who has used a chamber pot under the bed may not be able to use appropriately the commode at the bedside.

When incontinence persists despite diligent investigation and treatment the comfort and dignity of the individual becomes of paramount concern. Every effort should be made to avoid the impact of the consequences upon the person's ego. Protective garments are commercially available and should be used to provide appropriate protection at all times. Continence should be the expected behaviour rather than accepted passively as a normal consequence of demented behaviour (see also Chapter 7).

Personal appearance

Personal appearance is another factor to be considered in the care of an elderly person with dementia. Each person should be encouraged to participate in personal care activities.

Clothing is a constituent of personality and, often, expresses the way a person feels about him/herself as well as about other people. Care givers should be highly cognisant of the effects of clothing and grooming. Every effort ought to be made to assist the person to maintain normal standards. Compliments should reinforce success; tact and gentleness should modify failure. Inappropriateness needs to be corrected carefully to ensure that a moment of lucidity is not destroyed by the individual becoming aware of foolishness.

If a hairdresser is available, both men and women have an opportunity to maintain a satisfactory standard of hair grooming. When a hairdresser is not able to perform this function other staff or care givers need to act instead. Again, an adult standard should be maintained. Cute bows and pigtails may do little more than reinforce confusion. The availability of strategically placed, suitably illuminated mirrors is essential if people, whether confused or not, are to maintain an awareness of their appearance.

Movement and activation

Humans are active beings depending upon movement and stress for survival. Elderly people have a need for movement, for exercise and activity. Immobilisation, in itself, may add to the dementing process by decreasing circulation of the blood and therefore oxygen to the brain. Prolonged sitting is a common form of enforced immobilisation in people who are unable to move independently. It is inhumane to expect a person to sit without significant postural changes for more than an hour, probably even less. Unfortunately, many wards in nursing homes and hospitals clearly demonstrate the staff's lack of appreciation of this need for movement. Without assistance to change position many elderly people slump and slide into grotesque postures which are, apparently, tolerated because of the individual's state of mind.

In defence of staff it must be said that the standard of seating provided for frail, elderly people in many institutions is unsuitable. In general the design of chairs is inappropriate. Well designed chairs varying in height and width are available, but these tend to be more expensive. Some purchasers appear to think that all elderly people are the same size and height and have the same needs. A concerted effort is required to demand a higher standard of well designed appropriate and affordable furniture for use by those who are ageing.

Care givers have a responsibility to protect frail elderly people from injury. This responsibility to protect, however, does not mean that each person must be cocooned from all risk. A study of injury patterns may indicate some common factors that relate more to ineffective organisation than to a person's state of mind. A lack of occupying activity is one factor that may be modified with positive benefit, and may remove the need for physical restraint (Johnston 1989). Further, detailed assessment may reveal problems that contribute to instability. Hypotension is a very significant potential problem causing some elderly people to fall when suddenly changing postures. It is advisable, therefore, to suggest that they move slowly, sitting on the edge of bed or chair with feet firmly on the floor for a few minutes before standing. Carers have an important role in monitoring responses to changed medication regimens.

Each person has a level of activity that is characteristic for him or her and which is developed over a lifetime. Physically able but mentally disabled elderly people must be assessed carefully to determine their usual level of activity. A suitable programme may then be developed. Permitting a person to pace an area in caged-lion fashion is not acceptable.

The physical environment for such people needs to be designed, adapted or modified to promote a person's ability to move in safety. Functional competence and the environment have a reciprocal interaction which must be understood and appreciated by those responsible for the care and well-being of an elderly person. While the environmental principles that have been described in earlier chapters continue to apply there are a number of features that are particularly significant in relation to sufferers from dementia. Most importantly, the physical environment must promote orientation and diminish disorientation. Although the following is directed towards the institutional environment many of the principles, will apply in the home.

Space identification

Because of confusion and sensory disabilities many elderly people need to be assisted to remain orientated in space. Personal space needs to be clearly defined and identified readily by the owner as well as by others who may live in close proximity. There are a variety of ways in which a person can be assisted in identifying his or her territory, whether it be in a single room or in a shared room or ward. These include:

- Different coloured bedspreads
- Personal pictures and ornaments
- Personal furniture such as a chair or dressing table
- Different coloured carpet or vinyl tiles on the floor
- Wall paint or paper individual to the area, and door and door handles coloured according to choice with large print name, or distinctive picture.

Personal space in communal areas is also important, especially as an expression of territory. Many staff become very frustrated with their inability to alter the around-the-wall chair arrangements in sitting rooms. When the probable reasons are understood it may be possible to bring about more positive changes. People who prefer to sit in a row around the walls with little or no interaction with others may be declaring their right to the only possible form of privacy in conglomerate living. If the environment is arranged to enable periods of privacy away from others as well as periods of social activity in the company of others, it may be possible to alter this seemingly traditional nursing home pattern of arranging chairs.

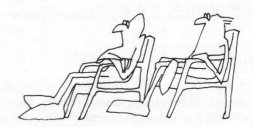

Specific spaces ought to be clearly assigned for particular functions if orientation is to be promoted. Very few people normally eat, sleep, bathe, eliminate and socialise in the same room. Homes usually provide different areas for each of these activities. Furnishings and fittings help to define the functions of each area. An institution must attempt to do the same thing, especially if effective care for those with dementia is to be attempted. Such spaces must be clearly identified as being for a specific purpose.

Toilets require particular attention when considering space identification. All doors of toilets that are to be used by the residents ought to be painted the same bright, very distinctive colour throughout the building. For example, if ladies' toilet doors were all painted bright deep pink (pink being the traditional female colour) confused ladies may learn to find this important room by colour. The doors to male toilets could be painted bright deep blue. Colour may be supplemented by large print signs and clear symbols. Some of the modern graphics currently in vogue cause people, in general, to wonder about the sex the figure is supposed to portray. Their value for dementing people is questionable.

Lighting

Careful planning for lighting is essential because many elderly people have visual handicaps. Glare is often painful and forces people into passivity because they are unable to cope with it, and sudden changes in light levels can cause disorientation. Night-time darkness may also present special problems as shadows and shapes can be identified incorrectly. The problems associated with personal bedside lights must, therefore, be weighed against the risks of mobility in confusion-increasing darkness.

Corridors

There has been extensive research into the disorientating effects of long corridors. Generally, a corridor of more than 40 metres, with shining floors and bright patches created by ceiling lights, and without clearly defined exits or rest bays may

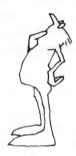

appear to be a long tunnel. This creates anxiety in people who may not have the ability to rationalise their perceptions. The impact of such corridors on a confused person being pushed at speed in a wheelchair by unseen and unheard staff is enormous.

Protection

Many old people, particularly those with dementia, are prone to wander if there are no signals to remind them of their space limitations. Some people may well leave the area if there are no barriers to prevent them. A carefully planned environment which facilitates freedom of movement within an area that is safe is an essential ingredient of the care programme.

Elderly people who wander are best accommodated on the ground floor with free access to a garden area. Features such as a shrubbery and flower beds can be used effectively to conceal fences which restrict departures from the garden, or it may be possible to have a rose garden with a figure of eight pathway providing a pleasant and secure environment.

Restricted areas within the living unit should be kept to a minimum and de-emphasised by painting doors the same colour as walls, placing signs above the usual vision line and, perhaps, using bilateral door handles. These door handles are usually beyond the ability of a confused person because they require two hands working in opposite directions, and avoid the undesirable and unsafe alternative of locking doors.

The environment in which a person functions is not limited to the arrangement of the physical aspects. The organisation with its schedules, rules and staff behaviour is a most significant environmental feature. The organisational environment is dynamic, changing and adapting, over time. Because of its dynamic nature the organisational environment may have profound effects upon an elderly person. It is, therefore, important that those responsible for management ensure flexibility in meeting individual needs and the wishes of relatives.

STAFF TRAINING

Consistency of staffing ought to be an important goal of the organisation. It is difficult to maintain a team approach if the membership is constantly changing. It is even more difficult for an old person to develop essential relationships with staff if the interaction lacks continuity. A team that is encouraged to extend its collective knowledge through a unified education programme, which is motivated by a shared challenge, and which is stimulated by positive recognition is likely to become an attractive employment prospect.

A positive staff attitude toward elderly people with dementia needs to be developed. Few education programmes for health care workers, except perhaps those specifically directed toward mental health disciplines, prepare staff for working with demented and often physically frail old people. In-service and short-course education programmes should be encouraged to assist staff to develop the necessary knowledge and to enable the development of positive attitudes.

Many of the following points have been described as 'commonsense' but experience has shown that the application of 'commonsense' is not all that common. It is important to:

• Ensure that the person knows the names of the people with whom he/she has contact, especially staff. Large print name badges should be worn and introductions made at every contact to assist in orientation. A number of institutions have found that the use of the given names of staff is a positive approach enhancing positive relationships.

• Encourage the highest level of decision making for each elderly person. Choosing when to get up, when to have a bath, what to eat and what to wear should be the right of every person. Providing a person with a sense of control over his or her life is an important step in the restoration of orientation. However, giving choices will sometimes create a dilemma for the client so these choices must be straightforward and presented clearly. Prior assessment is important to determine the previous personality of the client and the likely responses.

• Promote as great a degree of privacy as possible at all times. Dementia must never be a licence for neglecting the right to privacy especially for toilet and bathing activities. Degradation will pervade the mists of dementia. Staff ought to seek permission, always, before entering a person's personal space or touching personal possessions. Such old people cannot be expected to respect the privacy of another's personal space or possessions if the staff set the negative example.

• Provide a sense of security by establishing routines that give the day structure: by removing uncertainty the staff assist each person to cope more effectively.

• Eliminate monotony and boredom. A structured routine needs to include novel experience and excitement. Special events such as parties and outings add 'spice to life'.

A tendency to forget experiences immediately should not be interpreted as proving that participation is a waste of time. Often the feeling of pleasure and sense of well-being remain even if the event is beyond recall. While variety and colour are important, they should be carefully designed to appeal to the individual without confusing them. While the person concerned usually enjoys appropriate activities that relate to past experiences, they may find unaccustomed activity rather threatening.

Gentle firmness is required in setting limits on undesirable behaviour. Scolding a person as though he or she were an infant must be avoided. People with Alzheimer's disease lose cognitive abilities while infants usually gain these. Staff should try to be constructive in criticism, which should not be given in the presence of others if alternatives are possible. A sense of shame may filter through the confusion causing further distress and anxiety.

Correct incorrect responses gently and tactfully. It may be appropriate to laugh with the person when correcting an apparent foolishness. It is, however, never appropriate to laugh at him or her. Permit the elderly person to complain or to criticise, and attempt to correct the problem if the complaint is reasonable. This will assist the elderly person to develop a sense of control. However, it is essential to avoid making promises which cannot be kept. Promote opportunities for elderly people to form beneficial relationships with others as they have done all their lives.

A person is stimulus orientated throughout life seeking stimulus from the environment and responding to it. It is important to remember that demented elderly people do not form a homogeneous group. Rather, they are individuals with varied degrees of physical and mental ability and disability, with wide ranging personality patterns, social and economic backgrounds, and past experiences. Each ageing individual has a characteristic, comfortable level of activation, or stimulus need, which is developed by a lifetime of living. With the onset of monotony in the environment boredom or reduced activation results. Activity is an essential feature of living. It must be at least moderately variable with occasional novelty if the characteristic level of activation is to be maintained. If the dementing person becomes distressed with too much stimulation, gradually decrease it and the stress response should subside.

ACTIVITY PROGRAMMES

An interesting, sometimes exciting, activity programme geared to the particular requirements of each individual is an inherent feature of a therapeutic environmental programme of care. It must not be imagined that a diagnosis of dementia signifies a diminished need for activation. On the contrary, a confused brain requires a significant increase in sensory stimulation to promote maximal brain function.

Before planning an activity programme staff need to be aware of the potential effects of various activities on each elderly person. Some activities may be used to excite, others to calm. Some activities may promote habit training, others may just be fun. Essentially, an activity must have a purpose and a goal which seems worthwhile if a person is to participate enthusiastically. It is important, in planning activities, to remember that these people are mature adults who can no longer function adequately. They must be treated as adults if appropriate motivation is to be achieved. Of course, many activities may need to be simplified, broken into component parts so that the particular person is able to cope. The range of activities that may form the basis of a planned programme is limited only by the imagination of the planners and the capacity of the participant to respond.

Housekeeping

Where possible a physically active but demented old person should be encouraged to assist with household chores, even if living in an institution. Making the bed, dusting, tidying personal possessions, or arranging flowers may all be achievable and satisfying tasks. If the standard is not adequate staff may rectify the situation in the absence of the person. Little can be more demoralising than having a briskly efficient staff member re-do a task which has just been completed; the stimulation of memories of an impatient mother correcting an inexperienced child may do little to assist an improvement in mental state.

Cooking can be a very satisfying activity for an elderly person. Preparing meals or baking a cake are activities that may be undertaken by individuals or small groups. Pancake making using electric frying pans can be fun if a kitchen is not available. Preparation of food can be an activity that is broken down into a number of stages and can be satisfying to both person and carer, e.g. peeling vegetables.

Gardening

Most people have participated in gardening activities during their lifetime, and gardening is an effective sensory stimulant. The perfume, colours and texture can bring about memories of the past. Fortunately, there is a growing acceptance of resident participation in the gardens for those who are in institutions. Raised garden beds provide easier access for able and disabled people alike.

Music

The planned use of music is of value as an integral feature of the care of such people. Music and musical activities may enhance the everyday existence of people with varying degrees of emotional disturbance. Most people respond to music but the success of music therapy depends upon the adaption of musical techniques to the physical and mental state of each person and to his/her ethnic origin. While music may be used effectively as a group experience it is the response of the individual that counts.

Many elderly people, even those with mental impairment, enjoy moving to music or dancing with each other or carers. For the non-ambulant, wheelchairs can be manipulated to music by staff or volunteers. Old dance tunes that are likely to be familiar are the most suitable, but they may need to be modified to exclude quick changes and rapid turns.

Arts and crafts

Absorbing, creative activities are essential for promoting the highest degree of alertness and interest. Careful assessment of abilities and needs is an essential preliminary requirement. Each person must be free to join in an activity of choice. Clay modelling can be pleasant to the touch and enables the expression of creativity. However,

care must be taken to ensure that the task is possible. Success is a primary aim if satisfaction without frustration is to be achieved. Creativity ought to be the basic goal, not productivity.

Many activities may need to be modified, adapted or simplified to be satisfying. An elderly lady, for example, may wish to continue her previous hobby of embroidery. Fine needlework using silks plus counting canvas squares to create pictures may no longer be possible. Coarse needlework using wool and repeated patterns may prove an acceptable substitute. The fact that such old people are often handicapped by psychomotor slowness, short attention span, forgetfulness and sensory impairments clearly demonstrates the need for the careful planning of their activities.

Sport and games

Participation, either directly or vicariously, in sporting activities or games is a feature of life for the majority of Australians. Confusion should not be seen as a barrier to continuing participation at whatever level possible. As in most activities, games may need to be modified or adapted to permit the individual person's functioning. Both the individual and the group can be catered for through a very wide range of activities.

Pets

Many old people, particularly those with dementia, find it difficult to relate adequately to others. It may be possible for them to develop a meaningful relationship with a pet, especially one which responds to human contact. Kittens, rabbits and small dogs may be features of life at home or in an institution. Singing canaries, talking budgerigars or cockatoos, and colourful fish may enhance the environment without too much extra effort for staff. The variety of animal projects undertaken by institutions is limitless. Chickens, ducks, sheep, goats and cows are examples of projects associated with some Australian nursing homes.

Television

Television may be a useful activity if its use is carefully planned. Unfortunately, it is common for some staff to assume that their responsibility for activities is met by switching the television set on and leaving people to watch. There are some basic rules for television viewing which should be observed by all staff:

- Only turn on the set if someone wishes to watch, and provide adequate lighting.
- Position chairs to ensure that those interested can see.
- Ensure that the picture is clear and adjust the sound.
- Assist the viewer to select appropriate programmes, and discuss them afterwards.
- Avoid other activities in the same area and turn off the television after use.

Religious observances

Participation in religious activities may have been an important feature of life for an individual. As much religious observance is based on ritual and tradition, the habits of a lifetime may be sufficiently strong to permeate the state of dementia. Where possible, the person concerned should be encouraged to return to his or her familiar church because this familiarity will strengthen the memories, and reinforce the choices made in earlier years. Chaplains and pastoral care workers can visit and be a source of great comfort to believers and sometimes non-believers.

Summary and conclusion

All elderly people with dementia and their carers deserve thorough assessment to determine their needs. Restoration to the optimum of bodily and mental health, or at least maintenance of the condition of the old person concerned should be the primary aim. Reality orientation offers a structured programme which reminds the confused individual of such basic information as person, place and time. It is vital to remember that these are adult people who have relatively recently failed to function adequately according to some quite arbitrary standards of behaviour. Much can be done by care givers to adapt the environment to meet individual need so that life becomes more bearable for everyone.

Further research is required to define the needs of people with dementia and to evaluate the programmes devised for them. Elderly people must be consulted and their wishes respected; such elderly people are quite capable of making their wishes known through their behaviour if care givers are prepared to spend time with them.

Geriatric services need clear policies and goals so that caring programmes are coordinated and carried out effectively. Only then will care givers feel adequately supported.

REFERENCES

Boies B 1974–5 An instructors guide to reality orientation, sensory awareness, remotivation, attitude therapy, and the team approach to care. The Erie County Office for the Aging, Buffalo

Carter J 1981 States of confusion: SWRC reports and proceedings. Social Welfare Research Centre, Sydney

Crary W, Johnson W 1970 Attitude therapy in a crisis intervention program. Hospital and Community Psychiatry May: 45–48

Feil N 1989 Validation: the Feil method. E. Feil Productions, Cleveland, Ohio

Flew A 1980 Looking after granny: the reality of community care. New Society 54: 56–58

Folsom J G 1973 Team method of treating senility may contain seed for medical revolution. Nursing Care Dec: 17–23

Folsom J, Boies B, Pommersenck K 1978 Life adjustment techniques for use with the dysfunctional elderly. Aged Care and Services Review 1 (4): 1–11

Fonda D, Wellings C 1987 Urinary incontinence. AECD, Melbourne

Johnston M 1989 Alzheimer's: living and coping with it. M. Johnston, Point Lonsdale, Victoria

Kiersnowski C, Martsolf D, O'Brien P 1976 Miss Greene thought we were torturing her. Nursing 76: 58–60

Levin E 1989 Elderly people with dementia and their carers: problems strains and community support systems. Proceedings 24th Conference Australian Association of Gerontology, Melbourne

Levin E, Sinclair I, Gorbach P 1989 Families services and confusion in old age. Gower, Aldershot

Mandelstam D 1977 Incontinence: disabled living foundation. Heinemann, London

Marshall E, Eaton D 1980 Forgetting but not forgotten: residential care of mentally frail elderly people. Uniting Church Australia Melbourne

Redfern S J (eds) 1986 Nursing elderly people. Churchill Livingstone, Edinburgh

Royal District Nursing Service 1989 Annual report. RDNS Melbourne

Royal District Nursing Service 1990 Annual report. Melbourne, RDNS

Stephens L (ed) 1975 Reality orientation. APA Hospital and Community Psychiatry Service, Washington DC

17. Residential continuing care

Doreen Bauer

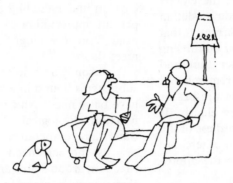

In Chapter 11, which covers the components of an extended care service, residential continuing care was described as the 'last resort' when measures to maintain a normal pattern of living at home were no longer possible or acceptable. At this point further assessment is important to determine the wishes of the person concerned, the type of care required, and the action necessary to resolve any outstanding issues.

Initial admission to either a hostel or nursing home should be on a temporary basis, because with socialisation, good nutrition and a review of medications, many people improve, and some may not in fact need to remain on a permanent basis at that time.

In planning the construction of hostels or nursing home units, it is desirable that they be small in scale and domestic in design. They are best located in residential areas, with preference of access for local people, and as much freedom of movement in and out for residents and their visitors as is possible.

RESIDENTIAL CARE

A vital component in the network of services for elderly people is specialised accommodation with appropriate support services, usually either hostels or nursing homes. These provide regular, ongoing supervision and assistance for people who are no longer competent, physically or mentally or both, and for whom attempts to maintain them at home have failed. People in these programmes will require, to varying degrees, help in performing normal functional activities, skilled technical nursing, and periodic attention from medical and allied health professionals. The majority of these people will need significant assistance and encouragement to participate in a life which has purpose and meaning. Although the residential care model has concepts of long-term and protracted processes it is essential that an overriding philosophy of dynamic, progressive care stimulates a positive approach at all times.

Nursing homes or the institutions that preceded them have been part of the social fabric within Australia since the mid 19th century. It is only in recent times that the former 'benevolent homes' ceased to be associated directly with destitution. The expectations of many old people today continue to be coloured by this history. Continuing care institutions do not, as a whole, enjoy a happy reputation, and very few people would willingly pack their lives into a suitcase and move into such an institution. While hostels and nursing homes are not considered highly desirable residences, many people experience great difficulty in finding a place when one is needed.

Some elderly or chronically ill people need extensive and protracted care which cannot be provided at home in a reasonable manner. There is a commonly expressed myth that Australia has a tradition of 'putting its old people away' in nursing homes. For less than 5% of the elderly population, however, has such accommodation been necessary. It is estimated currently that communities will need in the order of 40 nursing home beds and 60 hostel beds per thousand people over 70 years. It should be remembered that residential accommodation is a last resort for a small proportion of those who are elderly. It also needs to be recognised that, regardless of the development of domiciliary services, there are people for whom residential care is the appropriate service option.

There are a number of essential elements to be considered in a residential care service:

• Residential continuing care should be offered at a level commensurate with socially acceptable standards of life and living.

• The physical environment requires special provisions to maintain each person's ability to function maximally in all areas of physical, psychological and social endeavour.

• Because a meaningful and worthwhile life should be offered to each resident the psychosocial environment demands particular consideration.

• All aspects of the individual resident's personal care programme should be based on a thorough, ongoing assessment of needs.

• Since people are dynamic the care programme must be flexible, capable of modification and able to draw upon special skills to complement those of the primary care team.

• The support of the resident's family and the community is indispensable in the provision of quality care.

• If appropriate care is to be provided it is essential that the organisation supports and stimulates the staff employed to provide that care.

BASIC CONSIDERATION FOR AN ACCEPTABLE STANDARD OF LIFE

Continuing care ought to be offered at a level commensurate with socially acceptable standards of life and living. To meet this objective staff must have an understanding of the basic needs of people, an appreciation of the importance of those needs and a willingness to devise strategies to meet them.

A person is a complex structure of systems and subsystems bound in a functioning whole. People have basic needs which must be met to promote function. Biological needs are primary: food, water, air, temperature adjustment, exercise and rest. Psychosocial needs such as interpersonal satisfaction, group status and self-realisation are also elementary in assuring function. The methods chosen by a person to meet these lifelong needs have a significant cultural dimension. Cultures establish a set of rules expressed in terms of statuses and roles of expected behaviour. Within this frame the individual develops a pattern which makes him/her unique. In the residential continuing care programme this uniqueness must be highly valued in the caring process.

If a residential continuing care programme is to fulfill its expressed intent — providing a home and not just a biological existence — the psychological elements of living require particular attention. The manifestation of territorality is a basic feature of behaviour. People need to claim space and possessions as evidence of personal identity. 'Mine' in terms of accommodation, possessions and achievements is socially acceptable. Admission to an institution does not diminish the territorial drive even though its expression is limited. For many people the regular occupation of a chair in a very specific position is the only demonstration permitted. Single room accommodation with personal possessions is one method advocated for meeting this need. The majority of continuing care residents must, however, accept shared accommodation. Imaginative and caring staff may support the territorial drive by assisting the resident to define his/her living spaces and personalise then, and refrain from invading them without permission.

An adjunct of territorality is privacy. This has two aspects: freedom from the presence of others and, again, the sense of 'mineness'. The right to privacy is an elementary feature of our society, protected by law. Admission to a nursing home does not alter this right although its denial is a common occurrence. A resident's space and property, even if owned by the institution, must be considered private except in special circumstances. It costs little for staff to ask before burrowing in a drawer for a comb.

Perhaps the most critical aspect of privacy is related to protection of the body. Most cultures demand that people conceal their bodies, particularly the 'private parts'. In society it is unlawful for any person to invade the body privacy of another without consent. In an institution the physical or mental disabilities of a resident may necessitate staff invasion of body privacy. This should be undertaken with great care to protect the resident's dignity. It is particularly important that toilet and bathing privacy are respected at all times. Lack of privacy is a common feature of many institutions. It ought not to be tolerated. Staff who cannot accept or adjust to this basic element of living should be encouraged to participate in a sensitivity training programme, role-playing the resident subjected to indignity.

In conglomerate living it is essential for most people to have periods of aloneness. This need is variable but must be ascertained and catered for. Constant exposure to other people may be an untenable burden. Provision also should be made for private conversations and emotional expression whenever the resident chooses and with whomsoever the resident wishes. The denial by staff, or families, that an elderly or disabled person has a right to heterosexual companionship, in private, is unreasonable and unjust.

There are many other ways in which a person can be recognised as someone unique, someone of value and worth. It often takes great skill and understanding on the part of staff to achieve the appropriate balance for each individual. Staff, of course, must always recognise the presence of the resident and not cast the person into anonymity while conversing over him or her. The use of a person's preferred name is an important feature of human recognition. Formal names ought al-

ways to be used unless the individual staff member is invited to do otherwise. This is a usual social custom which admission to long-stay care does not eliminate. Conversation requires eye contact if the participants are to recognise each other. The physical status of most residents has them seated when conversation takes place. When one party in a conversation stands over another physical or psychological stress may result. This is particularly so when disability prevents ready postural alteration in the seated person. Staff need to sit or kneel when talking to a resident. The traditional concept that sitting down means laziness or work avoidance should be discouraged most vigorously by administrators and supervisors. Staff need also to be aware of the difficulty in conversing when sitting beside another person if posture cannot be changed. It is not uncommon to see people sitting in isolation

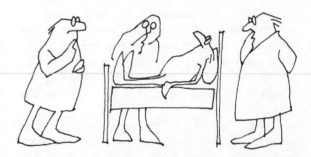

in rows. Many staff have found that it is not easy to alter established behaviour patterns especially when chair position has become fixed by territorial imperatives. Resourceful and caring staff, however, who are committed to a total living programme will find that it is possible to bring about change if the new pattern has desirable benefits.

Staff can do much to enhance the life of the resident by encouraging as much self-determination as possible. Many staff believe that allowing the resident the greatest degree of freedom to choose, to exercise a measure of control over his/her life may disrupt the apparently efficient operation of the unit. There are, however, many aspects of institutional life which may be subject to individual choice: what to wear, what to eat, when to go to bed, whether to be sociable or solitary, to participate in an

activity or not. Some staff have found that resident participation in planning and decision
making is not only possible and practical, it is
stimulating for staff and residents.

Many residents need a lot of encouragement
to assert themselves because admission, in itself,
has resulted from an inability to exercise self-
control. The burden of care became too great
for home carers. Regardless of the reasons, the
resident frequently interprets the admission as
rejection because he or she has become a
nuisance. Later, in the institution, many residents will go to great lengths to ensure that
they do not become nuisances to staff. Fear of
further rejection may outweigh the need for self-
determination. Caring staff will take specific
precautions to reassure and positively guarantee
acceptance of independence.

Freedom to choose also means freedom to
refuse and freedom to complain without fear
of reprisal or recrimination. Too many institutionalised elderly people sink into despair
without a whimper because they are too frightened to complain. Managers and supervisors
should view complaints with understanding and
action. They should also view lack of complaint
with suspicion.

Another aspect of freedom is acceptance of
personal risk. A living person cannot be cocooned
from all the potential hazards in life. Staff who
work in institutions need to be assisted to understand the difference between the resident's right
to live with risk and staff negligence. Fractured
minds caused by restraints are at least as disastrous as fractured hips. Preventing residents from
exercising their functional independence skills
because they might have an accident should
only be undertaken after careful consideration of
all the implications. The use of physical
restraints such as belts and ties, cot sides and
trays should be the subject of thoroughly examined organisational policies which demand
specific assessment procedures before permitting
implementation.

Freedom, however, must be tempered with
stability and security. It may be necessary to
establish a schedule for a particular resident to
help him/her maintain his/her orientation. Such
a schedule should be developed in response to

the needs of the individual. It should not be a
blanket process for a whole group nor should it
have its genesis in staff convenience. A schedule,
however, does not mean that life must be routine
and monotonous. Novelty and surprise are essential features of life and must be encouraged in
the caring process.

Caring staff will not allow the routine of the
nursing home to dominate the individual totally
but will find ways of permitting the resident to
express his/her individuality while protecting
his/her dignity and self-respect. Staff can readily
test the validity of their approach by assuming
the resident's role.

An impression of continuing care which the
present service fosters is the notion that people
in care are sick. Although many of the people
admitted to institutions have disabilities resulting
from chronic diseases the majority are not actually
ill. It is often difficult to convince staff that this
is so when there is so much stress placed on the
hospital model of care. The people are usually
patients, their accommodation is in wards, nurses
wear uniforms and strict adherence to traditional
hospital ward routines and schedules is normal.
This is despite the fact that many institutions providing this form of care are known as hostels or
nursing homes. De-emphasising the hospital concept is important if an appropriate attitude is to
grow. The use of the term 'resident' to refer to
the patient or, still too frequently, inmate is one
step in this direction.

A positive attitude toward continuing care
must also be fostered in society. The illusory high
walls that separate institutions from the community must be demolished. Ideally, elderly
people should be maintained within the community which contains familiar people and life.
Admission to an institution must not demand the
abdication of community membership, rights and
responsibilities. The location of the institution is
of primary importance. To be effective it should
be sited in a local community centre. Large cen-
tralised facilities are disasters in terms of human
costs when people are forced to move away from
the known community. They should be close to
public transport to facilitate visiting. They should
be close to shops, theatres, churches and hotels
to allow, if appropriate, resident participation in

these usual community activities. Too frequently, accommodation for the elderly is located in peaceful back streets where community life is a rare visitor. This reinforces the 'prison sentence' impression that many elderly people have of continuing care.

STAFFING

The key to appropriate residential care is the staff. Reconciling adequate numbers with budgetary constraints is a major problem for governments and managers. Administrators are unable to develop effective staff patterns without the cooperation of employees, professional bodies, unions and consumer representatives. Together they may be able to reach compromise to allocate, imaginatively, scarce and expensive human resources. Staffing, though, is much more than a numbers game. Suitable care demands people who have at least adequate knowledge and skills, people who are sensitive and adaptable. The contributions of staff who perceive continuing care only as the application of 'tender loving care' are quite different from those of staff who recognise the significance of assessment, goal setting, planning, evaluation, teaching and coordinating. Functioning in this latter capacity demands the highest level of professional competency.

Developing criteria for staffing patterns in residential care services has been the subject of some research in recent years, although considerable work still needs to be done. An obvious method is to determine the level of care required by a given number of residents. The more dependent the people the higher the number of staff required. There are, however, several serious flaws in this theory. First, will the dependency level for an individual elderly person be assigned after an attempt has been made to restore as much independence as possible? Secondly, there is a tendency to encourage dependency if it results in increased funding, either directly or through subsidies. This, of course, is directly contrary to the philosophy of geriatric care. Thirdly, effective programmes for frail or disabled elderly people who retain, even minimally, a degree of activity require more staff than do programmes for bed-fast, inactive people. Fourthly, physically independent but mentally frail elderly people require an intense ratio of staff. Dependency criteria, however, place inadequate stress on mental state.

Developing staffing standards for registered nurses and allied health professionals is a complex problem because of the tendency to view both hostels and nursing homes as a form of hospital. There is a need to alter the thinking of these health professions and their unions so that hostels and nursing homes will be viewed, first, as specialised accommodation. Some residents, just as some people in the community, will have need for skilled nursing, physiotherapy, occupational therapy and so on. These needs should be met by the appropriate personnel in a similar manner to those in the community. It must be borne in mind, however, that the criteria for admission to a nursing home are based on assessment of the individual's need for actual nursing care. Such residents are at risk and do require professional overview and supporting staff with the ability, skills and knowledge to meet their needs adequately in a relaxed and friendly atmosphere. Admission to a nursing home or hostel does not entitle residents automatically to access to a full range of therapeutic services, and staff providing such services must be able to demonstrate the cost-effectiveness of their activity, or its intrinsic value to the recipients concerned.

With regard to cost-effectiveness, for example, a person who is dependent in feeding may require an hour of direct nursing care each day for meals and snacks. Assessment may reveal the dependency to have a remediable cause such as an inability to use normal cutlery, an inability to manage at an inappropriate table, or an inability to see what is on the tray. Correction of such problems by an occupational therapist in one or two sessions may promote independence in feeding, thus saving an hour of nursing time each day. Multiply this hour by the number of feeding-dependent residents and the benefit of the occupational therapist becomes significant.

The significance of the effect on the morale of such residents in being helped to achieve this degree of independence is, of course, of major importance also.

An adequate number and disciplinary mix of personnel are only part of the staffing picture. The quality of the staff will have a significant effect upon the standard of the care provided. Quality is, to a large degree, dependent upon education. The growth in gerontological knowledge in the past decade has been substantial. The flow of information which proves theories and discards fallacies, presents ideas and fosters discussion is constant.

Unfortunately, continuing care residents are not benefiting from this information as rapidly as they should. Frequently, new research knowledge remains hidden in the highly technical or jargon language of the specialised professional journals. Most staff are not university graduates with the ability to interpret research reports. They have, however, a need for this information to be interpreted and presented in a practical way. For example, research has indicated that falls in elderly people may be precipitated by the failure of visual spatial perception. Some practical implications of this knowledge which must be presented to every staff member are the necessity for adequate illumination and the clear marking of hazards such as steps.

The number of staff who have access to appropriate education programmes is limited at present. There are not enough formal courses available because geriatrics is being recognised only slowly as a special area of care. This applies through the full range of disciplines. Governments, through health and education authorities, must be encouraged to attend to this urgent need. It will be disastrous if educational programmes are delayed until the numbers of elderly people requiring care are so great that the problems force rearguard action.

Improved educational opportunities will lead to the enhancement of the self-image of continuing care staff. The status of 'chronic' work is still not equal to that of 'acute' care. The challenges of meeting the often complex needs of frail or ill aged people require great skill and talent, at least equal, if not superior, to those required in a computerised intensive care unit. Education is an essential part of any attempt to upgrade the standard of continuing care. The greatest inhibiting force to quality care is individual acceptance of the status quo. Too many staff believe that experience alone is a satisfactory teacher. When these people occupy key positions in institutions they are unable to bring appropriate leadership qualities to bear on subordinate staff for the benefit of the residents.

An essential area of education which must receive priority is that of interdisciplinary understanding. Every member of the staff needs to recognise and accept that he or she is dependent upon other people for the successful care of the resident. No one person or discipline can bring the range of skills and talents required by each individual resident. The advent of paramedical staff into what was a nursing domain has not always been harmonious because of inadequate, if any, attempts to achieve understanding. Understanding is a two-way process which can only be built upon knowledge of the role and function of each discipline coupled with an appreciation of cooperative or team action.

An in-service education programme should be a significant priority in every nursing home. Key personnel must be prepared, again through education, to assume an enthusiastic leadership role in such a programme. Lectures, discussion groups, reading and audiovisual programmes should be part of the working life. Professional staff, especially, have an inescapable responsibility to seize every opportunity to share knowledge with co-workers for the greater benefit of the residents.

CONTINUING CARE INSTITUTIONS

The people who require continuing care are individuals with unique sets of needs. Experience has indicated that there are three broad sets — mental, physical or a combination of both. Further, each set may be divided into frail and independent classes. Each of these six categories of need requires different environmental and programme emphases.

Unfortunately, many continuing care facilities are unable to categorise and place people with similar needs together. Generally, there is considerable variety of major needs which makes the task of planning very complex. It is, also, often unsatisfactory for the people themselves to try to share their lives with others whose needs are very different.

It is important in a planned extended care service that a range of special units be developed to cater for particular need groups. These units may be separate facilities or sections within one building. People would then be admitted, following assessment, to the specific programme area that would best suit their needs.

Such a concept presupposes two things. First, that reliable data are available in each community upon which to base plans for the types and sizes of the units. Secondly, that there is community-wide acceptance of the importance of informed assessment of individual need before admission to any service or accommodation and that all organisations agree to participate in planning wise and flexible use of accommodation and resources. Such an approach would not be easy because it would involve a coordinated commitment by diverse public, voluntary and private agencies. Since all have the same basic objectives the organisational difficulties may not prove insurmountable.

Generally, there are two types of continuing care institutions, each with subgroups according to the type of resident or the type of programme.

Hostels

Domestic level supervisory care facilities (hostels or special accommodation houses) are for frail but reasonably physically independent people who need some assistance to cope with living. Most residents are mobile, perhaps with a frame or sticks, sometimes in a wheelchair. Some residents may need help with aspects of daily living functions such as putting on shoes or bathing. Occasionally, the degree of assistance may increase, temporarily, when the resident is briefly unwell. Some people may require assistance to develop, or participate in, a meaningful lifestyle. The hostel must, therefore, provide or ensure access to a wide range of social, recreational, or religious activities.

Bed-sitting rooms with small group dining and lounge areas are usual. The environment should simulate a normal home with the use of resident's personal property being encouraged.

Specially designed, protective environments make hostel living a most appropriate solution to the needs of the mentally frail.

Supervision by suitably caring staff is essential on a 24 hour basis. The skilled services of medical, nursing and paramedical staff should be available only when specifically required.

Nursing homes

Nursing home care is that required by people with physical or mental disabilities which force them into dependency in one or more areas of functional activity. Programmes of care involve the provision of personal and nursing services which promote the highest level of independent activity; psychosocial stimulus to assist in the maintenance of a meaningful life; and appropriate support and care during the dying process. While such care entails, to a major degree, the provision of nursing services to maintain the comfort and well-being of individuals, it has a very definite, dynamic treatment and restorative element. Stress is often placed on the maintenance of function which may result in the neglect of recognition of need for review and reassessment and the important diagnostic, preventive, treatment and rehabilitation skills that are an integral part of an appropriate extended care programme. In other words, 'tender loving care' is only one aspect of the care required.

Continuing care in Australia is provided in nursing homes, mental hospitals, residential centres for the intellectually disabled, hospitals and hospices.

FLEXIBILITY OF USE

Admission to a continuing care facility is not necessarily a permanent sentence. People, and their needs are not static. A well organised extended care service must promote a progressive care philosophy and a flexible approach to bed use.

Holiday admissions

Many families are able to maintain an elderly person at home when they have access to temporary admissions for holiday relief. Without such opportunities the burden of care may become intolerable.

The benefits of holiday beds are not always recognised in economic terms because a bed represents money no matter who occupies it. When one considers, though, that one bed could cater for some 12 elderly people the benefits become clear.

Experience has shown that the most satisfactory results occur when the caring family actually goes away from home for this period. A family that remains at home to experience the usual environment without the problems imposed by the dependent elderly person often finds it difficult to resume responsibility. In any event, admission should always be preceded by the development of definite discharge plans for a specified time.

Planned intermittent admissions

It may not be possible for an elderly person to remain at home with relatives on a continuing basis. The burden of care may increase progressively until it becomes unendurable. If the family is able to cope for short periods the provision of an intermittent admission programme may be a very satisfactory solution. By sharing the care responsibility between a family and a continuing care facility permanent admission may be avoided.

Experience in many places has indicated that six-weekly exchanges of responsibility are viable without causing too much distress to the elderly person. Very clear guidelines for the programme with strict adherence to the schedule is important, although there must be some flexibility to enable admission to acute or subacute treatment beds should the need arise. The organisation of the use of a group of intermittent admission beds is best carried out by a social worker in conjunction with a domiciliary liaison district nurse or health visitor.

Night admissions

Some elderly people are able to cope reasonably well in their own homes during the day but have serious problems at night. Fear and nocturnal confusion are quite common for elderly people who live alone. Rather than force admission to full-time care it may be possible to bring the elderly person into the nursing home at night.

Discharge to home or lower levels of care

The chronic or acute illness which precipitates admission to a continuing care facility is rarely static. Improvement is common enough to demand a positive attitude to discharges. Frequently, superimposed conditions such as depression are correctable. Successful treatment may result in improvement in independence to such an extent that a return to home may be possible. Alternatively, transfer to a lower level of care may be appropriate.

Decisions to transfer or to be discharged are frequently made by the resident or the family. Such a decision must be viewed positively by staff even if felt to be inappropriate. Support could be sought from domiciliary services through the extended care liaison nurse and the patient's own local doctor, as the person should be encouraged to make decisions about his or her own life, to benefit from this realisation, or to even learn from mistakes. The extended care service must maintain contact and provide appropriate support and readmission should this prove necessary.

Transfers between levels of care

A person with a chronic illness may be subject to acute flares of that illness or to new acute medical conditions. The general orientation of the care unit in which the person resides may not be able to provide the more intensive level of care required temporarily. It may be necessary to arrange a transfer to a more appropriate area of care until the acute stage is resolved. Some elderly people, however, do not respond well to environmental changes. A temporary increase in staff in the 'home' unit may be a more suitable solution during an acute episode.

Transfers to restorative care should be reasonably frequent in a continuing care facility. Slow deterioration or a sudden increase in dependency may indicate the need for appropriate short-term rehabilitation procedures to improve the person's level of functioning. Again, the transfer may be of the person or of staff.

Some elderly people and their families wish to allow death to occur within the familiar surroundings of home. A supportive continuing care programme will facilitate such requests. It may be necessary to mobilise extra domiciliary resources during this time.

ADMISSION

At the present time a very high percentage of elderly people live out their lives within their own homes with the support of relatives, with some being admitted to hospital for a short terminal phase. Many more could remain at home if adequate supportive services were available *as* and *when* required.

Admission to a continuing care facility is a most serious step in the life of a person and the family. There seems no escaping the last resort connotations that accompany acceptance of this decision. Because of this it is absolutely essential that the decision is soundly based on the considered evaluation of an informed medical and social assessment.

Whenever possible, admission should be preceded by a formal orientation programme conducted by the staff who will later care for the person. Staff may undertake a home or hospital visit to establish a relationship and try to paint an accurate picture of life in the hostel or nursing home. A prospective hostel resident could well visit the unit to meet other residents in a social atmosphere such as afternoon tea. With these visits the elderly person can be assisted to prepare, a little more positively, for the move.

It would be of value to arrange a short-term admission whether to hostel or nursing home in the first instance to enable review after one or two-months, before long-term decisions are made.

The actual admission and settling in process requires very special care on the part of all staff. Most new residents are likely to feel depressed, rejected, perhaps angry, or even frightened by such a change.

The manner of their introduction into the world of the continuing care facility may be most

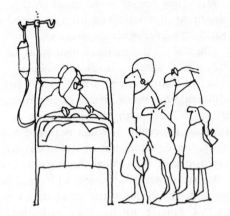

significant in their ability to cope or not with their futures. Admission time is also vitally important for families. If they are involved, actively and purposefully, in the process they will be encouraged to see themselves as a necessary part of the older person's new life. Meeting other residents, becoming familiar with the environment and observing activities are all important aspects of the admission process.

Admission assessment

Despite the fact that a thorough assessment was undertaken prior to the decision for admission it is necessary for staff to develop a detailed profile of the new resident, usually with quite different emphases. The admission assessment, and consequent initial planning, takes time. A planned orientation programme should accompany this process so that the new resident is not harried and pressured by continual tests and questions and then left alone to await results.

An admission assessment should be a planned activity. The depth of examination will, of course, depend upon the level of knowledge and experience of the staff. Where possible, the multidisciplinary team should participate in the data collection. Facilities that do not have direct access to all the disciplines should seek assistance in the preparation of a comprehensive assessment procedure which can be implemented by the available staff.

The following areas should be assessed in adequate detail to provide a complete picture of the new resident:

1. Historical review — to assist in the development of a satisfying lifestyle based on the resident's previous experiences.

2. Clinical — the medical history is, of course, a vital element in the assessment process. The continuing care resident requires the diligent supervision of his or her medical status at all times with the application of appropriate intervention when required and the cessation or alteration of treatment when it is inappropriate. A medical diagnosis is not an accurate reflection of a person's physical or mental capacity because the same diagnosis varies in character, intensity and duration with individuals.

3. Mobility — within the new environment to determine the level of ability, the potential for improvement and the possible assistance required.

4. Function — daily living tasks within the new environment must be comprehensively reviewed to discover abilities and disabilities, to test solutions for improving independence.

5. Communication — skills in language, hearing, reading, writing and television viewing as well as non-verbal communication methods require examination to determine limitations which may hinder activity and to experiment with possible solutions to problems.

6. Nutrition — the nutrition needs of the new resident must be determined as well as his/her preferences.

7. Social — the situation regarding the family and its involvement or not is very important. Other social and financial matters may have significant implications for the new resident.

8. Emotional — the psychological state of the new resident will have a major effect on any programme. Simple tests and measurements should be part of the assessment process.

9.. Mental state — an assessment of the new resident's memory skills, especially, will provide essential data for determining the overall management programme. Again, simple tests and measurements should be available.

10. Cultural background — has significant implications for explaining behaviour as well as for assisting staff to make appropriate approaches to the care of the new resident.

11. Religious needs — must be known if suitable arrangements are to be made for spiritual support if, and when, required.

12. Activity — ascertainment of the resident's personal level of activity, both generally and at times during the day, is important for planning a suitable and satisfactory daily care plan.

13. Recreation — a picture of previous interests and present aspirations will assist the resident and staff in planning appropriate social and recreative activities.

14. Wishes — of paramount importance are the expressed wishes of the resident because these will guide his/her responses to any programme and may significantly affect the programme's priorities.

Planning

The admission assessment will have identified needs, wants and problems. From this documented data a care plan can be developed. As far as possible, this plan should involve contributions from the resident and the family as well as all members of the team who may be available in the facility. Traditionally, each discipline prepared a separate care plan for their particular contribution with little direct reference to others involved in the process. A comprehensive 'resident care plan' will provide a more reliable guide for everyone. This plan should indicate, in writing, the problem, need or want, the goals, the procedure options, and who is responsible for implementation.

Setting realistic goals and establishing priorities are, frequently, the most difficult aspect of planning. They are, though, absolutely essential if the resident, the family and staff are to know the aim of their efforts. The most common criticisms of continuing care concern the all too apparent aimlessness of many residents. Rows of bland faces slumped in chairs along a wall are vivid evidence.

The short- and long-term goals of the care plan should provide for the maintenance of an acceptable quality of life. The resident should be assisted to attain and maintain his/her maximum level of physical independence within his/her limitations. This goal must be worth the effort to achieve. The ability to walk is not worth the effort of practice if he/she has no where to walk purposefully — to the toilet, in the garden, to the shops. There is no purpose, however, in pursuing the goal of walking if the physical capacity to do so is lost. Being dragged around by two staff is not desirable function. The mobility goal of more dignified wheelchair use should be the aim. This modification in the mobility goal must not be seen as the reason for similarly downgrading all other goals, thus leaving the resident immobile, inactive and non-creative in his/her bedside chair.

In setting goals it is important that staff allow the resident to participate. Staff, alone, tend to set goals based on their perceptions of what the elderly person ought to want without due regard for the characteristics that make every individual unique. It is easy to label a person as 'uncooperative' because he/she refuses to conform to the pattern established by others. Many elderly people who have been forced by circumstances to enter an institution need to have the opportunity to experience success before they can make a positive contribution. Failure has been a major feature of their recent lives, admission being its ultimate expression. Thus, the initial goals may need to be quite small so that achievement of success will motivate higher aspirations. Frequently, suggestions of rejection of activity stem from the resident's fear of being a nuisance because nuisances get rejected. By working toward the long-term goal of participation through success-ensuring intermediate goals and involving other successful residents in the process much can be achieved.

Many residents of both hostels and nursing homes have problems related to confusion and are, therefore, unable to participate effectively in all areas of planning. To the extent that they are able they should be encouraged and assisted to do so. Where they are unable it is important that an advocate participate on their behalf. It is not enough for the staff to assume this advocacy role, it must be delegated to someone who is only concerned with the resident's interests. Preferably, this will be a member of the family who has knowledge of the resident's previous lifestyle, interests, habits, history, likes and dislikes.

Desirable goals and the resources for meeting them may, often, be in conflict. Insufficient staff, inadequate funds or an unsatisfactory environment may limit the possible goals of the programme. Imaginative staff will often be able to circumvent these problems by readjusting priorities and fully utilising all available resources. Passive submission is untenable.

A care plan is a dynamic tool used by staff to facilitate comprehensive care. A documented plan provides the clear basis for evaluating or testing the effects of each part of the process. When plans are left vague and stored in the memory, it is difficult, if not impossible, for changing staff to maintain a common approach. It is also difficult to measure progress in the absence of documentation. Evaluation is a constant process because people, especially chronically ill or disabled elderly people, are not static objects. The caring process, illustrated by the care plans, must be flexible and adaptable to meet the changing needs of the resident.

Frequently, staff who do not have direct access to a range of health care disciplines become concerned that they do not have the necessary skills to implement a comprehensive programme. If planning is viewed as a problem-solving task with staff thinking about the problem rather than the complex medical diagnoses that usually accompany the resident, attempts at solutions will be more realistic.

For example, Mr Grey's major problem may be shortness of breath on exertion, the medical diagnosis being congestive cardiac failure. Mr Grey wishes to remain as independent as possible in all activities but is limited by the shortness of breath. The care plan must provide for increased time for Mr Grey to accomplish tasks, must ensure that he is always within his range of a toilet, and must allow him to intersperse physical activity with sedentary occupations. He may need to be encouraged, tactfully, to accept assistance in accomplishing some tasks to ensure that he has the energy to indulge in more pleasant activities. Walking to the sunroom, for instance, may be viewed as essential exercise. It is, however, not worth the energy expenditure if Mr Grey is too fatigued to join the card party. A short wheelchair journey should not be seen as failure.

18. Care of dying people

Sister Margaret Ryan

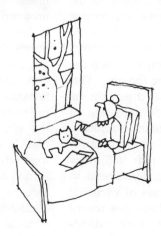

An appropriate introduction to the subject of care of dying people is found in the report of the Victorian Palliative Care Education and Training Committee (1989):

Death is a significant event, not just for those who die, but for all those involved; family, friends and the many professionals and non-professionals who are involved as care givers.

When people die from a terminal illness, such as cancer, there will be difficulties for everyone. The ill person may suffer considerable pain and discomfort from a range of symptoms. Family and friends share this suffering and everyone grieves. Palliative care aims to make this experience less difficult and less painful for all those involved.

Palliative care challenges much of what is now fundamental to the health care system. It calls for a shift of focus from the illness to the patient. It calls for a move away from high technology medicine with treatment aimed at the prolongation of life. It focuses clearly on death as an experience in the continuum of one's life and aims to maintain quality of life to the end. This means offering choice about how those last months, weeks and days are lived, enhancing the person's dignity and ensuring the person is as comfortable as possible.

These appear to be simple and straightforward requests and yet for many who have died from a terminal illness, the experience has been quite different.

Those involved with palliative care are demonstrating that it is possible to die better. This different approach to care challenges the traditional way people have worked with terminally ill people. The ability to accept dying and stop trying to cure, the ability to be comfortable in the presence of death, the ability to support others in times of grief, the ability to help rather than take over, all have to be taught.

Those working in palliative care should receive education and training which aims to develop appropriate skills and knowledge to develop them as secure, sensitive and competent human beings. It should aim to bring about an understanding that all people need to feel in control of what is happening to them and need to maintain a sense of dignity. It should aim to produce care givers who are flexible in the way they work and are able to do things they might not have done in the traditional health care setting.

In the wake of the giant technological advances of recent years there is a quieter crusade for more appropriate care of people whose illnesses remain beyond the furthest boundaries of the curative process. This movement has been strengthened by significant improvements in pain control as well as the relief of other distressing symptoms which may be present in the terminally ill person. Serious consideration of legal and ethical issues is needed in terminal care to allow some discretion in the pursuit of extreme life support measures. There is also a need to accept the basic right of an ill person, spouse or parent to make informed decisions on care.

The wealth of research into the psychological process associated with dying and grieving is portraying patterns of needs more clearly. Australians, like the people of many other Western nations, are beginning to realise that the cost of replacing family and neighbourhood care with salaried service is too high in both financial and human terms.

These insights into the care of dying people have resulted in an increasing awareness that death has become institutionalised away from society. Many people die behind screens in acute hospitals and nursing homes. Few die within the normal matrix of the neighbourhood community. Because of this it is quite common to find adults who have not seen a dead person, who have not lingered with a dying person. Most Australians of recent generations have lived in communities where birth and death have been the business of people dressed in white secreted within the walls of formidable brick buildings. Increasingly, however, people are questioning their lack of involvement and the philosophy of hospice care is gathering momentum.

There is growing support for the concept of integrating hospice care into the mainstream of hospital and community health services. This move towards a more considered approach to the care of dying people generally, is seen as more important than setting up special facilities for terminal illness. The significance of special hospitals for dying people, however, is not to be minimised because they have helped enormously to focus attention on what is possible, which was for so long ignored.

HOSPICE CARE

Hospice or palliative care as defined by the Victorian Palliative Care Council (1989)

is an approach to treatment of a person with a terminal illness. It recognizes that at some point there is a change from a focus which is aimed at curing the disease, to that of controlling and alleviating symptoms. The care aims to enable the person to live in dignity, peace and comfort throughout the duration of their illness. It therefore involves total care of the patient responding to physical, psychological, emotional, social and spiritual needs. Fundamental to this is the control of distressing symptoms.

The target population for hospice care is not defined clearly. Indeed, an attempt to establish a 'definitely' terminally ill group is an unrealistic exercise.

The category of person requiring the care of a hospice programme is the 'probably' terminally ill person about whom medical practitioners agree that curative measures are exhausted, but for whom a periodic review of clinical status should be undertaken. A 'six months prognosis' has been suggested in hospice literature. However, intervention by hospice workers relates more to the state and rate of deteriorating health than to hazardous estimates of time.

GOALS OF HOSPICE CARE

The care of a dying person requires a high order of comprehensive and sensitive care with support for family and friends. While the implications of impending death bring special needs to the care planning process it is essential to remember that hospice care is the terminal phase of continuing care. The principles of appropriate continuing care with the emphasis upon upholding dignity and worth, and identifying and meeting needs of the individual person, are the foundation of such care. Particular goals may be added to reinforce the special significance of the hospice programme. These hospice care goals include the following objectives:

- To facilitate and sensitise community support for home care for a person who chooses to die at home, with particular consideration of cultural and religious needs

- To facilitate appropriate institutional support as necessary, and to educate care givers to ensure that the needs of the dying person and family are met
- To provide appropriate assistance to caring families, to encourage mutual support among those who are grieving and, when necessary, to facilitate counselling of the bereaved.

Hospice programmes have been extensively documented. There are four cornerstones common to most of the programmes described.

1. Every community should have access round the clock to comprehensive palliative care services, including medical, nursing and social work support.
2. Inpatient beds must be available to supplement home care for:

(a) initial and periodic assessment
(b) temporary admissions for relative relief
(c) final phase care, if required.

3. Bereavement support and counselling services should be readily available throughout the dying process if the dying person or family require them.
4. Education programmes must be promoted for staff and the public, especially to assist individuals in coming to terms with attitudes toward their own death.

Additionally, a planned hospice care programme should have:

- Clear objectives that are understood and supported by the community health and welfare workers
- Designated geographical boundaries within which the demographical and sociocultural characteristics of the population in need are clearly understood by service staff
- Identification of community resources and development of close working relationships.

An overriding aim of a hospice care programme should be a commitment to maintaining the dying person as an active participant in life. People need to be in touch with the earth, trees and flowers, to remain aware of the transition of time and the change in seasons. Piped music, murals and fish tanks on the tenth floor of a hospital cannot have the same effect. Further, in death a person takes leave of family, friends and home. The break should not be forced upon anyone prematurely in the name of care.

BEREAVEMENT CARE

Bereavement care commences before the death of the family member. It is needed from the moment the impending loss emerges in the awareness of family members and friends. It should be carried through in allowing the bereaved to express their grief fully at the moment of death in the manner of their choosing and cultural background, be they at home, in nursing home or hospital. What will happen spontaneously in the home should be allowed spontaneously in the institutional setting.

Bereavement care requires an alertness of hospital or nursing home staff to relatives, especially an alone family member leaving after the death of a patient. Staff must know to whom or to where the grieving person is going. Maybe to no-one, no-one at all.

Families may need assistance with funeral arrangements and costs, in managing family finances and in winding up the practical affairs of the deceased. Particular support may be needed for a grieving spouse with personal problems such as disabilities due to chronic disease, alcoholism or loneliness. Widowers may be unaccustomed to shopping and cooking, widows may be unused to arranging for household repairs or managing the maintenance of a car. The hospice care programme has responsibility for ensuring that problems are identified and solutions organised. It may be simply a matter of heightening the visibility of existing services and strengthening neighbourly support. It may, however, be necessary to mobilise more intense intervention and counselling resources.

HOSPICE CARERS

The philosophy of team activity is highly relevant in a hospice programme. The dying person and the family (kin or adopted) constitute the primary team supplemented by friends and neighbours, health and welfare staff, pastoral and legal professionals. A team programme does not mean that a body of professional helpers should cross the family threshold. It does mean that the primary carers have direct and immediate access to the advice and help of a wide range of disciplines governed, through a team commitment, to a common philosophy. One person rarely has a sufficiently strong grasp of the broad dimension of the problems a dying person and the family may be facing.

Staff need to:

• Be able to recognise a certain fluidity in community attitudes and be flexible in meeting various and changing social circumstances.

• Have interpreters available to communicate in the dying person's language. This is very important in the many Australian neighbourhoods where almost any language may be heard.

• Have well developed clinical skills and experience such that they are able to recognise subtle changes in the clinical status of the dying person.

• Be sensitive to the needs of the dying person and the family and able to share, emotionally but without losing effectiveness, in this very caring process.

Such staff abilities are rarely inborn. Staff education and sensitivity training must become an essential feature of all continuing care programmes, large or small, organised or informal.

Since people cannot be governed into dying during office hours it is essential that hospice staff, especially in domiciliary care programmes, be available when needed, very often in the quiet pre-dawn. The current constraints on public spending will probably project a significant amount of the team action back onto voluntary community resources. Carefully selected, trained and supported volunteers could be an integral part of a hospice home care programme, and provide support if a family so desires. Church or voluntary charitable organisations and ethnic social groups may form the wellspring from which volunteers can be drawn.

One of the major concerns of effective terminal care is the declining energy resources of the ill person. There must be recognition that any intervention, by friend, family or professional, constitutes 'work of a sort' for the ill person.

Good professional teamwork recognises limits for each ill person on intervention in a 24 hour cycle, and sets priorities on team members' contributions.

Good terminal care recognises the need for limited efficient use of the ill person's resources of energy, so that he or she can make the best use of the time left for living.

Priorities need to be decided by the patient in consultation with the family and professional team to allow the best use of resources within the limitations of the situation to achieve the patient's perception of quality living.

Conclusion

Hospice or palliative care does need specialist leadership and centres of excellence for practitioner training; however, the challenge of good care for all dying people embraces the totality of the health care system.

What constitutes 'total care' of a patient needs careful thought in respect to every individual. Indeed, 'total care' may be a misnomer as a description of a care giver's response to suffering in another. What is being sought is a breadth of vision and fidelity in practitioners, and what is readily proven is that, where goals are clearly defined, teamwork enhances the individual effort. Because a particular helping person may not have a sufficiently broad grasp of the dimensions of problems an ill person and his/her family might be facing, the sharing of knowledge is important. So that where a community nurse can be advised by an occupational therapist, family counsellor by nurse, doctor by family counsellor, minister or priest by doctor, the intervention by the individual is likely to be more carefully planned and effective, and appropriate assistance more readily available. It is important to reiterate that a team programme does not mean a body of professional helpers should cross the family threshold; nor does it mean that confidential family histories are freely available to all staff members. It does relate, more specifically, to the discipline and development of the care being offered.

At present, it does not seem possible to do more than indicate a starting point in hospice care with a few basic guidelines to give direction along the way:

- Let the programme be guided by the people who need the care
- Let there be a quiet attempt to correct the excessive tendency to institutionalise the dying

- Let such care be open to peer review and the broad stream of health care education and development.

In this way optimal care of the dying may be fully implemented and the care of people suffering chronic illness improved.

REFERENCES

Victorian Palliative Care Council 1989 Palliative care services in Victoria. Section I. Health Department Victoria, Melbourne
Victorian Palliative Care Education and Training Committee 1989 Palliative care services in Victoria. Section II. Health Department Victoria, Melbourne, p 49

19. Challenges

Marion Shaw

This final chapter seeks to raise issues that need to be addressed and which represent challenges for all members of society, remembering that each of us in turn will progressively age. It reflects on the developments in geriatric medicine during the last 50 years as changes in some areas of health care, particularly those concerned with ageing, develop slowly, or in a haphazard fashion, with direction being lost from time to time. Attempts must be made to avoid the constant need to 'reinvent the wheel' by reviewing the past and planning for the future.

HISTORY

In Britain in the early 1940s Dr Marjory Warren, deputy medical superintendent at the West Middlesex Hospital, was made responsible for an infirmary with 600 beds. The 'inmates' were designated 'chronic sick', and received no more than simple custodial care. From the outset Dr Warren questioned the necessity for such a level of passive dependence and immobility. There had been little review of physical condition on an individual basis, and there were no written medical histories. Dr Warren commenced by examining all patients, and recording their problems and functional potential. This process took many months to complete, but the knowledge gained enabled her to introduce progressively programmes of personalised treatment and simple rehabilitation. Day clothes were obtained, and patients were encouraged to leave their beds and be dressed. An encouraging proportion of the patients regained to a marked degree their independence in mobility and in the normal activities of daily living, while the majority received at least substantial benefit.

Dr Warren was a pioneer also in the treatment and rehabilitation of those who suffered 'stroke'. She built up a meticulous organisation, which over subsequent years came gradually to be accepted by her colleagues as not merely a better but, indeed, the best alternative to the custodial care of many disabled old people.

In 1988, Dr Lefroy suggested that although this system has, during the subsequent half century, come to be an integral part of Britain's health service, its acceptance elsewhere has been slow and sporadic.

In the early 1950s another notable pioneer, Dr Lionel Cosin, was appointed to Cowley Road Hospital in Oxford, a former 'workhouse' which also was fully occupied by 'chronic sick' people. Dr Cosin's enthusiasm, teaching ability and infectious activity gained the full support of his staff in getting patients out of bed, dressed in day clothes, talking and active. Many who had been accepted as long-term 'chronic sick' were even able, following rehabilitation, to return to the community, provided that appropriate planned support and periodic review were instituted.

Dr Cosin visited patients in their own homes, and also persuaded general practitioners to refer to him people showing signs of chronic confusion. He treated and managed to return many of these also to the community. Dr Cosin had many ideas: for example, he introduced in his special day hospital a circular corridor with access to a central enclosed garden, where dementing people could wander in safety. At the same time he introduced the concept of a half-way house (linked with the rehabilitation inpatient unit), in which by spending time with the patient prior to discharge, both a supporting relative and the patient could learn to manage the residual disability. During this period, functions carried out by staff were gradually assumed by the relative. In this way both the patient and relative gained confidence before discharge. He was also an early advocate of planned intermittent admission (respite care).

This type of comprehensive service, based on informed diagnosis and psychosocial assessment of need, supported by a multidisciplinary team and encompassing liaison between general practitioner, acute hospital, psychiatric services, and care in the community, was pioneered in the 1950s and 1960s by a number of physicians and social workers both in Britain and in Australia. Both Dr Marjory Warren and, later, Dr Lionel Cosin visited Australia on a number of occasions by invitation, and helped greatly in the dissemination of ideas in this regard.

In Australia the most notable development commenced in 1950, when Dr Dick Gibson and his close associate Grace Parbery, a social worker, undertook a survey in the Hunter Valley region into the domiciliary care needs of those who had suffered disabilities as a consequence of contracting poliomyelitis. This led to a realisation of the parallel need by many elderly disabled people for rehabilitation and community support. A regional geriatric service was then developed, which was subsequently described as 'at least as creative as that of Marjory Warren in England, the only comparable service at that time'. It was known as the Royal Newcastle Geriatric Service, the first such service in Australia to be linked with an acute hospital.

Even though this service was of proven value, many physicians in other parts of Australia (though appreciating the need for similar systems of care based on acute hospitals, with links through rehabilitation units and day hospitals to services in the community) found many obstacles that hindered their achieving similar systems of care in their own areas. Hence, the reference in the introduction to this chapter to 're-inventing the wheel', or at least needing to set out again to prove to funding and professional bodies the value of such services.

In 1973, after several years of lobbying by Dr John Shepherd, then medical superintendent of Mount Royal Hospital in Melbourne, funds were released through the Victorian Hospitals and Charities Commission to enable the establishment of a pilot project to serve the local government area of Brunswick, which had a population of 60 000 with approximately 10% over the age of 65 years. The project was under the direction of Dr Boyne Russell, a specialist geriatrician, and the intention was to provide a comprehensive service in the manner referred to previously. Details of the project were contained in a report released by Mount Royal Hospital (Russell 1976). The very real value of the comprehensive and coordinated service was again proven. It has continued and been further developed, and has been used as a model in many other areas. Arrangements were made from the outset to ensure access for teaching purposes for medical students and others from related health disciplines.

Over the years effective services on similar lines have been established in these ways in Britain, in European countries, in Australasia and elsewhere. In some instances, however, the maintenance of the service has relied on the ability of committed and persuasive advocates able to influence and gain the support of committees and funding bodies. In such situations there is a risk that such services may decline or even be discontinued should the key person retire or move elsewhere.

There can be no assurance of an integrated system of health care for ageing and disabled people without acceptance of the holistic approach embodied in the teaching of geriatrics, as part of the mainstream of medicine and health care. The special needs of older people must be addressed in all basic health professional education programmes, and students should have realistic exposure to needs and problems within the community as well as within acute care situations. There has been considerable progress in this regard within Australia in recent years.

MATTERS OF CONCERN IN AUSTRALIA

Ageing of the population

This matter has been well covered in Chapter 2, and the demographic changes likely to occur are demonstrated in Figure 2.1. The expected marked increase in the next two decades in the percentage of the population over 75 years of age adds weight to the need to develop effective systems of care, while at the same time promoting healthy attitudes to ageing to enhance independence.

Research

The increasing number of 'old old' people also heightens the urgency for objective research in the clinical, biological and sociological fields of gerontology and geriatrics. It is very important, however, that research undertaken previously be studied and utilised to ensure that findings of significance are implemented and evaluated progressively. Knowledge of research, or pilot projects of proven value, needs to be disseminated through teaching programmes, literature and the media.

Maintenance of health

Maintenance of health and independence are prime objectives in ageing, but a number of factors can affect these aims adversely: premature retirement, inadequate housing, inadequate income, poor nutrition, social isolation and transport systems that may not meet the needs of those who are impaired.

Present health system overall

The following quotation is taken from a paper given by Dr Sydney Sax at a conference in 1985, and remains applicable:

The misfit between present medical services and current patterns of illness suggests that the supply of services is unsatisfactory. It responds to the open-ended pressures imposed by fee-for-service practitioners in a system where recipients of services face little or no price. Concurrently, we grapple with an increasing prevalence of chronic conditions which have multiple causes that defy interruption at single specific points. Their prevention and management should involve the co-ordinated contributions of several professionals in comprehensive care packages, and not only the episodic provision of single but often repeated items of service.

Resources for such modern practice are limited by budgets; those summoned by access to medical benefits schedules, on the other hand, are not seen to have significant limits. What are the obstacles to change? One of them lies in the division of responsibility between different levels of government for different aspects of our health services. What incentives have State Governments had to pay salaried staff to run assessment, rehabilitation and community care programs while the Commonwealth was paying fees for medical services which on their own had little effect in curtailing the rate of admission to Commonwealth supported nursing homes?

Though admittedly the Federal Government is now allocating funds to establish assessment teams and community care programmes, this does not alter the fact that practitioners in the acute field remain geared to episodic provision of service and swift turnover in the use of hospital beds.

There is a need for research into the conflicts in the present health system which militate against the health care needs of people with chronic disease or disability.

COORDINATION OF CARE

Old people can and do recover from acute illness and major surgery, provided their special needs are recognised and a rehabilitation programme planned. The proportion of acute patients in the higher age range is likely to continue rising, and a holistic approach to the planning of care on discharge from hospital is essential. This involves close liaison with families, general practitioners, community nurses and access to other options of an extended care service as necessary.

It should be borne in mind that the individual client or patient needs to be well informed, and has every right to be well informed and consulted on matters that affect or concern him or her.

Many families, who at present recoil in dismay at the problems presented by an increasingly dependent relative and see institutional care as the only answer, would be pleased to cooperate in helping that person to continue living at home if they were involved in the planning of care, were taught management skills, and given an assurance of appropriate support or professional help when required. The knowledge that immediate help would be available if a crisis developed would be reassuring. Shared care with planned intermittent admissions to residential care for agreed periods, with day centre support when at home, can be invaluable, because this affords relief to the family and continuing contact with professional staff and the extended care service.

Health care of ageing people calls for an individual and understanding approach. Health, economic and social factors interrelate, and action cannot be effective if it focuses only on one apparent problem or 'diagnosis'.

Pathological changes that could benefit from treatment are often overlooked because either people themselves or health professionals attribute perceived problems to the ageing process and assume their inevitability. Behavioural disorders including dementia, mobility problems and incontinence are cases in point. Underlying reasons need to be sought. *Something* (at best, cure; at least, appropriate care and management) *can always be done.*

EDUCATION

As stated previously, the subject of gerontology and geriatrics should be included as a core component in the basic curriculum of all health professional studies. Ongoing postgraduate programmes should be available for all who are currently engaged in the hospital and community health fields, especially physicians, nurses, social workers and therapists who are immediately involved.

Doctors, nurses, social workers and therapists must:

- Understand the normal physical, social and psychological changes of ageing in order to maintain functional ability at the achievable optimum
- Appreciate the importance of informed assessment of the needs of individual people, to enable appropriate action.

Doctors, nurses and therapists must:

- Know the characteristic presentation of common pathology in the elderly in order to question, explore or intervene in serious clinical problems confronting them
- Understand the effects on ageing people of therapeutic agents such as drugs, in order to ensure appropriate use, recognise toxicity, and be aware of possible side-effects.

While nurses appreciate how the principles of patient assessment facilitate the process of nursing, and understand the treatment, management and care needed by patients who are acutely ill, they must also understand the principles of rehabilitation and restorative care embodied in the treatment plans and aims of doctors, therapists and social workers with whom they are working, so that a consistent and coordinated approach to the patient and family can be assured. For example:

- The role of the specialist physician or geriatrician concerned with medical assessment, diagnostic definition of problems and assets, and the planned coordination of treatment programmes.
- The approach of the physiotherapist in teaching or enabling movement and mobility; the early basic instruction following a stroke (to bridge, to sit and to roll); transfer from bed to chair; the walking pattern for hemiplegic or amputee; the prevention of contractures, pressure sores or lung congestion as well as the many other details essential for achievement of the restoration of function, however limited the degree.
- The role of the occupational therapist, which is not only craftwork, but enabling people to function by developing their potential by devising means or providing aids; retraining them in the basic skills of daily living; visiting a patient's home to create or advise on the creation of a safe and appropriate environment within which a disabled person can function independently; and assisting in vocational retraining.

• The skills of the speech pathologist in enabling communication, understanding, for instance, the difference between receptive and expressive dysphasia, and the management of swallowing problems inherent in dysarthria.

• The special value of music therapy, which contributes to the physical, psychological and functional well-being, aids communication, stimulates the withdrawn and releases sadness or the dysphoria of depression.

There are many others who contribute, not least the relatives who form by far the largest group of providers of care and support for aged or dependent people.

GROUPS WITH SPECIAL NEEDS

Aborigines

The special needs of Aboriginal people and other groups from varied ethnic backgrounds must not be overlooked. This single label 'Aborigines' can cover a wide range of possibilities and actualities (Berndt 1981). The needs of Aborigines vary widely within communities, and the differences are even greater between those living in urban areas and in remote or country regions.

In 1984, the Aboriginal Health Organisation in South Australia conducted research aimed at identifying the health and social needs of the elderly, and the physically and emotionally disadvantaged Aboriginal people in metropolitan Adelaide. This study identified a group of Aboriginal people who displayed the health and social characteristics of aged people, but at a chronologically much younger age (Divakaran-Brown 1985).

Wide ranging research tailored to the characteristics of each situation is required to identify the best means of providing community health services and care as appropriate to the varied needs identified in a manner acceptable to those concerned.

Multicultural groups

The special needs of people from varied ethnic backgrounds as they enter old age require consideration also. Many of those now in Australia migrated to join younger relatives, and even those who arrived 30 or 40 years ago, may well have retained the thought patterns and precepts ingrained in their youth. With increasing age there could be a tendency for many to revert to the language and mores of their early years. Meanwhile, younger relatives, who may have adapted more thoroughly to other patterns of living, and become engrossed in the struggle to establish themselves, might lack the time and understanding required to provide the family support for ageing parents, which in the past was traditional.

Thus, such older people could feel doubly at a loss. Unable to benefit from the family protection which they were accustomed to expect, they feel betrayed and abandoned, left to the mercy of strangers to whom their language and customs are unknown, and at a loss as to how to communicate their needs or to elicit help and sympathy.

The availability of interpreters and nurses from similar ethnic backgrounds would be of great value, but there could be difficulty in providing adequate numbers. Therefore, those providing care for such people must try to acquire knowledge and understanding of their cultures, and to be tolerant and sympathetic to their needs.

Data from two surveys which present insight into the unmet needs of older Australians from non-English-speaking backgrounds are detailed in Chapter 2.

SUMMARY

This chapter commenced by looking back 50 years, as it is important to remain aware of the reasoned approach of the pioneers in geriatric medicine during that time, and to continue to build on their sound and practical groundwork.

With the continuing increase in the numbers of old people there is a heightening awareness of the need to promote health and independence, to promote positive images of ageing and to identify and reduce the inequities in health status among elderly people.

In an era of tightening monetary policy it is even more necessary to devise means of delivering efficient and cost-effective services. To achieve this end it is important to ensure that all those concerned are appropriately trained and well motivated, and that the quality of such services is subjected to periodic review and evaluation.

As the greatest resource of any country is its people, means need to be devised to encourage and assist them to be self-supporting as far as is possible, particularly within families, and to encourage neighbourhood groups to be more involved in the good of the community at large.

REFERENCES

Berndt C H Ageing in Aboriginal society. In: Howe A L (ed) 1981 Towards an older Australia. University of Queensland Press, Brisbane

Divakaran-Brown C 1985 Premature ageing in the Aboriginal community. Proceedings of the 20th Annual Conference, Australian Association of Gerontology, Melbourne

Lefroy R B 1988 R.M. Gibson Travelling Fellowship Lectures. Australian Association of Gerontology, Melbourne

Russell B 1976 A geriatric community care service in Brunswick. Mount Royal Hospital, Melbourne

Sax S 1985 Perspectives on the development of gerontology in Australia. Proceedings of the 20th Annual Conference, Australian Association of Gerontology, Melbourne

Bibliography

Agate J 1972 Geriatrics for nurses and social workers. Heinemann, London

Anderson W F 1988 Practical management of the elderly, 5th edn. Blackwell Scientific, Oxford

Barnes J 1974 Effects of reality orientation classroom on memory loss, confusion and disorientation in geriatric patients. The Gerontologist 14(2)

Barraclough F, Pinel C 1978 Geriatric care for nurses. Heinemann Medical, London

Bauer D 1989 Foundations of physical rehabilitation. Churchill Livingstone, Melbourne

Brocklehurst J C (ed) 1985 Textbook of geriatric medicine and gerontology, 3rd edn. Churchill Livingstone, Edinburgh

Bugen L 1979 Death and dying. Larry C Bown, Iowa

Burnside I M (ed) 1976 Nursing and the aged. McGraw Hill, New York

Canter D 1977 The psychology of place. Architectural Press, London

Carver V, Liddiard P (eds) 1978 An ageing population. Hodder and Stoughton, London

Chalmers G L 1980 Caring for the elderly sick. Pitman Medical, London

Coni N, Davison W, Wedster S 1988 Lecture notes in geriatrics, 3rd edn. Blackwell Scientific, Oxford

Copp L A (ed) 1981 Care of the aging (Recent advances in nursing). Churchill Livingstone, Edinburgh

Drummond L, Kirchhoff L, Scarborough D 1978 A practical guide to reality orientation: a treatment approach for confusion and disorientation. The Gerontologist 18(6)

Du Bois 1980 The hospice way of death. Human Sciences Press, New York

Fonda D, Wellings C 1987 Urinary incontinence. AECD, Melbourne

Ford B 1979 The elderly Australian. Penguin Australia, Melbourne

Hamilton M, Reid H F (eds) 1980 A hospice handbook. Eerdmans, Michigan

Harris C, Ivory P 1976 An outcome evaluation of reality orientation therapy with geriatric patients in a state mental hospital. The Gerontologist 16(6): 496–503

Havard M 1990 A nursing guide to drugs, 3rd edn. Churchill Livingstone, Melbourne

Howe A L (ed) 1981 Towards an older Australia. University of Queensland Press, Brisbane

Isaacs B (ed) 1985 Recent advances in geriatric medicine — 3. Churchill Livingstone, Edinburgh

Johnstone M 1987 Restoration of motor function in the stroke patient, 3rd edn. Churchill Livingstone, Edinburgh

Kamal A 1987 A colour atlas of stroke: cerebrovascular disease and its management. Wolfe Medical, Ipswich

Kratz C R 1978 Care of the long term sick in the community. Churchill Livingstone, Edinburgh

Kubler Ross E 1970 On death and dying. Tavistock Press, London

Lamerton R 1975 Care of the dying. Penguin, Middlesex

Lefroy R, Page J, Sang M 1988 A special hostel for the care of people with dementia. University of Western Australia, Perth

Levenson A J 1978 Neuropsychiatric side effects of drugs in the elderly. Raven Press, New York

Levin E, Sinclair I, Gorbach P 1989 Families services and confusion in old age. Gower, Aldershot

Norton D, McLaren R, Exton-Smith A N 1975 An investigation of geriatric nursing problems in hospital. Churchill Livingstone, Edinburgh

Oberleder M 1969 Emotional breakdown in elderly people. Hospital and Community Psychiatry 27(5)

Parkes C M 1975 Bereavement. Penguin, Middlesex

Plane T 1981 Palliative care manual for home nursing. Mt Carmel Hospital, Sydney

Redfern S J (ed) 1986 Nursing elderly people. Churchill Livingstone, Edinburgh

Russell C 1981 The ageing experience. George Allen & Unwin, Melbourne

Simpson M 1979 The facts of death. Prentice Hall, New York

Sine R D, Holcomb J D, Liss S E, Wilson G B 1980 Basic rehabilitation techniques. Blackwell Scientific, Oxford

Stephens L (ed) 1975 Reality orientation. APA Hospital and Community Psychiatry Service, Washington, DC

Stewart M C 1971 My brother's keeper, 2nd edn. Health Horizon, London

Wells T J 1980 Problems in geriatric nursing. Churchill Livingstone, Edinburgh

Index